Clinical Respiratory Physiology

Editors

DENIS E. O'DONNELL
J. ALBERTO NEDER

CLINICS IN
CHEST MEDICINE

www.chestmed.theclinics.com

June 2019 • Volume 40 • Number 2

ELSEVIER

1600 John F. Kennedy Boulevard • Suite 1800 • Philadelphia, Pennsylvania, 19103-2899

http://www.theclinics.com

CLINICS IN CHEST MEDICINE Volume 40, Number 2
June 2019 ISSN 0272-5231, ISBN-13:978-0-323-67837-7

Editor: Colleen Dietzler
Developmental Editor: Casey Potter

Clinics in Chest Medicine (ISSN 0272-5231) is published quarterly by Elsevier Inc., 360 Park Avenue South, New York, NY 10010-1710. Months of issue are March, June, September, and December. Periodicals postage paid at New York, NY and additional mailing offices. Subscription prices are $377.00 per year (domestic individuals), $726.00 per year (domestic institutions), $100.00 per year (domestic students/residents), $423.00 per year (Canadian individuals), $902.00 per year (Canadian institutions), $484.00 per year (international individuals), $902.00 per year (international institutions), and $230.00 per year (international and Canadian students/residents). International air speed delivery is included in all Clinics subscription prices. All prices are subject to change without notice. **POSTMASTER:** Send address changes to Clinics in Chest Medicine, Elsevier Health Sciences Division, Subscription Customer Service, 3251 Riverport Lane, Maryland Heights, MO 63043. **Customer Service: Telephone: 1-800-654-2452** (U.S. and Canada); **1-314-447-8871** (outside U.S. and Canada). **Fax: 1-314-447-8029. E-mail: journalscustomerservice-usa@elsevier.com (for print support); journalsonlinesupport-usa@elsevier.com (for online support).**

Reprints. For copies of 100 or more of articles in this publication, please contact the Commercial Reprints Department, Elsevier Inc., 360 Park Avenue South, New York, NY 10010-1710. Tel.: 212-633-3874; Fax: 212-633-3820; E-mail: reprints@elsevier.com.

Clinics in Chest Medicine is covered in *MEDLINE/PubMed (Index Medicus), Current Contents/Clinical Medicine, EMBASE/ Excerpta Medica, Science Citation Index,* and *ISI/BIOMED.*

Contributors

EDITORS

DENIS E. O'DONNELL, MD, FRCPI, FRCPC, FERS
Professor, Respiratory Investigation Unit, Division of Respirology, Kingston Health Science Center & Queen's University, Kingston, Ontario, Canada

J. ALBERTO NEDER, MD, PhD, FRCPC, FERS
Professor, Laboratory of Clinical Exercise Physiology, Division of Respirology, Department of Medicine, Kingston Health Science Center, Queen's University, Kingston, Ontario, Canada

AUTHORS

PIERGIUSEPPE AGOSTONI, MD, PhD
Department of Clinical Sciences and Community Health, Cardiovascular Section, University of Milano, Centro Cardiologico Monzino, IRCCS, Milano, Italy

DANILO C. BERTON, MD, PhD
Professor, Division of Respirology, Federal University of Rio Grande do Sul, Porto Alegre, Brazil

ASTRID BLONDEEL, PT, MSc
Researcher, PhD candidate, Department of Rehabilitation Sciences, Laboratory of Pneumology, KU Leuven–University of Leuven, Respiratory Division, University Hospitals Leuven, Leuven, Belgium

LAURENT BROCHARD, MD
Medical and Surgical Intensive Care Unit, Keenan Research Centre, Li Ka Shing Knowledge Institute, St. Michael's Hospital, Interdepartmental Division of Critical Care Medicine, University of Toronto, Toronto, Ontario, Canada

KIM-LY BUI, MPT
Centre de Recherche, Institut Universitaire de Cardiologie et de Pneumologie de Québec, Université Laval, Québec, Canada

RICHARD CASABURI, PhD, MD
Rehabilitation Clinical Trials Center, Los Angeles Biomedical Research Institute at Harbor-UCLA Medical Center, Torrance, California, USA

IVAN CUNDRLE Jr, MD, PhD
Department of Anesthesiology and Intensive Care, St. Anne's University Hospital, Faculty of Medicine, Masaryk University, International Clinical Research Center, St. Anne's University Hospital, Brno, Czech Republic

HELEEN DEMEYER, PT, PhD
Postdoctoral Fellow, Department of Rehabilitation Sciences, Laboratory of Pneumology, KU Leuven–University of Leuven, Respiratory Division, University Hospitals Leuven, Leuven, Belgium

JEROME A. DEMPSEY, PhD
John Robert Sutton Professor (Emeriti) of Population Health Sciences, University of Wisconsin-Madison Medical School, Population Health Sciences, John Rankin Laboratory of Pulmonary Medicine, Madison, Wisconsin, USA

ASLI GOREK DILEKTASLI, MD
Rehabilitation Clinical Trials Center, Los
Angeles Biomedical Research Institute at
Harbor-UCLA Medical Center, Torrance,
California, USA; Faculty of Medicine,
Department of Pulmonary Medicine, Uludağ
University, Turkey

JORDAN A. GUENETTE, PhD
Centre for Heart Lung Innovation, St. Paul's
Hospital, Faculty of Medicine, Department
of Physical Therapy, Division of Respiratory
Medicine, University of British Columbia,
Vancouver, British Columbia,
Canada

MATTHEW D. JAMES, BSc
Department of Medicine, Queen's University,
Kingston Health Sciences Centre, Kingston,
Ontario, Canada

WIM JANSSENS, MD, PhD
Professor of Medicine, Department of
Chronic Diseases, Metabolism and Aging,
Laboratory of Pneumology, KU
Leuven-University of Leuven, Respiratory
Division, University Hospitals Leuven,
Leuven, Belgium

BRUCE D. JOHNSON, PhD
Department of Cardiovascular Diseases, Mayo
Clinic, Rochester, Minnesota, USA

PIERANTONIO LAVENEZIANA, MD, PhD
Sorbonne Universités, Université Pierre
et Marie Curie Université Paris 06, Institut
National de la Santé et de la Recherche
Médicale, Unité Mixte de Recherche
S_1158 Neurophysiologie Respiratoire
Expérimentale et Clinique, Service des
Explorations Fonctionnelles de la Respiration,
de l'Exercice et de la Dyspnée Hôpital
Universitaire Pitié-Salpêtrière (AP-HP),
Département Respiration, Réanimation,
Réhabilitation, Sommeil, Pôle PRAGUES,
Groupe Hospitalier Pitié-Salpêtrière Charles
Foix, Assistance Publique-Hôpitaux de Paris,
Paris, France

FRANÇOIS MALTAIS, MD
Centre de Recherche, Institut Universitaire
de Cardiologie et de Pneumologie de
Québec, Université Laval, Québec,
Canada

KATHRYN M. MILNE, MD, FRCPC
Department of Medicine, Queen's University,
Kingston Health Sciences Centre, Kingston,
Ontario, Canada; Department of Medicine,
Clinician Investigator Program, University of
British Columbia, Vancouver, British Columbia,
Canada

YANNICK MOLGAT-SEON, PhD
Centre for Heart Lung Innovation, St. Paul's
Hospital, Department of Physical Therapy,
Faculty of Medicine, University of British
Columbia, Vancouver, British Columbia,
Canada

PAULO T. MULLER, MD, PhD
Professor, Division of Respirology, Federal
University of Mato Grosso do Sul, Campo
Grande, Brazil

**J. ALBERTO NEDER, MD, PhD, FRCPC,
FERS**
Professor, Laboratory of Clinical Exercise
Physiology, Division of Respirology,
Department of Medicine, Kingston Health
Science Center, Queen's University, Kingston,
Ontario, Canada

ANDRÉ NYBERG, RPT, PhD
Department of Community Medicine and
Rehabilitation, Section of Physiotherapy, Umeå
University, Umeå, Sweden

**DENIS E. O'DONNELL, MD, FRCPI, FRCPC,
FERS**
Professor, Respiratory Investigation Unit,
Division of Respirology, Kingston Health
Science Center & Queen's University,
Kingston, Ontario, Canada

LYLE J. OLSON, MD
Department of Cardiovascular Diseases, Mayo
Clinic, Rochester, Minnesota, USA

MICHAEL I. POLKEY, MB ChB, PhD, FRCP
Consultant Physician, Department of
Respiratory Medicine, Royal Brompton &
Harefield NHS Foundation Trust, London,
United Kingdom

JANOS PORSZASZ, MD, PhD
Rehabilitation Clinical Trials Center, Los
Angeles Biomedical Research Institute at
Harbor-UCLA Medical Center, Torrance,
California, USA

ROBERTO RABINOVICH, PhD
ELEGI and COLT Laboratories, Queen's Medical Research Institute, The University of Edinburgh, Department of Respiratory Medicine, Royal Infirmary of Edinburgh, Edinburgh, United Kingdom

ALCIDES ROCHA, MD, PhD
Heart Failure-COPD Outpatients Service and Pulmonary Function and Clinical Exercise Physiology Unit (SEFICE), Division of Respirology, Federal University of Sao Paulo, Sao Paulo, Brazil

FERNANDA M. RODRIGUES, PT, MSc
Researcher, PhD Candidate, Department of Rehabilitation Sciences, Laboratory of Pneumology, KU Leuven–University of Leuven, Respiratory Division, University Hospitals Leuven, Leuven, Belgium

CHRISTOPHER J. RYERSON, MD
Centre for Heart Lung Innovation, St. Paul's Hospital, Division of Respiratory Medicine, Faculty of Medicine, University of British Columbia, Vancouver, British Columbia, Canada

DIDIER SAEY, PT, PhD
Centre de Recherche, Institut Universitaire de Cardiologie et de Pneumologie de Québec, Université Laval, Québec, Canada

ELISABETTA SALVIONI, PhD
Centro Cardiologico Monzino, IRCCS, Milano, Italy

MICHELE R. SCHAEFFER, PhD
Centre for Heart Lung Innovation, St. Paul's Hospital, Department of Physical Therapy, Faculty of Medicine, University of British Columbia, Vancouver, British Columbia, Canada

CURTIS A. SMITH, PhD
Professor (Emeriti), University of Wisconsin-Madison Medical School, Population Health Sciences, John Rankin Laboratory of Pulmonary Medicine, Madison, Wisconsin, USA

WILLIAM W. STRINGER, MD
Rehabilitation Clinical Trials Center, Los Angeles Biomedical Research Institute at Harbor-UCLA Medical Center, Torrance, California, USA

MARTIN J. TOBIN, MD
Professor of Medicine, Division of Pulmonary and Critical Care Medicine, Hines Veterans Affairs Hospital, Loyola University of Chicago Stritch School of Medicine, Hines, Illinois, USA

THIERRY TROOSTERS, PT, PhD
Professor, Department of Rehabilitation Sciences, Laboratory of Pneumology, KU Leuven–University of Leuven, Respiratory Division, University Hospitals Leuven, Leuven, Belgium

JAMES R. VALLERAND, PhD
Undergraduate Medical Education, Cumming School of Medicine, University of Calgary, Calgary, Alberta, Canada

SANDRA G. VINCENT, BScH
Department of Medicine, Queen's University, Kingston Health Sciences Centre, Kingston, Ontario, Canada

JASON WEATHERALD, MD
Division of Respiratory Medicine, Department of Medicine, Cumming School of Medicine, University of Calgary, Libin Cardiovascular Institute of Alberta, Calgary, Peter Lougheed Centre, Calgary, Alberta, Canada

MAGDY YOUNES, MD, FRCPC, PhD
Distinguished Professor Emeritus, Department of Medicine, University of Manitoba, Winnipeg, Manitoba, Canada

Contents

Accuracy in diagnosis trumps all other elements in clinical decision making. If diagnosis is inaccurate, management is likely to prove futile if not dangerous. Knowledge of physiology provides a periscope for identifying abnormalities beneath the skin responsible for clinical manifestations on the surface. Expert diagnosticians suspect disorders based on pattern recognition and automatic retrieval of knowledge stored in memory. A superior diagnostician looks at the same findings other clinicians see but thinks of causes that others have not imagined. Solving clinical mysteries depends on a clinician's power of imagination, not the capacity to recite an algorithm or apply a protocol.

On mechanical ventilation, the lungs is subjected to the action of 2 pumps with independent control systems. The patient's control system responds to actions of the ventilator via programmed mechanisms that alter respiratory output in response to lung volume changes; blood gas tensions; and, in conscious patients, to ventilator-induced changes that are different from those expected by the patient's control system. By contrast, the ventilator responds to the patient's actions according to operational characteristics of the specific ventilator mode. That patient and ventilator responses are not coordinated results in complex breathing patterns that may adversely affect the clinical outcome.

We examine recent findings that have revealed interdependence of function within the chemoreceptor pathway regulating breathing and sympathetic vasomotor activity and the hypersensitization of these reflexes in chronic disease states. Recommendations are made as to how these states of hyperreflexia in chemoreceptors and muscle afferents might be modified in treating sleep apnea, drug-resistant hypertension, chronic heart failure–induced sympathoexcitation, and the exertional dyspnea of chronic obstructive pulmonary disease.

Lung diffusing capacity for carbon monoxide (D_{LCO}) remains the only noninvasive pulmonary function test to provide an integrated picture of gas exchange efficiency in human lungs. Due to its critical dependence on the accessible "alveolar" volume

(Va), there remains substantial misunderstanding on the interpretation of DLco and the diffusion coefficient (DLco/Va ratio, Kco). This article presents the physiologic and methodologic foundations of DLco measurement. A clinically friendly approach for DLco interpretation that takes those caveats into consideration is outlined. The clinical scenarios in which DLco can effectively assist the chest physician are discussed and illustrative clinical cases are presented.

Respiratory muscle weakness is relatively rare in clinical practice; therefore, it is seldom a clinician's first thought. However, it should always be considered where a patient has unexplained breathlessness, respiratory failure, or experiences difficulty weaning from mechanical ventilation. Diaphragm weakness can often be ruled out by careful application of history, examination, and noninvasive bedside tests, although more quantitative tests exist. Where the predominant problem is respiratory muscle weakness, these tests convey useful prognostic information, which can be used for the management of an individual patient and to enrich study populations allowing reduced sample size in clinical trials.

The pathogenesis of obstructive sleep apnea (OSA) has undergone major revisions since it was first described in 1978. This article focuses on new advances. Although it is still necessary to have a collapsible airway to develop OSA, it is primarily the response to obstruction that determines OSA severity and clinical presentation. Identifying factors that determine whether the response is stable or unstable through phenotyping is a promising approach that may lead to pharmacologic therapy in selected patients.

We examine 2 means by which the healthy respiratory system contributes to exercise limitation. These include the activation of respiratory and locomotor muscle afferent reflexes, which constrain blood flow and hasten fatigue in both sets of muscles, and the excessive increases in pulmonary vascular pressures at high cardiac outputs, which constrain O_2 transport and precipitate maladaptive right ventricular remodeling in endurance-trained subjects.

Dyspnea, the most common symptom in chronic obstructive pulmonary disease (COPD), often becomes disabling in advanced stages of the disease. Chronic dyspnea erodes perceived health status and diminishes engagement in physical activity, often leading to skeletal muscle deconditioning, anxiety, depression, and social isolation. Broader understanding of the pathophysiologic underpinnings of dyspnea has allowed us to formulate a sound rationale for individualized management. This review examines recent research and provides historical context. The overarching objectives are to consider current constructs of the physiologic mechanisms of activity-related dyspnea and identify specific targets amenable to therapeutic manipulation in patients with COPD.

The Relevance of Limb Muscle Dysfunction in Chronic Obstructive Pulmonary Disease: A Review For Clinicians

Kim-Ly Bui, André Nyberg, Roberto Rabinovich, Didier Saey, and François Maltais

Chronic obstructive pulmonary disease (COPD) is often accompanied by extrapulmonary manifestations such as limb muscle dysfunction. This term encompasses several features, including atrophy, weakness, and reduced oxidative capacity. Clinicians should become accustomed with this manifestation of COPD because of its relevance for important outcomes such as exercise tolerance and survival. Measuring muscle strength and mass can be performed with simple and valid tools that could be implemented in clinical practice. One identified, limb muscle dysfunction is amenable to therapy such as exercise training that has been repeatedly shown to improve muscle mass, strength, and oxidative capacity in COPD.

Physiologic Effects of Oxygen Supplementation During Exercise in Chronic Obstructive Pulmonary Disease

Asli Gorek Dilektasli, Janos Porszasz, William W. Stringer, and Richard Casaburi

Supplemental long-term oxygen therapy (LTOT) is a well-established therapy that improves mortality in patients with chronic obstructive pulmonary disease (COPD) with resting hypoxemia. In the large number of patients with COPD who do not have severe resting hypoxemia but who desaturate with exercise, the clinical benefits that can be obtained by supplemental O_2 therapy during exercise is an area of interest and active research. A summary of current evidence for benefits of supplemental O_2 therapy and a review of physiologic mechanisms underlying published observations are reviewed in this article.

Strategies to Increase Physical Activity in Chronic Respiratory Diseases

Thierry Troosters, Astrid Blondeel, Fernanda M. Rodrigues, Wim Janssens, and Heleen Demeyer

Physical activity is important to maintain health. Patients who reduce their physical activity are at increased risk of developing comorbidities and faster decline in health. Interventions to enhance physical activity require a behavior change from patients and these interventions have become increasingly popular in chronic obstructive pulmonary disease. However, few interventions have shown long-term effects and all focused on enhancing physical activity rather than the maintenance thereof. In patients with very low exercise tolerance or with significant symptom burden, enhancing physical activity may be difficult and interventions should first focus on enhancing exercise tolerance.

Exercise Pathophysiology in Interstitial Lung Disease

Yannick Molgat-Seon, Michele R. Schaeffer, Christopher J. Ryerson, and Jordan A. Guenette

Interstitial lung disease (ILD) is a heterogeneous group of disorders that primarily affect the lung parenchyma. Patients with ILD have reduced lung volumes, impaired pulmonary gas exchange, and decreased cardiovascular function. These pathologic features of ILD become exacerbated during physical exertion, leading to exercise intolerance and abnormally high levels of exertional dyspnea. In this review, the authors summarize the primary pathophysiologic features of patients with ILD and their effect on the integrative response to exercise.

Chronic obstructive pulmonary disease (COPD) and heart failure with reduced ejection fraction (HF) frequently coexist in the elderly. Expiratory flow limitation and lung hyperinflation due to COPD may adversely affect central hemodynamics in HF. Low lung compliance, increased alveolar-capillary membrane thickness, and abnormalities in pulmonary perfusion because of HF further deteriorates lung function in COPD. We discuss how those negative cardiopulmonary interactions create challenges in clinical interpretation of pulmonary function and cardiopulmonary exercise tests in coexisting COPD-HF. In the light of physiologic concepts, we also discuss the influence of COPD or HF on the current medical treatment of each disease.

The heart and lungs are intimately linked. Hence, impaired function of one organ may lead to changes in the other. Accordingly, heart failure is associated with airway obstruction, loss of lung volume, impaired gas exchange, and abnormal ventilatory control. Cardiopulmonary exercise testing is an excellent tool for evaluation of gas exchange and ventilatory control. Indeed, many parameters routinely measured during cardiopulmonary exercise testing, including the level of minute ventilation per unit of carbon dioxide production and the presence of exercise oscillatory ventilation, have been found to be strongly associated with prognosis in patients with heart failure.

Periodic breathing (PB) during exercise is a slow, prominent, consistent fluctuation in ventilation and derived parameters that may be persistent for the entire exercise or present only in the early phases of exercise. It is associated with a negative prognosis, particularly if concomitant with PB during sleep. Little is known about exercise-induced PB physiology, but hyperventilation is likely due to an increased sympathetic activity combined with an enhanced stimulation of intrapulmonary, chemoreceptors and metaboreceptors, low cardiac output leading to increased circulatory delay, and cerebrovascular reactivity to CO2, all with have a definite role.

Cardiopulmonary exercise testing can be a useful tool for clinicians working with pulmonary hypertension (PH) patients. Exercise magnifies numerous cardiopulmonary decompensations, which can help inform diagnoses, assess degrees of physical impairment, evaluate exertional dyspnea, and estimate prognoses for PH patients. Supervised exercise training also holds promise in PH, because it is safe for patients and feasible and may improve key prognostic outcomes that relate to improvements in quality of life and survival. Still, few clinical trials have evaluated the potential therapeutic effects of exercise training, and future trials may benefit from integrating programming that focuses on light-intensity endurance, strength, and respiratory training.

Denis E. O'Donnell, Kathryn M. Milne, Sandra G. Vincent, and J. Alberto Neder

Unexplained dyspnea presents a significant diagnostic challenge. Dyspnea arises when inspiratory neural drive (IND) to the respiratory muscles is increased and the respiratory system fails to meet this increased demand. Cardiopulmonary exercise testing (CPET) is a valuable tool to unravel the causes of exertional dyspnea in the individual. Moreover, analysis of breathing pattern, operating lung volumes and flow-volume loops allows characterization of abnormal dynamic mechanical response to increased IND - an important source of breathing discomfort. We illustrate the clinical utility of this approach which examines respiratory sensation, ventilatory control, respiratory mechanics and cardio-circulatory responses in cases of unexplained dyspnea.

CLINICS IN CHEST MEDICINE

SERIES OF RELATED INTEREST

Clinics in Sports Medicine
https://www.sportsmed.theclinics.com/

THE CLINICS ARE AVAILABLE ONLINE!
Access your subscription at:
www.theclinics.com

Preface
Why Clinical Physiology Remains Vital in the Modern Era

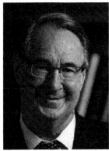

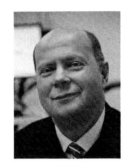

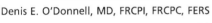

Denis E. O'Donnell, MD, FRCPI, FRCPC, FERS   J. Alberto Neder, MD, PhD, FRCPC, FERS

Editors

In 1955, a panel of famous physiologists led by Julius H. Comroe Jr[1] lamented the underutilization of basic principles of physiology in clinical practice. In the preface to their influential monograph, "The Lung, Clinical Physiology, and Pulmonary Function Tests," they wrote: *"Pulmonary physiologists understand pulmonary physiology reasonably well. Many doctors and medical students do not."* This sad reality inspired them to write their practical opus, devoid of turgid narrative and complex algebraic formulae and aimed at enlightening the reader *"by simple words and diagrams"* about those aspects of pulmonary physiology that are important to clinical medicine.

In the modern era, these existential concerns have become amplified, and there is a prevailing belief that many medical students, trainees, and clinicians lack a solid grounding in pulmonary physiology and its application in the clinical arena. Influential scientists bemoan the fact that the clinical physiologist represents "a vanishing phenotype" and that funding for research in integrated human physiology has dramatically diminished, and with it, educational opportunities for the next generation of clinicians. However, these dire predictions of an uncertain future have been solidly counterbalanced by the erudite contributors to this current issue of *Clinics in Chest Medicine* dedicated to Clinical Physiology. Their contributions demonstrate, beyond reasonable doubt, that this discipline is very much alive and indeed continues to

thrive and yield remarkable innovations in patient care.

The overarching aim of this issue is to highlight some truly transformative research in clinical physiology over the last few decades. These new revelations are succinctly presented by preeminent scientists, who offer a unique perspective on the clinical implications of these important advances. To set the stage, the practical importance of pulmonary physiology for proper clinical assessment and management of patients with respiratory diseases is emphatically underlined by a well-seasoned, master-clinician.

Refinement in mechanical ventilation strategies for patients in respiratory failure must rank among the greatest scientific achievements of modern times. Clearly, this is a great example of how direct application of physiologic principles can ultimately have a global impact on patient mortality and morbidity. The scholarly exposition of the physiologic basis for optimizing the interface of human and mechanical ventilator will be of great interest to clinicians treating patients with respiratory failure. Great strides have also been made in our understanding of the regulation of breathing in humans and the intricate compensatory responses mounted to physiologic stress and respiratory disease. This otherwise complex subject is lucidly deconstructed here to enlighten even the casual physiologist.

Reliable measurement forms the basis for the discipline of Clinical Physiology, and new insights

Clin Chest Med 40 (2019) xiii–xiv
https://doi.org/10.1016/j.ccm.2019.03.001
0272-5231/19/© 2019 Published by Elsevier Inc.

into the causes and consequences of physiologic dysfunction go hand in hand with advances in methodology. Measurement of the diffusing capacity of the lung for carbon monoxide is a well-established but often misunderstood physiologic measurement regularly used by clinicians. A fresh perspective is provided on the enduring clinical value of this simple measurement as exemplified by multiple case studies. In addition, advances in the comprehensive assessment of respiratory muscle function in patients with respiratory and neuromuscular diseases are adeptly presented by leading clinician-scientists.

Impressive gains have been made in our understanding of the pathogenesis of obstructive sleep apnea (OSA) and the heterogeneous physiologic underpinnings of this common disorder. This new knowledge will surely accelerate development of personalized management strategies for various clinical phenotypes of OSA and is germane to clinicians who treat such patients.

Cardiopulmonary exercise testing (CPET) provides a unique opportunity to evaluate the integrative functions of the metabolic, respiratory, cardiocirculatory, locomotor muscle, and neurosensory systems under conditions of measured physiologic stress. This field of study has recently been illuminated by new mechanistic insights into how harmonious integration of these multiple dynamic systems is achieved in health and how this becomes disrupted in cardiopulmonary diseases. Several articles in this issue have used CPET as the platform to explain the characteristic physiologic perturbations that shape the clinical presentation of patients with various respiratory and cardiocirculatory diseases. Chronic obstructive pulmonary disease (COPD), the most common chronic respiratory disease, received special consideration, and current constructs for the physiologic basis of exercise intolerance and its therapeutic reversal by supplemental oxygen and peripheral muscle training are clarified here. The growing evidence that reduced physical activity is a powerful predictor of poor survival and chronic morbidity in COPD prompted the inclusion of an important article on this topic.

Our knowledge of the underlying physiologic mechanisms of exercise limitation in various cardiopulmonary diseases has substantially expanded in recent years. This new information is presented in separate articles by leading experts in each of the following diseases: (1) pulmonary hypertension, (2) interstitial lung disease, (3) congestive heart failure (CHF), and (4) combined COPD and CHF. Finally, in an effort to consolidate this diverse information and to further reinforce the clinical utility of CPET, several illustrative case studies are presented. These show that, faced with challenging clinical presentations, CPET is well poised to unravel the complex mechanisms of dyspnea and exercise intolerance that can remain elusive even after extensive clinical investigations.

Denis E. O'Donnell, MD, FRCPI, FRCPC, FERS
Respiratory Investigation Unit
Division of Respirology and Sleep Medicine
Kingston Health Science Center &
Queen's University
Kingston, ON K7L 2V6, Canada

J. Alberto Neder, MD, PhD, FRCPC, FERS
Laboratory of Clinical Exercise Physiology
Division of Respirology and Sleep Medicine
Richardson House
102 Stuart Street
Kingston, ON K7L 2V6, Canada

E-mail addresses:
odonnell@queensu.ca (D.E. O'Donnell)
alberto.neder@queensu.ca (J.A. Neder)

REFERENCE

1. Comroe JH Jr, Forster RE II, DuBois AB, et al. The lung clinical physiology and pulmonary function tests. Chicago: Year Book Publishers; 1955. p.viii + 219.

Why Physiology Is Critical to the Practice of Medicine
A 40-year Personal Perspective

Martin J. Tobin, MD

KEYWORDS

• Diagnosis • Clinical reasoning • Intuition • Physical examination • Hyperventilation syndrome

KEY POINTS

- Accuracy in diagnosis trumps all other elements in clinical decision making. If diagnosis is inaccurate, management is likely to prove futile if not dangerous.
- The ability to apprehend clues that other clinicians miss depends on mental set (the prepared mind). Knowledge of physiology provides a periscope for identifying abnormalities beneath the skin responsible for clinical manifestations on the surface.
- Expert diagnosticians suspect disorders based on pattern recognition and automatic retrieval of knowledge stored in memory. Experts make decisions based on intuition rather than conscious analytical reasoning. Intuition is the fruit of years of book learning, analytical reasoning, and clinical practice.
- When making routine decisions, physicians typically do not cite mechanistic understanding, but they call on physiologic principles when confronted with challenging cases.
- A superior diagnostician looks at the same findings other clinicians see but thinks of causes that others have not imagined. Solving clinical mysteries depends on a clinician's power of imagination, not the capacity to recite an algorithm or apply a protocol.

My thoughts on the importance of physiology in clinical decision making represent a personal viewpoint based on more than 40 years of evaluating patients in outpatient clinics, hospital wards, and intensive care units (ICUs) while concurrently undertaking mechanistic physiologic research in patients and healthy subjects. The review is far from exhaustive, and I focus on items that stump present-day trainees and would have been far less challenging to residents in the early 1980s when I was hired as an assistant professor. The essay can be looked on as an *apologia pro vita sua*.

PROLOGUE

The 3 most important things in clinical medicine are diagnosis, diagnosis, diagnosis. As with a syllogism in logic, when the major premise is wrong, the elegance of ensuing deductions is irrelevant. The pivotal importance of diagnosis should be evident especially to pulmonologists. Despite deep understanding of the basic biology (chemistry, molecular biology) of venous thromboembolism and a slew of sophisticated diagnostic techniques, pulmonary embolism is the most frequently missed fatal diagnosis.

Conflict of Interest: M.J. Tobin receives royalties for 2 books on critical care published by McGraw-Hill, Inc, New York.

Dedication: This essay is dedicated to Professor Muiris X. FitzGerald, MD, University College Dublin, Ireland. M.J. Tobin served as M.X.F.'s registrar 1979-1980, and his approach to patient assessment and clinical decision making has served as the author's template throughout his career.

Division of Pulmonary and Critical Care Medicine, Hines Veterans Affairs Hospital, Loyola University of Chicago Stritch School of Medicine, Hines, IL 60141, USA

E-mail address: mtobin2@lumc.edu

Clin Chest Med 40 (2019) 243–257
https://doi.org/10.1016/j.ccm.2019.02.012
0272-5231/19/© 2019 Elsevier Inc. All rights reserved.

Fatal pulmonary embolism is found in more than 10% of autopsies. In 4 autopsy series, the diagnosis was missed in 55% to 70% of patients,[1–4] and in more than 80% of patients who had chronic obstructive pulmonary disease (COPD).[4] Mortality was 4 to 6 times higher in patients in whom the diagnosis was missed.[4] When promptly diagnosed and treated, pulmonary embolism rarely kills.

If formulation (and dissemination) of clinical-practice guidelines was the solution to a perplexing problem, fewer than 5% of pulmonary emboli should be missed. No other topic has attracted greater attention from the founders of evidence-based medicine (EBM), and it has been the subject of more guidelines than any other topic: the American College of Chest Physicians has published 10 editions of voluminous guidelines since 1986.

Elegant algorithms for the management of venous thromboembolism are of no value to patients if their doctor never suspects the diagnosis. This is the crucial stumbling block. For decades, physicians have been admonished to keep a high index of suspicion. Scolding is clearly not working. The fundamental problem is that symptoms of venous thromboembolism are far from unique, and many patients have atypical presentations. Most importantly, physiologic features are not consistent and are not readily detected at the bedside.

Every clinical encounter involves a search for clues that lead to a correct diagnosis. The task is to separate wheat from chaff, to spot pertinent clues and eschew distracting siren calls. Being able to ground one's thinking in physiology provides a roadmap that helps travelers reach the right destination. Pulmonary embolism presents a salutary example of what happens when clinical suspicion is not aroused by physiologic findings. It is not simply a case of being unable to navigate the road to the desired terminus; without a diagnostic trigger, physicians are not able to find the entry point, the feeder road, to get on to the correct highway.

> The search for the correct diagnosis remains the most crucial endeavor to assure the best possible care to patients.

MENTAL SET

When I stand at the bedside of a patient with a glaringly obvious physical sign, residents commonly cannot identify it. "To see what is in front of one's nose," Orwell averred, "needs a constant struggle."

Anatomy teaches that we see with the retina and visual cortex. This is true nominally, but incomplete. Immanuel Kant argued persuasively that the mind does not passively receive sense data.[5] Instead, it actively digests and structures what is being perceived. All cognition is channeled through the mind's categories, involving "a priori" forms of time and space. We look at what is in front of our eyes, but we discern with what is behind them, particularly through the prism of memory. "We see," mused Goethe, "only what we know."

In the *American Journal of Respiratory and Critical Care Medicine* series "How it *really* happened,"[6] most authors said their major discovery arose through serendipity. Many demurred that they did not discover anything, they were simply lucky. However, as Pasteur shrewdly observed, "Chance favors *only* the prepared mind."[7] The person making the serendipitous connection is already primed to appreciate its significance. An accidental event acquires significance only when it catches the attention of someone capable of putting it into scientific context. As with discovery in science, the same concepts apply to spotting clues in patients with obscure presentations.

The reason one clinician apprehends clues that other physicians miss depends on mental set: the set of beliefs that determines what a person perceives (the prepared mind).[8] Physiologic mechanisms provide a periscope for identifying what is wrong with a patient: pinpointing abnormalities in the machinery beneath the skin that are responsible for signs on the surface. A mental set forged through detailed knowledge of physiologic mechanisms selects and shapes what it is a clinician notices. Without a mental set, the obvious becomes invisible. The clinician is distracted and blinded by a blizzard of other possible diagnoses.

The word "physiology" has the same etymologic root as "physics": the study of things of nature. Many look on physiology as the application of physics to living organisms.[9] Ernest Rutherford, father of nuclear physics, quipped: "All science is either physics or stamp collecting," implying that soft activities such as surveys and categorization represent uninspired drudgework.

> A physiological mindset influences what a physician perceives and enables a physician to distinguish critically important processes from distracting findings.

WORK OF BREATHING

The most difficult cognitive challenge for intensivists is deciding whether (or not) patients can be managed without recourse to an endotracheal tube. This dilemma arises at the point of placing a patient on the ventilator,[10] and it recurs at the point of deciding whether the ventilator can be discontinued.[11]

The dominant reason to institute mechanical ventilation is increased work of breathing, and it is also the principal cause of weaning failure.[12] Given the supreme importance of respiratory work, one might expect that inserting esophageal-balloon catheters would be routine in the ICU. It is not. This is not because catheter insertion is technically challenging or the discomfort it produces (doctors have little hesitancy in performing far more painful procedures). Instead, interpretation of the tracings is formidable.[13] Precise calculation of intrinsic positive end-expiratory pressure is taxing in patients contracting their expiratory muscles. Lining up esophageal-pressure tracings against the chest-wall recoil line to construct a Campbell diagram requires nuanced judgment. These skills are not found in the quiver of most intensivists. Instead of attempting such calculations, clinicians can profit more by becoming skilled in performing a sequence of carefully performed steps on physical examination.

In judging whether work of breathing is increased, I rely on palpation of the sternomastoid muscle more than any other sign. This emphasis is not widely accepted. There is no mention of sternomastoid activity in the chapter on physical examination by Dr Murray in *Murray and Nadel's Textbook of Respiratory Medicine*; indeed, palpation is explicitly judged "the least productive" part of physical examination of the respiratory system and "is not routinely performed by many physicians."[14,15]

Patients with COPD rarely contract their sternomastoids when in a stable state. Insertion of electromyography (EMG) needle electrodes into the sternomastoids of 40 patients with severe COPD (forced expired volume in 1 second [FEV$_1$], 0.69 ± 0.18 L; 17 having hypercapnia) revealed activity in only 4 (10%).[16] Conversely, sternomastoid contraction is common in patients experiencing acute respiratory failure. In a study of patients being weaned from mechanical ventilation, my colleagues and I recorded (EMG wire) activity of the sternomastoid in all of 11 weaning failure patients but in only 3 of 8 weaning success patients (the latter activity was modest).[17] Sternomastoid activity became evident within the first minute of the T-tube trial in 8 failure patients but only 1 success patient, signifying that it is a sensitive harbinger of respiratory deterioration.

McFadden and colleagues[18] observed visible sternomastoid contraction in 59% of patients experiencing acute asthma attacks. It was the only sign (or symptom) that identified severe pulmonary impairment (dyspnea and wheezing were

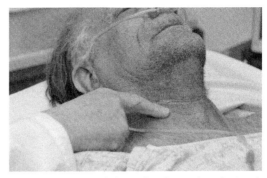

Fig. 1. Placement of the index finger (gently, barely touching) on the body of the sternomastoid muscle to judge the presence of phasic contraction and qualitatively determine its magnitude (mild, moderate, marked).

much less reliable). In patients with sternomastoid activity, FEV$_1$ was less than half that in patients without contraction (0.65 ± 0.26 vs 1.34 ± 0.56 L).

In the nineteenth century, French physicians considered sternomastoid contraction to be of such importance they dignified it the respiratory pulse.[19]

When gauging sternomastoid activity, I do not rely on inspection. Patients with minimal adipose tissue exhibit prominence of the sternomastoids without increased contractile activity, "sculpting," akin to the jutting sternomastoid in Michelangelo's *David*. Assessment requires placing the index finger, gently, barely touching, on the body of the sterno-mastoid, the finger pad mimicking an EMG electrode (**Fig. 1**). The examiner needs to focus solely on phasic muscle activity; tonic activity is used for posture and has no respiratory significance.

The second sign in judging work of breathing is tracheal tug, downward motion of the trachea with each inspiratory effort. Again, this sign should not be ascertained by inspection. Instead, the tip of the index finger should be placed on the thyroid cartilage (**Fig. 2**). Healthy subjects exhibit no

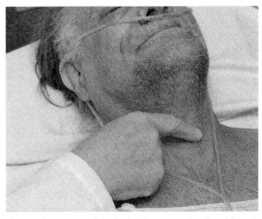

Fig. 2. Placement of the index finger on the thyroid cartilage to judge the presence of tracheal tug and qualitatively determine its magnitude (mild, moderate, marked).

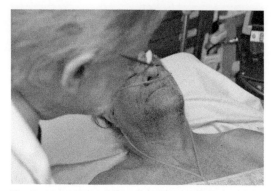

Fig. 3. Inspection of the suprasternal fossa to judge the presence of recession with each inspiration and qualitatively determine its magnitude (mild, moderate, marked).

tracheal tug. The degree of tug varies among patients, but its presence is always significant.[20] Because the respiratory muscles are not directly attached to the trachea, tugging is the result of the diaphragm pulling the entire mediastinum downwards with each inspiratory effort (like Quasimodo pulling the bell in Notre Dame) and, thus, signifying a marked increase in respiratory work.

The third sign involves careful inspection (not palpation) of the suprasternal fossa (**Fig. 3**). As swings in intrapleural pressure become more negative, the suprasternal fossa is visibly excavated with each inspiration. My colleagues and I demonstrated that recession of the suprasternal fossa, quantified using surface inductive plethysmography (a loop of wire fixed to the skin and excited by an oscillator circuit), was directly proportional to swings in esophageal pressure.[21] Supplementary evidence of increased pleural-pressure swings is obtained by inspecting the ipsilateral and contralateral hemithorax for intercostal recession[22] (**Fig. 4**).

Last, I check for diaphoresis, reflecting autonomic activation consequent to physiologic stress. I slowly move my index finger across the patient's forehead and then inspect the finger pad for moisture (this is more reliable than simply inspecting the brow for sweat) (**Fig. 5**).

With these 5 signs (sternomastoid contraction, tracheal tug, suprasternal-fossa recession, intercostal recession, diaphoresis), I form a judgment of whether work of breathing is increased or not and to what extent. There is no yardstick a physician can rely on for this assessment; discernment depends on having made the determination previously in thousands of patients (and storing them in the temporal lobe). The presence of signs of increased work is not necessarily bad (and absence is not necessarily good). If a patient has significant respiratory acidosis (or hypoxemia) and no signs of elevated respiratory work, the combination signifies respiratory depression. For clinicians harking after simple black-and-white rules, they do not exist and are never likely to exist. The signs need to be placed in overall context. There is no substitute for wisdom and experience when taking care of seriously ill patients.

Investigators have attempted to quantify physical signs and reported poor correlations with pulmonary function.[23,24] Such studies exemplify the McNamara fallacy (in logic): reaching conclusions based solely on quantitative data, discounting qualitative factors. Physical examination is a craft learned through apprenticeship. The essence of physical examination is its tacit coefficient; the explicit measurable components may be the least relevant.[10] As Georges Braque cautioned: "The only valid thing in art is that which cannot be explained."

The measurement I crave most in deciding whether to institute mechanical ventilation is

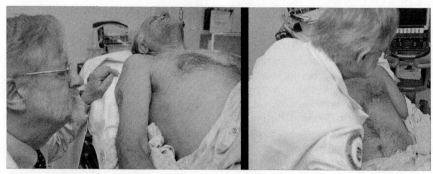

Fig. 4. (*Left*) Inspecting the ipsilateral intercostal spaces to judge for the presence of inspiratory recession. (*Right*) Sometimes recession is easier to detect upon inspecting the profile of the contralateral hemithorax. When inspecting each hemithorax, the clinician should also check for Hoover sign, a paradoxic inward motion of the lower rib cage during inspiration, signifying a flattened and disadvantaged diaphragm. (See Ref.[22])

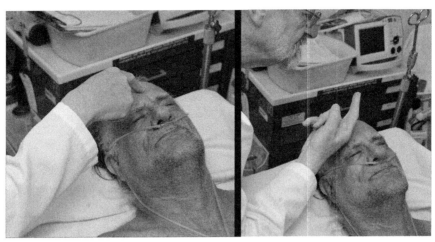

Fig. 5. To judge for the presence of diaphoresis, slowly move the index finger across the patient's brow and then inspect the finger pad for moisture.

spontaneous tidal volume (V_T).[25] This value cannot be gleaned from inspection, palpation, or auscultation.[26] In intubated patients, spontaneous V_T is visible on the ventilator screen, furnished by the pneumotachograph in the circuit. On switching ventilator assistance to zero, patients make little respiratory effort for 30 to 90 seconds because their respiratory centers are depressed consequent to relative hypocapnia and persisting mechanoreceptor stimulation. V_T increases gradually until it reaches a steady state. Eyeballing breath-by-breath values on the ventilator screen, the first 2 digits of the V_T should be higher than the respiratory frequency (f) (eg, 290 and 25); if lower, this signifies a frequency/tidal volume ratio (f/V_T) greater than 100.[27] Patients commonly perform better than the charted f/V_T simply because respiratory therapists obtain measurements long before a patient has attained a steady state. (Further discussion on this topic is provided in The Control of Breathing during Mechanical Ventilation).

In nonintubated patients, it is virtually impossible to get reliable measurements of V_T. It has long been recognized that employment of instrumentation requiring use of a mouthpiece alters breathing pattern.[28] (The Heisenberg principle is an omnipresent cofounder when evaluating respiration in patients.) Clinicians rely instead on respiratory rate. Although rate is a cardinal vital sign, most physicians do not know its normal value, imagining 20 breaths/min to signify tachypnea. That threshold has been enshrined in SIRS criteria of sepsis guidelines.[29] The average respiratory rate in health is 17 breaths/min with a normal range of 12 to 22 breaths/min.[30]

Respiratory rate needs to be placed in the context of a patient's physiologic characteristics.[25] Patients with stiff lungs (low compliance)

achieve a lower oxygen cost of breathing by breathing fast and shallow.[31] With elevated resistance, work is minimized by slow deep breathing. Rather than managing patients according to a protocol, each patient's unique physiologic characteristics need to be taken into account when making decisions regarding mechanical ventilation.

Recordings of peak airway pressure, plateau pressure, inspiratory flow, and delivered volume on a ventilator over 2 to 3 minutes provides greater insight into a patient's respiratory status than can be gleaned from an hour in a pulmonary function laboratory. Meaningful interpretation of the tracings (and their nuances) requires substantial grounding in physiology. I will not dwell on these recordings because I have discussed them too many times in the past: at length[12,32] and succinctly.[33–35]

> To reach a clinical judgment as to whether work of breathing is increased or not, the physician should palpate the sternomastoid muscles, palpate the cricoid cartilage to assess for tracheal tug, inspect the suprasternal fossa and intercostal spaces, and check for diaphoresis.

GAS EXCHANGE

Pulse oximetry has become the most widely used instrumentation after the sphygmomanometer. Although blood pressure is easily interpreted (given its linearity), the sigmoid shape of the O_2-disassociation curve can render pulse-oximeter interpretation similar to hieroglyphics. This is compounded by O_2 therapy. One of the commonest orders is "Titrate supplemental oxygen to keep O_2 saturation above 92%." The order is viewed so benignly that it is included in preprinted admission orders.

When properly used, pulse oximetry is invaluable in alerting staff of a significant deterioration in a patient's condition.[36] An unexpected decrease in oximetry to 88% (equivalent to Pao_2 55 mm Hg) alerts staff of the need to determine the cause of a patient's deterioration. Because of the flatness of the upper O_2-dissociation curve, a patient with a saturation of 95% (equivalent to Pao_2 75 mm Hg) while receiving oxygen therapy may incur considerable deterioration in respiratory function yet exhibit minimal decrease in oximetry.[37]

When supplemental oxygen is administered, tissue oxygenation is optimally achieved at an oxygen saturation of 90%.[38] To allow for biological fluctuation, it is reasonable to aim for an oximetry target of 92%. Physicians should always specify the upper boundary of the target: rarely is it advisable to accept oximetry higher than 94% (equivalent to Pao_2 70 mm Hg). A saturation of 97% to 99% (often seen with supplemental oxygen) is consistent with a Pao_2 anywhere between 90 and 500 mm Hg.[37] A 92% target minimizes the risk of oxygen complications (O_2-induced hypercapnia) while enabling oximetry to warn of significant deterioration in respiratory function (see also Physiologic Effects of O_2 Supplementation during Exercise in Chronic Obstructive Pulmonary Disease).

Using Pao_2 in assessment of gas exchange requires knowledge of fractional inspired oxygen concentration. This is instantly available in intubated patients, but unknowable in nonintubated patients receiving supplemental O_2. Nostrums such as 2 L/min by nasal cannula is equivalent to 24% inspired O_2 concentration are delusive because of variable entrainment of air between patients. With a nasal cannula set at 2 L/min, inspired oxygen concentration ranges anywhere between 24% and 35%.[39]

Calculation of alveolar-to-arterial O_2 gradient can be invaluable in decoding veiled presentations.[32] Proving rapid-onset pulmonary edema can be challenging in ventilated patients. Pulmonary infiltrates commonly preexist, making it impossible to see superimposition of new edema. Hearing crackles is confounded by ventilator noise. I have taken care of patients who repeatedly failed T-tube trials for no obvious reason. The sole consistent finding was decrease in Pao_2 associated with an increase in alveolar-arterial oxygen gradient; the finding of critical obstruction at coronary angiography, followed by stenting, led to rapid weaning and extubation.

Hypoxemia poses greater danger to patients than does hypercapnia. $Paco_2$, however, provides deeper insight into what is going wrong with a patient than does Pao_2.

The respiratory controllers (respiratory centers, neurons and muscles that produce alveolar ventilation) maintain a stable $Paco_2$ across wide fluctuations in CO_2 production (further discussion on this topic is provided in Update on Chemoreception: Influence on Cardiorespiratory Regulation and Patho-Physiology).[12] CO_2 production can vary 10-fold during exercise, yet $Paco_2$ remains virtually unchanged. This stability is achieved by exquisite sensitivity of the chemoreceptor system, typically expressed as change in minute ventilation during CO_2 rebreathing. The normal range is 0.5 to 8.0 L/min/mm Hg (1.5–5.0 in 80% of subjects).[12] Thus, an increase in $Paco_2$ of 3 mm Hg should cause minute ventilation to increase by 10 L per minute (or double). Failure to observe such an increase signifies significant respiratory impairment, because the patient either will not breathe (secondary to significant respiratory center depression) or cannot breathe (consequent to mechanical load or muscle weakness).

I was recently consulted about a young woman admitted to a medical ward with acute pancreatitis, for which she was receiving morphine at frequent intervals. Five days after admission, the patient experienced a cardiac arrest that resulted in irreversible hypoxic brain injury. An arterial gas, obtained 2 days before the arrest, revealed pH 7.29, $Paco_2$ 44 mm Hg, Pao_2 76 mm Hg, bicarbonate 18 mEq/L, and oxygen saturation 93%. In the progress notes, the resident noted "Patient saturating well on 2 L of oxygen with nasal cannula. Pco_2 levels within normal limits. Continue present management."

It is true that the patient's $Paco_2$ was within the normal range. However, the recorded $Paco_2$ signaled considerable compromise. The marked metabolic acidosis was producing substantial stimulation of the central chemoreceptors.[12] Consequently, $Paco_2$ should have been much lower than 44 mm Hg, more like 31 to 35 mm Hg. The $Paco_2$ of 44 mm Hg signified considerable respiratory depression. When staff further increased the dosage of morphine, they markedly increased the patient's susceptibility to further respiratory depression, hypoventilation, and hypoxemia.

At the other extreme, high $Paco_2$ is commonly accepted as sufficient to explain change in mental status. Readers can still profit by reading the 1956 article by Sieker and Hickam,[40] which provides details on 25 patients exhibiting varying degrees of hypercapnia and mental disturbance. If $Paco_2$ was less than 90 mm Hg (and pH >7.25), patients exhibited no change in mental state or only minimal drowsiness and intermittent confusion. Conversely, a semicomatose or comatose state was observed in every instance when $Paco_2$ was greater than 130 mm Hg (and pH <7.14). For $Paco_2$ between 90 and 130 mm Hg (and pH between 7.25 and 7.14), patients varied between consciousness and deep coma.

In patients proving difficult to be weaned from mechanical ventilation, it is profitable to relate $Paco_2$ to minute ventilation. If $Paco_2$ exceeds 45 mm Hg and minute ventilation exceeds 10 L/min, the pairing points to elevated dead space. The higher the minute ventilation (and higher $Paco_2$), the greater the dead space. Such patients will have great difficulty in making progress in weaning until improvements in lung disease lead to a decrease in dead space. There is rarely a unique therapy that dependably lowers dead space, and tincture of time is the safest prescription.

Interpretation of arterial blood gases is challenging enough without having ratiocination subverted by inaccuracies in venous blood gases.[41]

Evaluation of gas exchange involves relating arterial oxygen saturation to the shape of the oxygen-disassociation curve, relating arterial oxygen pressure (Pao_2) to inspired oxygen concentration, and relating arterial carbon dioxide pressure ($Paco_2$) to prevailing minute ventilation.

HISTORY AND PHYSICAL EXAMINATION

For patients attending a general-medicine clinic, studies show that correct diagnosis is made on the basis of history in about 82% of patients, by physical examination in 9%, and laboratory investigation in the remaining 9%.[42,43] Contributions differ with subspecialty referrals. Special investigations are more important than history or physical examination in patients presenting with gastrointestinal or endocrine problems.[44] Robust data on pulmonary clinics do not exist.

When taking a patient's history, it is imperative to ask open-ended questions, enabling the patient to drive the transfer of information. A new fashion has emerged among residents wherein they relate that a patient "endorses" something or other.

Information gleaned from leading questions runs the risk of not only being worthless, but also dangerous.

The commonest symptom I encounter in clinic is dyspnea (further discussion on this topic is provided in The Pathophysiology of Dyspnea and Exercise Intolerance in COPD).[45] Most referrals to my clinic have COPD or asthma, but a substantial number have dyspnea out of proportion to pulmonary function. Many of these patients have hyperventilation syndrome (psychosomatic dyspnea), yet trainees (and attendings) miss this diagnosis even when it stares them in the face.

The combination of substantial dyspnea with normal (or near normal) pulmonary function serves as an alert. The diagnosis is made primarily on history taking. The physician must listen in silence, allowing the patient to speak freely without interruption. Skillful listening involves hearing what a patient wants to communicate, as contrasted with getting the patient to tell you what you want to hear. Interrupting a patient's account early in the encounter backfires.

The characteristics of the dyspnea is different: patients typically describe a sense of being unable to take a deep enough (satisfying) breath, greater difficulty in breathing in than out, a sense of oppression (suffocation) in the chest. Unlike patients with pulmonary or cardiovascular dysfunction, dyspnea in hyperventilation syndrome has a less clear-cut relationship to exercise and is less likely to improve with rest. Chest pain is frequent and sometimes mimics angina pectoris. Some patients attribute symptoms to a life-threatening disorder, such as myocardial infarction, and, fearing death, rush to the emergency room.[46] Erroneous attribution sets off a vicious circle, causing more dyspnea and anxiety, leading to a sense of doom.[47,48]

Physical examination helps by excluding organic disease. While interacting with the patient, the clinician should be on the lookout for sighs. Healthy people take up to 4 sighs per hour,[30] whereas up to 100 sighs per hour are seen with anxiety[49] (Fig. 6).

Empathetic interaction (while elucidating the history) and explanation of what is causing the symptoms is the primary therapy. Patients have a long history of alarming symptoms for which no clinician has been able to offer an explanation. Many doctors consider these patients hysterical or anxious. Patients fear their symptoms will be considered imaginary, which further contributes to their distress.

When I make the diagnosis, I explain to patients that the cause of their symptoms is hyperactivity of the respiratory control system. I

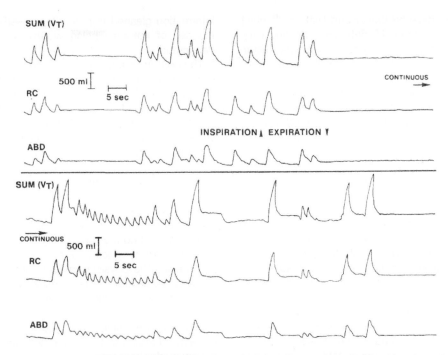

Fig. 6. Chaotic breathing pattern in a patient with chronic anxiety. Deep sighing respirations alternate with periods of rapid, shallow breathing and prolonged apneas at different lungvolumes. ABD, abdominal excursion; RC, rib cage excursion; SUM(VT), the sum of rib cage and abdominal excursion, equivalent to tidal volume.

explain that people differ in the number of signals sent from receptors in their lungs to the respiratory centers and that patients with hyperventilation syndrome are more aware of these signals than are people without dyspnea. Research shows that these patients have elevated respiratory motor output and other abnormalities of respiratory control.[47,48,50]

I emphasize to patients that the condition does not signify a psychiatric disorder (patients resent any insinuation that their symptoms are "mental" in nature). I communicate that they have a "lung condition" that is likely to continue, and the primary treatment is for a patient to understand its origin (increased signals to respiratory centers). I emphasize that despite repeated feelings of imminent demise, the condition never threatens life. The aim is to break the vicious circle that drives the symptoms by providing the patient with insight into the physiologic basis of the condition.[46–48] I never prescribe pharmacotherapy. Talking to the patient, words, is the most effective therapy.

A physician making the diagnosis of previously undetected hyperventilation syndrome has a greater opportunity of alleviating dyspnea than in patients with any other pulmonary disorder (as illustrated in Case # 7 in Unraveling the Causes of Unexplained Dyspnea: The Value of Exercise Testing).

Inspection, palpation, percussion, and auscultation constitute a time-hallowed quartet. I rely on inspection more than the other 3 and find inspection the component most often misapplied by trainees. Clinicians commonly miss Cheyne-Stokes respiration because they do not engage in a few minutes of silent inspection. Many devote less than 1 minute to inspection: axiomatically, the diagnosis of Cheyne-Stokes respiration cannot be made.

In patients with respiratory disorders, it is invaluable to surreptitiously creep up and watch their breathing pattern (**Fig. 7**). Spying is best accomplished when the patient is in a state of reverie or asleep (further discussion on this topic is provided in Pathogenesis of Obstructive Sleep Apnea). This golden opportunity is undone when some clodhopper announces loudly "we just want to watch your breathing."

The importance of palpation in assessing work of breathing has already been emphasized.

Elucidation of the cause of dyspnea requires asking open-ended questions, relating the degree of patient discomfort to the severity of pulmonary dysfunction, and surreptitiously observing the patient's pattern of breathing.

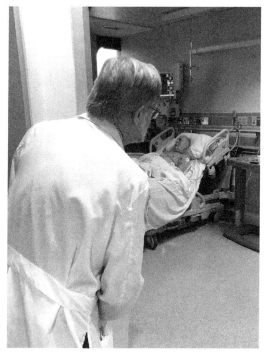

Fig. 7. Watching breathing pattern surreptitiously in order to evade the cofounding influence of the Heisenberg principle, wherein the technique of measurement changes the very entity being measured.

CLINICAL JUDGMENT

The naming of illnesses has become ostensibly less onerous because of widespread use of tags linked with *ICD* codes that empower clerks to claim reimbursement but are empty of cognitive content. Examples include *hypoxic respiratory failure*, an elastic term that begs more questions than it answers, *ventilator-dependent respiratory failure*, an appellation that connotes predestined defeat, and *acute respiratory distress syndrome (ARDS)*, a ragbag that subsumes multiple idiosyncratic conditions. When clinicians affix jejune epithets like these, they delude themselves into believing they have reached a diagnosis, whereas the designations obfuscate more than they illuminate. In a patient presenting with infiltrates and hypoxemia, a physician may diagnose ARDS and conclude that ARDS is causing the hypoxemia. Given that ARDS is defined by hypoxemia, the reasoning is circular (and vacuous).

For intensivists, the major challenge is to make decisions grounded on careful characterization of the patient: delineations derived from physiologic assessment (it is not based on procalcitonin titers or playing musical chairs with antibiotics). Rather than simply appending a diagnostic label, the cognitive task is: "What is *really* wrong with this patient, and how can I fix it?" A surgeon has steel, but a pulmonary and critical care physician has only thoughts. Fresh thinking that breaks free from circular reasoning and clichés is vital. Each patient is unique: not the next specimen on a conveyor belt awaiting treatment by protocol.[51]

We teach medical students (and we should) to search for all relevant information, weigh it, and formulate it into a differential diagnosis. However, expert clinicians do not use differentials when arriving at most diagnoses. Instead, they aim for a bull's-eye. On a list of 5 differentials, the 4 that do not match the actual diagnosis are of no value to a patient.

Cognitive-psychology research reveals that experts solve problems rapidly, *augenblick*, at the blink of the eye. Decisions are automatic, often nonverbal.[52] Much of daily practice consists of seeing patients who closely resemble previously seen cases. Diagnoses are based on pattern recognition and automatic retrieval from a well-structured network of stored knowledge.[53] Experts are generally not aware of solving problems and making conscious deliberations; rather, they do what normally works.[54]

The hallmark of an expert is sound intuition, which can be defined as a judgment that appears quickly in consciousness, whose underlying reasons we are not fully aware of, and is strong enough to act on.[55] Intuition is characterized by use of heuristics, mental shortcuts learned through experience, which saves time and effort.[56]

Intuition overlaps with tacit knowledge, as contrasted with explicit (conscious) knowledge. The central epistemological thesis of tacit knowledge is: "We can know more than we can tell and we can tell nothing without relying on our awareness of things we may not be able to tell."[57]

In *Thinking, Fast and Slow*, the Nobel laureate, Daniel Kahneman, brings together 5 decades of research on human decision making.[58] Kahneman presents human thinking as involving 2 independent systems. (Dual-process terminology has mutated, and the present preferred nomenclature is type 1 and type 2 processing.[59]) Type 1 is amazingly fast, intuitive, and effort free; it operates automatically with no sense of voluntary control. Type 2 does the slow work of forming judgments based on conscious thinking and deductive reasoning.[58] Doctors like to believe they mostly use type 2, but all humans use type 1 for about 95% of daily decisions.[60]

Evidence in support of dual-process theory is substantial and includes anatomic localization based on functional MRI. Intuition-based decisions by experts are associated with activation of the precuneus of the parietal lobe and the caudate nucleus of the basal ganglia.[61]

A second Nobel laureate, Herbert Simon,[62] did extensive research on perception of experts by studying what might seem to be the least intuitive of fields: chess. To develop the intuitive skill of a chess master required at least 10,000 hours of dedicated practice (5 hours a day for 6 years). From hours of intense concentration, a chess master becomes familiar with thousands of combinations and sees pieces on the board differently from the rest of us. Simon concluded that intuition is a form of pattern recognition: "The situation has provided a cue; this cue has given the expert access to information stored in memory, and the information provides the answer. Intuition is nothing more and nothing less than recognition."[62] Simon reduces the magic of intuition to the everyday phenomenon of memory.

Memory holds the vast repertoire of skills we acquire over a lifetime of practice. In a recent article, I discuss the differences in comprehension of material presented on paper versus online, and that material read online is stored in a weaker form of memory than material on paper.[63,64] Given the importance of memory for expertise, trainees are best advised to lay down the foundations for their storehouse of knowledge by deep reading on the printed page as opposed to scanning online resources. It is memory that enables wise decisions and skilled performance, involving the ability to deal with vast amounts of information swiftly and efficiently.[65,66]

The idea of intuition appeals to the lazy who think that true expertise is nothing more than a random guess or inspiration of a mystic. Guessing involves reaching a conclusion when one does not have sufficient knowledge or experience to do so. True intuitive skill (type 1) is the fruit of many years of deliberative analytical thinking (type 2): it is knowledge hard earned and shaped by experience.

> Experts reach diagnoses based on pattern recognition and automatic retrieval of knowledge stored in memory. Experts make decisions based on intuition (or tacit knowledge) employing mental shortcuts learned through repeated experience.

The following case illustrates the role of intuition, tacit knowledge, and memory. A nurse sees a patient fighting the ventilator and calls a resident to evaluate. The resident finds no obvious cause for distress and plans to administer lorazepam. An expert looks at the airway-pressure waveform and spots a bump at end-inspiration, causing her to suspect activation of the expiratory muscles during inflation (**Fig. 8**).[67] During pressure support, the switch between inflation and exhalation is delayed in COPD because of prolonged time constant. The delay fosters activation of the expiratory muscles while the ventilator is still trying to push gas into the patient.[68] On switching from pressure support to assist control, the patient stopped fighting the ventilator.

The bump at end-inspiration activated information stored in the expert's memory, causing a particular diagnosis, expiratory-muscle activation, to spring to mind. The expert was not so much thinking as reacting. Over years, experts build up a bank of experiences, stored in memory, that shapes how they perceive new information. The skill is not the result of conscious reasoning, but pattern recognition: a feat of perception and memory, not analysis.[62]

Although a clinician suspects a diagnosis within milliseconds (type 1), he or she still subjects the thought to analytical reason (type 2). The initial intuition may not feel right. When a decision carries considerable risks, a prudent physician asks: "What else might this be?" There are no pure type 1 or type 2 tasks in medicine, and no single approach can be applied across all diagnostic problems. The final judgment is typically a synthesis of the 2 systems.[69] An enlarged distal phalanx suggests clubbing, but the nail fold must be brought to eye level to check if the angle approaches 180°.

Speed in making decisions will arouse suspicion that a clinician is slipshod. The doctor conducting laborious rounds is viewed as more dependable and conscientious. However, the critical point is not the means used to reach a decision, but whether the decision is the right one (and that is why creative imagination is the key ingredient: see later discussion). Several experimental studies show that experts reach correct diagnoses very rapidly (type 1), and slowing down and deliberate use of type 2 reasoning do not improve accuracy.[70–74] This does not mean that trainees should be encouraged to make speedy diagnoses: diagnoses rarely need to be made with alacrity. That is not the point. Among experts, the speed at which they reach a diagnosis is linked with accuracy, and longer processing time is associated with more, not fewer, errors.[69] The irony here is that payment to physicians is proportional to time spent, rather than accuracy of decisions.

Mistakes that result from use of heuristics (type 1 mental shortcuts) are termed cognitive biases, and more than 100 have been described.[60] "Availability bias" is the disposition to consider a diagnosis more likely if it readily come to mind. "Premature closure" is the tendency to stop

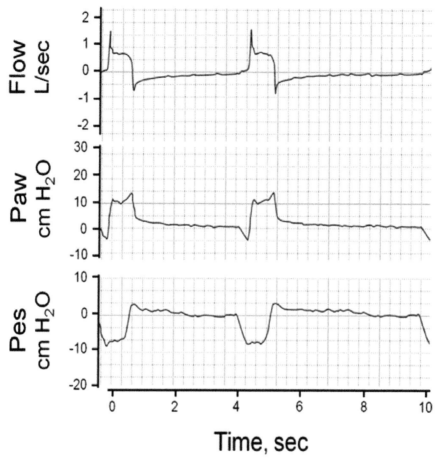

Fig. 8. A patient with COPD receiving pressure support 10 cmH₂O, with tracings of flow (inspiration directed upward), airway pressure (Paw), and esophageal pressure (Pes). The increase in airway pressure above the preset level resulted from activation of expiratory muscles.

decision making too soon and fail to gather additional critical information.

Some researchers claim that cognitive biases are responsible for more diagnostic errors than are deficiencies in knowledge.[75,76] If, however, a physician is not aware that positive airway pressure fosters persistence of a bronchopleural fistula, the problem is knowledge deficit, not a faulty thinking process. Despite repeated chidings about cognitive biases, experimental studies evince that knowledge is the key determinant of diagnostic accuracy.[70,74,77,78]

Some investigators recommend use of specific rethinking steps (metacognition) to minimize the normal human predisposition to cognitive biases, these are termed debiasing strategies.[75] Reflecting on one's decision making is commendable, but studies disclose that systematic employment of debiasing strategies does not reduce diagnostic errors.[79–81] It makes little sense to posit that diagnostic errors originate primarily with type 1[75,76] or type 2 processing because

both operations are involved in most medical judgments.

Physicians acquire 2 types of knowledge: *formal* (book learning) and *experiential* (from clinical encounters). Book knowledge provides the foundation on which experiential knowledge is constructed. Although physicians may not cite mechanistic understanding in routine decisions, they revert to physiologic principles when confronted with obscure or ambiguous situations.[53] In a study of complex electrolyte problems, nephrology faculty made more extensive use of physiologic principles than residents and reached correct diagnoses more than 90% of the time contrasted with 25% for residents.[82] Pathophysiologic knowledge relating to disease mechanisms serves as a theoretic framework for the organization and recall of clinical knowledge, and it persists longer in memory than information devoid of physiologic underpinning.[83]

Every so often, clinicians encounter problems whereby knowledge is incomplete, and they need to reason from first principles. In such a situation, it is better to base deductions on physiologic mechanisms as opposed to probabilistic outcomes based on chance.[84] The number of physiologic principles necessary for managing patients is endless: examples are listed in **Box 1**.

Box 1
Some physiologic principles that apply to patient management

- A fragile respiratory control system predisposes to life-threatening hypercapnia when supplemental oxygen is targeted to oxygen saturation greater than 94% (see also Update on Chemoreception: Influence on Cardiorespiratory Regulation and Patho-Physiology).

- Patients with sleep apnea are vulnerable to profound hypoventilation after small doses of sedatives (see also Update on Chemoreception: Influence on Cardiorespiratory Regulation and Patho-Physiology and Pathogenesis of Obstructive Sleep Apnea).

- A decrease in pulmonary artery pressure after pharmacotherapy may signify right-ventricular failure rather than improvement of pulmonary hypertension (see also Clinical and Physiological Implications of Negative Cardiopulmonary Interactions in Coexisting COPD-Heart Failure).

- In patients with elevated respiratory motor output, the default inspiratory-flow setting on a ventilator results in an increase in work of breathing (see also The Control of Breathing during Mechanical Ventilation).

- Patients with a prolonged time constant (COPD) typically recruit expiratory muscles during the inflation (inspiratory) phase of pressure support (see also The Control of Breathing during Mechanical Ventilation).

- Using low V_T on a ventilator is necessarily accompanied by shortening of mechanical inspiratory time, and, when this decreases below neural inspiratory time, double triggering (and delivery of high V_T) is inevitable (see also The Control of Breathing during Mechanical Ventilation).

- Airway pressures during compression of a bag-valve mask (Ambu) frequently reach 100 cm H_2O and can be responsible for cardiac arrest during resuscitation attempts (see also Clinical and Physiological Implications of Negative Cardiopulmonary Interactions in Coexisting COPD-Heart Failure).

A third Nobelist, Peter Medawar,[85] founding father of transplantation immunology, wrote more sagaciously about intuition than any other hands-on scientist. He emphasized that transformative advances in science depend on imaginative intuition (type 1), not the use of apparatus and the ritual of fact finding (type 2). Much writing on clinical reasoning cleaves to the 2-step hypothetic-deductive method, whereby a hypothesis is first advanced and then ruled in (or out). Clinical expertise resides more in dreaming of fertile hypotheses (type 1) than in doing tests (type 2).[86] Confronted with an inscrutable case, the imperative is to look at findings that other clinicians have seen and think of causes none have imagined.

In the past, it was believed that expertise was closely related to years of experience. In reality, the 2 are poorly correlated (skill commonly decays over time).[87] Expert performance, however, can be traced to active engagement in deliberate practice. Superior diagnostic performance is linked with repeated exposure to challenging cases, involving unusual presentations that draw on a rich understanding of pathophysiologic principles.[88] Repeated engagement with thousands of difficult cases, and ability to recall these from memory, is strongly related to expertise.[54,59,89]

Doctors are familiar with the truism that each patient is unique. Likewise, the reasoning of experts is unique because memory of cases is, by nature, idiosyncratic.[90] There is a positive-feedback loop between type 1 processing and expertise: the acquisition of expertise results in a better developed type 1 and sophisticated use of type 1 is what distinguishes an expert from a nonexpert.

If I were to pick the biggest deficiency in trainees, it is lack of imagination. Even worse is failure to appreciate the importance of creativity in solving vexing problems. When a physician is challenged with an enigmatic case, what he or she yearns more than anything else is to figure out what is happening beneath the patient's skin. Cracking these riddles depends on a clinician's power of imagination (type 1 processing). The solution of conundrums never rests in the capacity to recite some algorithm or apply a protocol. Unraveling mysteries depends on a clinician's capacity to imagine internal biologic happenings that explain external clinical findings. This is where physiology comes in. Faced with a perplexing patient, my mind conjures simulacra of machines with chambers and tubes, cogwheels, and pumps, and what happens when a spanner gets thrown into the works.

A superior diagnostician looks at the same findings that other clinicians see but thinks of causes that other clinicians have not imagined. Solving clinical mysteries depends on a clinician's power of imagination, the capacity to imagine internal biologic happenings that explain perplexing clinical manifestations.

CODA

When launching EBM, the founders specified their goal was to deemphasize all reasoning based on pathophysiologic rationale in the practice of medicine.[91] They have surpassed expectations of even the most starry-eyed devotee. Trainees of the 2010s possess a fraction of the pathophysiology known by residents of the 1980s. What did we get in exchange? The promise that grading of articles (into a hierarchy) would improve patient care, an epistemological strategy that had been demolished by far brighter brains (Karl Popper and critics of the logical-positivism movement) more than 40 years before.[92,93] Randomized controlled trials are invaluable in evaluating drugs and other therapies, but provide zero help with the principal impediment in all clinical encounters: perceiving the right diagnosis concealed beneath confounding camouflage (pulmonary embolism). Creative thinking depends on neurons nourished by scientific understanding, not on grading of articles. From the nineteenth-century onward, the epoch of Virchow, Bernard, and Starling, the practice of medicine had been grounded on physiologic principles. To barter science for sophistry is an exchange that even Faust would not have contemplated.

REFERENCES

1. Goldhaber SZ, Hennekens CH, Evans DA, et al. Factors associated with correct antemortem diagnosis of major pulmonary embolism. Am J Med 1982; 73(6):822–6.
2. Rubinstein I, Murray D, Hoffstein V. Fatal pulmonary emboli in hospitalized patients. An autopsy study. Arch Intern Med 1988;148(6):1425–6.
3. Morgenthaler TI, Ryu JH. Clinical characteristics of fatal pulmonary embolism in a referral hospital. Mayo Clin Proc 1995;70(5):417–24.
4. Pineda LA, Hathwar VS, Grant BJ. Clinical suspicion of fatal pulmonary embolism. Chest 2001;120(3):791–5.
5. Tarnas R. The passion of the western mind: understanding the ideas that have shaped our world view. New York: Ballatine; 1991. p. 341–6.
6. Tobin MJ. Introducing the "How it *really* happened" series. Am J Respir Crit Care Med 1999 Dec; 160(6):1801.
7. Bernard C. An introduction to the study of experimental medicine. New York: Dover Publications, Inc.; 1927. p. 38.
8. Butterfield H. The origins of modern science 1300-1800. London: G Bell and Sons; 1949. p. 205.
9. Haldane JS. An address on the relation of physiology to physics and chemistry. Br Med J 1908;ii: 693–6.
10. Laghi F, Tobin MJ. Indications for mechanical ventilation. In: Tobin MJ, editor. Principles and practice of mechanical ventilation. 3rd edition. New York: McGraw-Hill Inc.; 2012. p. 129–62.
11. Tobin MJ, Jubran A. Weaning from mechanical ventilation. In: Tobin MJ, editor. Principles and practice of mechanical ventilation. 3rd edition. New York: McGraw-Hill Inc.; 2012. p. 1185–220.
12. Tobin MJ, Laghi F, Jubran A. Ventilatory failure, ventilator support and ventilator weaning. Compr Physiol 2012;2(4):2871–921.
13. Tobin MJ. Respiratory mechanics in spontaneously-breathing patients. In: Tobin MJ, editor. Principles and practice of intensive care monitoring. New York: mcgraw-hill inc.; 1998. p. 617–54.
14. Murray JF. History and physical examination. In: Murray JF, Nadel JA, editors. Textbook of respiratory medicine. Philadelphia: WB Saunders; 1988. p. 431–51.
15. Fitzgerald FT, Murray JF. History and physical examinations. In: Mason RJ, Broaddus VC, Murray JF, et al, editors. Murray and Nadel's textbook of respiratory medicine. 4th edition. Philadelphia: Elsevier-Saunders; 2005. p. 493–510.
16. De Troyer A, Peche R, Yernault JC, et al. Neck muscle activity in patients with severe chronic obstructive pulmonary disease. Am J Respir Crit Care Med 1994;150(1):41–7.
17. Parthasarathy S, Jubran A, Laghi F, et al. Sternomastoid, rib cage, and expiratory muscle activity during weaning failure. J Appl Physiol (1985) 2007;103(1): 140–7.
18. McFadden ER Jr, Kiser R, DeGroot WJ. Acute bronchial asthma. Relations between clinical and physiologic manifestations. N Engl J Med 1973;288(5):221–5.
19. Maitre B, Similowski T, Derenne JP. Physical examination of the adult patient with respiratory diseases: inspection and palpation. Eur Respir J 1995;8(9): 1584–93.
20. Campbell EJM. Physical signs of diffuse airways obstruction and lung distension. Thorax 1969; 24(1):1–3.
21. Tobin MJ, Jenouri GA, Watson H, et al. Noninvasive measurement of pleural pressure by surface inductive plethysmography. J Appl Physiol (1985) 1983; 55:267–75.
22. Laghi F, Tobin MJ. State-of-the-art: disorders of the respiratory muscles. Am J Respir Crit Care Med 2003;168(1):10–48.

23. Godfrey S, Edwards RH, Campbell EJM, et al. Repeatability of physical signs in airways obstruction. Thorax 1969;24(1):4–9.

24. Spiteri MA, Cook DG, Clarke SW. Reliability of eliciting physical signs in examination of the chest. Lancet 1988;1(8590):873–5.

25. Tobin MJ. Non-invasive monitoring of ventilation. In: Tobin MJ, editor. Principles and practice of intensive care monitoring. New York: McGraw-Hill Inc.; 1998. p. 465–95.

26. Semmes BJ, Tobin MJ, Snyder JV, et al. Subjective and objective measurement of tidal volume in critically ill patients. Chest 1985;87(5):577–9.

27. Yang KL, Tobin MJ. A prospective study of indexes predicting the outcome of trials of weaning from mechanical ventilation. N Engl J Med 1991;324(21):1445–50.

28. Perez W, Tobin MJ. Separation of factors responsible for change in breathing pattern induced by instrumentation. J Appl Physiol (1985) 1985;59(5):1515–20.

29. Bone RC, Balk RA, Cerra FB, et al. Definitions for sepsis and organ failure and guidelines for the use of innovative therapies in sepsis. The ACCP/SCCM Consensus Conference Committee. American College of Chest Physicians/Society of Critical Care Medicine. Chest 1992;101(6):1644–55.

30. Tobin MJ, Chadha TS, Jenouri G, et al. Breathing patterns. 1. Normal subjects. Chest 1983;84(2):202–5.

31. Brack T, Jubran A, Tobin MJ. Dyspnea and decreased variability of breathing in patients with restrictive lung disease. Am J Respir Crit Care Med 2002;165(9):1260–4.

32. Tobin MJ. State-of-the-art: respiratory monitoring in the intensive care unit. Am Rev Respir Dis 1988;138(6):1625–42.

33. Tobin MJ. Respiratory monitoring. JAMA 1990;264(2):244–51.

34. Tobin MJ. Mechanical ventilation. N Engl J Med 1994;330(15):1056–61.

35. Tobin MJ. Advances in mechanical ventilation. N Engl J Med 2001;344(26):1986–96.

36. Jubran A. Pulse oximetry. In: Tobin MJ, editor. Principles and practice of intensive care monitoring. New York: McGraw-Hill Inc.; 1998. p. 261–87.

37. Severinghaus JW. Simple, accurate equations for human blood O_2 dissociation computations. J Appl Physiol (1985) 1979;46:599–602 (revisions 1999, 2002, 2007).

38. Chittock DR, Ronco JJ, Russell JA. Oxygen transport and oxygen consumption. In: Tobin MJ, editor. Principles and practice of intensive care monitoring. New York: McGraw-Hill Inc.; 1998. p. 317–43.

39. Bazuaye EA, Stone TN, Corris PA, et al. Variability of inspired oxygen concentration with nasal cannulas. Thorax 1992;47(8):609–11.

40. Sieker HO, Hickam JB. Carbon dioxide intoxication: the clinical syndrome, its etiology and management with particular reference to the use of mechanical respirators. Medicine 1956;35:389–423.

41. Wallbridge PD, Hannan LM, Joosten SA, et al. Clinical utility of sequential venous blood gas measurement in the assessment of ventilatory status during physiological stress. Intern Med J 2013;43(10):1075–80.

42. Hampton JR, Harrison MJ, Mitchell JR, et al. Relative contributions of history-taking, physical examination, and laboratory investigation to diagnosis and management of medical outpatients. Br Med J 1975;2(5969):486–9.

43. Peterson MC, Holbrook JH, Von Hales D, et al. Contributions of the history, physical examination, and laboratory investigation in making medical diagnoses. West J Med 1992;156(2):163–5.

44. Sandler G. Importance of the history ventilatory failure is in the medical clinic and the cost of unnecessary tests. Am Heart J 1980;100(6 Pt 1):928–31.

45. Tobin MJ. Dyspnea: pathophysiologic basis, clinical presentation, and management. Arch Intern Med 1990;150(8):1604–13.

46. Saisch SG, Wessely S, Gardner WN. Patients with acute hyperventilation presenting to an inner-city emergency department. Chest 1996;110(4):952–7.

47. Gardner WN. The pathophysiology of hyperventilation disorders. Chest 1996;109:516–34.

48. Howell JBL. Behavioural breathlessness. Thorax 1990;45:287–92.

49. Tobin MJ, Chadha TS, Jenouri G, et al. Breathing patterns. 2. Diseased subjects. Chest 1983;84(3):286–94.

50. Folgering H. The hyperventilation syndrome. In: Altose MD, Kawakami Y, editors. Control of breathing in health and disease. New York: Marcel Dekker; 1999. p. 633–60.

51. Tobin MJ. Generalizability and singularity. The crossroads between science and clinical practice. Am J Respir Crit Care Med 2014;189(7):761–2.

52. Elstein AS. What goes around comes around: return of the hypothetico-deductive strategy. Teach Learn Med 1994;6(2):121–3.

53. Schmidt HG, Rikers RM. How expertise develops in medicine: knowledge encapsulation and illness script formation. Med Educ 2007;41(12):1133–9.

54. Dreyfus H, Dreyfus S. Mind over machine: the power of human intuition and expertise in the era of the computer. New York: The Free Press; 1986. p. 30–1.

55. Gigerenzer G. Gut feelings: the intelligence of the unconscious. London: Penguin; 2007. p. 16.

56. Croskerry P. A universal model of diagnostic reasoning. Acad Med 2009;84(8):1022–8.

57. Polanyi M. The tacit dimension. New York: Anchor; 1967. p. 4.

58. Kahneman D. Thinking, fast and slow. New York: Farrar, Straus and Giroux; 2011.

59. Evans JS, Stanovich KE. Dual-process theories of higher cognition: advancing the debate. Perspect Psychol Sci 2013;8(3):223–41.

60. Croskerry P, Singhal G, Mamede S. Cognitive de-biasing 1: origins of bias and theory of debiasing. BMJ Qual Saf 2013;22(Suppl 2):ii58–64.

61. Wan X, Nakatani H, Ueno K, et al. The neural basis of intuitive best next-move generation in board game experts. Science 2011;331(6015):341–6.

62. Simon HA. What is an "explanation" of behavior? Psychol Sci 1992;3(3):150–61.

63. Tobin MJ. Put down your smartphone and pick up a book. BMJ 2014;349:g4521.

64. Tobin MJ. Author's response to comments on "Put down your smartphone and pick up a book. BMJ 2014. Available at: http://www.bmj.com/content/349/bmj.g4521/rapid-responses.

65. Mayer RE. Applying the science of learning to medical education. Med Educ 2010;44(6):543–9.

66. Mayer RE. What neurosurgeons should discover about the science of learning. Clin Neurosurg 2009;56:57–65.

67. Jubran A, Van de Graaff WB, Tobin MJ. Variability of patient-ventilator interaction with pressure support ventilation in patients with chronic obstructive pulmonary disease. Am J Respir Crit Care Med 1995;152(1):129–36.

68. Parthasarathy S, Jubran A, Tobin MJ. Cycling of inspiratory and expiratory muscle groups with the ventilator in airflow limitation. Am J Respir Crit Care Med 1998;158(5 Pt 1):1471–8.

69. Norman GR, Monteiro SD, Sherbino J, et al. The causes of errors in clinical reasoning: cognitive biases, knowledge deficits, and dual process thinking. Acad Med 2017;92(1):23–30.

70. Norman GR, Rosenthal D, Brooks LR, et al. The development of expertise in dermatology. Arch Dermatol 1989;125(8):1063–8.

71. Sherbino J, Dore KL, Wood TJ, et al. The relationship between response time and diagnostic accuracy. Acad Med 2012;87(6):785–91.

72. Ilgen JS, Bowen JL, McIntyre LA, et al. Comparing diagnostic performance and the utility of clinical vignette-based assessment under testing conditions designed to encourage either automatic or analytic thought. Acad Med 2013;88(10):1545–51.

73. Norman G, Sherbino J, Dore K, et al. The etiology of diagnostic errors: a controlled trial of system 1 versus system 2 reasoning. Acad Med 2014;89(2):277–84.

74. Monteiro SD, Sherbino JD, Ilgen JS, et al. Disrupting diagnostic reasoning: do interruptions, instructions, and experience affect the diagnostic accuracy and response time of residents and emergency physicians? Acad Med 2015;90(4):511–7.

75. Croskerry P. The importance of cognitive errors in diagnosis and strategies to minimize them. Acad Med 2003;78(8):775–80.

76. Graber ML, Franklin N, Gordon R. Diagnostic error in internal medicine. Arch Intern Med 2005;165(13):1493–9.

77. Hatala R, Norman GR, Brooks LR. Impact of a clinical scenario on accuracy of electrocardiogram interpretation. J Gen Intern Med 1999;14(2):126–9.

78. Groves M, O'Rourke P, Alexander H. Clinical reasoning: the relative contribution of identification, interpretation and hypothesis errors to misdiagnosis. Med Teach 2003;25(6):621–5.

79. Sherbino J, Yip S, Dore KL, et al. The effectiveness of cognitive forcing strategies to decrease diagnostic error: an exploratory study. Teach Learn Med 2011;23(1):78–84.

80. Sherbino J, Kulasegaram K, Howey E, et al. Ineffectiveness of cognitive forcing strategies to reduce biases in diagnostic reasoning: a controlled trial. CJEM 2014;16(1):34–40.

81. Smith BW, Slack MB. The effect of cognitive debiasing training among family medicine residents. Diagnosis (Berl) 2015;2(2):117–21.

82. Norman GR, Trott AL, Brooks LR, et al. Cognitive differences in clinical reasoning related to postgraduate training. Teach Learn Med 1994;6:114–20.

83. Woods NN, Neville AJ, Levinson AJ, et al. The value of basic science in clinical diagnosis. Acad Med 2006;81(10 Suppl):S124–7.

84. Hacking I. The taming of chance. Cambridge (England): Cambridge University Press; 1990.

85. Medawar P. Induction and intuition in scientific thought: Jayne lectures to the American Philosophical Society. In: Medawar P. Pluto's republic: incorporating the art of the soluble and induction and intuition in scientific thought. Oxford (England): Oxford University Press; 1984. p. 99–103.

86. Norman GR, Coblentz CL, Brooks LR, et al. Expertise in visual diagnosis: a review of the literature. Acad Med 1992;67(10 Suppl):S78–83.

87. Ericsson KA. Deliberate practice and acquisition of expert performance: a general overview. Acad Emerg Med 2008;15(11):988–94.

88. Ericsson KA. An expert-performance perspective of research on medical expertise: the study of clinical performance. Med Educ 2007;41(12):1124–30.

89. Norman G. Research in clinical reasoning: past history and current trends. Med Educ 2005;39(4):418–27.

90. Norman G, Young M, Brooks L. Non-analytical models of clinical reasoning: the role of experience. Med Educ 2007;41(12):1140–5.

91. Evidence-Based Medicine Working Group. Evidence-based medicine. A new approach to teaching the practice of medicine. JAMA 1992;268(17):2420–5.

92. Tobin MJ. Counterpoint: evidence-based medicine lacks a sound scientific base. Chest 2008;133(5):1071–4.

93. Magee B. Popper. Glasgow (Scotland): Fontana Press; 1973. p. 46–8.

The Control of Breathing During Mechanical Ventilation

Magdy Younes, MD, FRCPC, PhD[a],*, Laurent Brochard, MD[b,c]

KEYWORDS

- Patient–ventilator interactions • Inspiratory time • Respiratory time constant

KEY POINTS

- Nonsynchrony between patients and ventilators is very common.
- Nonsynchrony takes different forms that vary with the ventilator mode, the mechanical properties of the respiratory system, the level of consciousness, the level of respiratory muscle effort, and the undistressed respiratory rate of the patient.
- Poor patient–ventilator interaction can result in serious complications that may adversely affect the outcome.

INTRODUCTION

The respiratory system of patients on mechanical ventilation (MV) is uniquely challenged; a single gas exchange system (the lungs) is controlled by 2 different pumps that interact in complex ways, depending on the ventilator mode, the mechanical properties of the respiratory system, and the level of consciousness. At one extreme, these interactions result in an ideal outcome: gas exchange is maintained at acceptable levels without distress and without inducing lung damage or diaphragmatic atrophy or injury. At the other extreme, the interaction may be associated with severe abnormalities in gas exchange, distress, lung injury, and/or diaphragm atrophy or injury. These complications adversely affect clinical outcome. Hence, it is critical that clinicians learn how to identify and respond to these abnormal interactions. Because of space limitation, only a brief overview of the complex mechanisms involved can be given. Interested readers can refer to several reviews for more detail.[1–13]

PHYSIOLOGIC PRINCIPLES UNDERLYING PATIENT–VENTILATOR INTERACTIONS
The Patient's Control System

The respiratory control system consists of respiratory centers in the brain stem; efferent pathways (spinal tracts and respiratory nerves), which transfer instructions from the centers to pump muscles; the thorax, which performs gas exchange and contains the pump muscles; and afferent sensory pathways, which inform the centers about the adequacy of gas exchange (chemoreceptors), the state of lung inflation (mechanoreceptors), and the presence of pathologic conditions in the lungs

Disclosure Statement: M. Younes is the inventor of a ventilator mode discussed here (proportional assist ventilation [PAV]). All related patents have expired and the author no longer receives any royalties from commercial institutions that provide this mode. L. Brochard's laboratory receives financial support or equipment from different companies for specific research projects: Medtronic Covidien (PAV+), Air Liquide (helium, cardiopulmonary resuscitation), Philips (sleep), Fisher Paykel (Optiflow Nasal High Flow), General Electric (ultrasound), Drager (Electrical Impedance Tomography), Sentec (transcutaneous CO2).
[a] Department of Medicine, University of Manitoba, 1001 Wellington Crescent, Winnipeg, Manitoba R3M0A7, Canada; [b] Medical and Surgical Intensive Care Unit, Keenan Research Centre, Li Ka Shing Knowledge Institute, St. Michael's Hospital, 209 Victoria Street, 4th Floor, Room 4-079, Toronto, Ontario M5B 1T8, Canada; [c] Interdepartmental Division of Critical Care Medicine, University of Toronto, Toronto, Ontario, Canada
* Corresponding author.
E-mail address: mkyounes@shaw.ca

Clin Chest Med 40 (2019) 259–267
https://doi.org/10.1016/j.ccm.2019.02.009

(nociceptors). In addition, this basic control system is subject to the influence of higher centers that, when the patient is conscious, provide additional inputs to the respiratory centers that can alter breathing in response to anxiety, excessive effort, pain, and other disturbances. The following features are particularly relevant to responses of the control system during MV (further discussion on this topic is provided in Update on Chemoreception: Influence on Cardiorespiratory Regulation and Patho-Physiology).

Mechanical properties of the thorax

The mechanical properties of the thorax underlie almost all abnormal interactions with ventilators. Gas exchange requires cyclic expansion and emptying of the thorax. This is achieved through cyclic activity of pump muscles and, during MV, cyclic changes in airway pressure. Clearly, tidal volume (V_T) and frequency are related to amplitude and frequency of the applied pressure. However, for any given amplitude of applied pressure V_T and flow-rate depend highly on the resistance and compliance of the thorax. Although also relevant during inhalation (see Pressure Support Ventilation section), it is simpler to illustrate their operation during exhalation:

Once inflated, the thorax must exhale what went in during inspiration before the next inspiration. Rate of emptying is primarily related to resistance and compliance of the respiratory system. It is intuitively obvious that for a given end-inspiratory volume (ie, peak alveolar pressure) rate of emptying is slower if airway resistance is higher. Likewise, for a given peak alveolar pressure at end inspiration, lung volume is higher if compliance is higher. Thus, more time is required to exhale this larger volume.

Without expiratory muscle activity to force air out at a faster speed, rate of emptying is a function of the product (resistance * (or x) compliance), generally referred to as the respiratory time constant. Because compliance units are in liters per centimeter of water (cmH_2O) and resistance units are in cmH_2O per liter per second, the product of the 2 has units of time. For a normal compliance of 0.1 L/cmH_2O and normal resistance of 5.0 $cmH_2O/L/s$, the time constant is 0.5 second. This means that volume and flow will reach one-third of their peak values at 0.5 second into exhalation and one-third of the latter values (ie, one-ninth of peak values) at 1.0 seconds, and so forth (**Fig. 1**). The thorax can, therefore, return to functional residual capacity (FRC) well within the normal expiratory time. However, if resistance is 12 $cmH_2O/L/s$, the time constant is 0.1×12, or 1.2 seconds. Three seconds are needed to reach

FRC. This expiratory time may not be available. The next inspiration would then begin before FRC is reached, resulting in what is called dynamic hyperinflation (DH). Slow emptying is responsible for many of the poor patient–ventilator interactions. By contrast, when the time constant is short (stiff lungs or relatively normal resistance), the lungs may respond too rapidly to the applied pressure, resulting in different abnormal interactions (see Control of Breathing with Different Ventilator Modes section).

> The respiratory control system consists of respiratory centers in the brain stem; efferent pathways (spinal tracts and respiratory nerves), which transfer instructions from the centers to pump muscles; the thorax, which performs gas exchange and contains the pump muscles; and afferent sensory pathways, which inform the centers about the adequacy of gas exchange (chemoreceptors), the state of lung inflation (mechanoreceptors), and the presence of pathologic conditions in the lungs (nociceptors).

Influence of higher centers Control of breathing during MV can differ substantially between wakefulness and sleep or obtundation. In sleeping or obtunded patient, control is dominated by chemoreceptors' feedback. Chemoreceptors' input increases whenever ventilation is inadequate (increasing $Paco_2$), resulting in greater inspiratory efforts and V_T. In addition, above a threshold chemical drive, the respiratory rate (RR) also increases. These responses moderate the increase in $Paco_2$. With overventilation, chemoreceptors' output decreases. Amplitude of respiratory efforts decrease but, unlike the case with hypercapnia, the RR does not decrease until a certain $Paco_2$, which is only slightly below normal $Paco_2$, is reached (apneic threshold). At this point, respiratory efforts suddenly cease completely (central apnea). Apnea continues until $Paco_2$ increases above the apneic threshold again. Thus, unless the ventilator responds to the weaker efforts by lowering applied pressure, overventilation continues until $Paco_2$ decreases below the apneic threshold and the patient then develops recurrent central apneas (see also Update on Chemoreception: Influence on Cardiorespiratory Regulation and Patho-Physiology and Pathogenesis of Obstructive Sleep Apnea).

During wakefulness, higher centers may alter this homeostatic response in 2 ways:

1. Respiratory efforts no longer cease when $Paco_2$ decreases below the apneic threshold. Thus, the mechanism by which chemical control

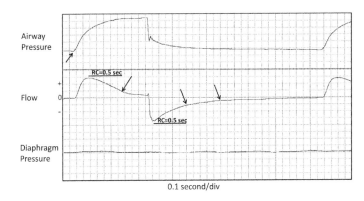

Airway
Pressure

RC=0.5 sec

Flow   0

RC=0.5 sec

Diaphragm
Pressure

0.1 second/div

Fig. 1. Time course of flow during inspiration during pressure support ventilation with minimal inspiratory effort. Note the minimal triggering effort in airway pressure (*up arrow*) and minimal inspiratory deflection in diaphragm pressure. The patient's time constant is 0.5 second. Flow decreases to one-third of its peak value with each elapsed time constant (*down arrows*), both in inspiration and expiration. div, division.

prevents severe hypocapnia (apnea) no longer operates and $Paco_2$ can decrease to very low levels.

2. Behavioral responses intrude into the control system. Typically, events are not perceived unless they are different from what is expected or desired. For example, the brain expects lung volume to increase when inspiratory muscle activity is ramping up during inspiration, and vice versa. Any deviation from this expected behavior, such as failure of the ventilator to trigger at the onset of inspiratory effort or to cycle-off when effort ends, is rapidly sensed and triggers defensive responses. These defensive responses are highly unpredictable and range from increasing efforts and use of expiratory muscles to entrain the ventilator to inspiratory efforts, to acquiescing to the ventilator and making only triggering efforts. The impact of these abnormal sensations on mood and sleep should also not be underestimated.

Determinants of desired breathing pattern

Breathing pattern is determined by the RR and the ventilation required to satisfy ventilatory demands. V_T is a dependent variable and is adjusted via chemical feedback to provide the required ventilation at the prevailing RR. There is a tendency in intensive care unit (ICU) medicine to equate a high RR with distress. Although the RR tends to increase when ventilatory demands are high, a high RR does not necessarily denote distress or high demand. The RR varies from 5 to 25 per minute in perfectly normal subjects. Adjustments to this basic (undistressed) RR are made in response to disease, body temperature, and emotional factors. An important difference between a high RR due to distress and one that is not, is whether the RR decreases if the ventilator assist is increased. If it does not, it can be assumed that it is not distress related.

An important feature of the patient's control system is that ventilation and V_T vary considerably as

the control system responds to changes in metabolic rate (eg, related to muscle activity), changes in higher centers' activity (eg, sleep, anxiety), fluctuation in blood gas tensions or blood pressure, and so forth. These fluctuations can be large and may occur over short (eg, breath by breath) or long intervals (eg, wake vs sleep). As previously indicated, higher centers expect sensory feedback to reflect these changes in demand. When normal subjects are placed on a ventilator delivering a constant V_T, and V_T is set to equal average V_T off the ventilator, they become uncomfortable, presumably because average V_T fails to meet V_T demand in some breaths. Comfort returns when V_T is set well above their normal average V_T, resulting in hypocapnia.

> *The breathing pattern is determined by the RR and the ventilation required to satisfy ventilatory demands. V_T is a dependent variable and is adjusted via chemical feedback to provide the required ventilation at the prevailing RR.*

CONTROL OF BREATHING WITH DIFFERENT VENTILATOR MODES

The ventilator settings essentially determine whether patient–ventilator interactions will be optimal or not, and what type of poor interactions will result. They are also tools by which clinicians can optimize interactions, with different patients requiring different settings to achieve optimal interaction.

Settings Relevant to Patient–Ventilator Interactions

Settings common to all modes

Settings common to all modes include trigger sensitivity and positive end-expiratory pressure (PEEP) level. PEEP level is important if DH exists.

By definition, with DH, alveolar pressure at end-expiration is above external PEEP (intrinsic or auto-PEEP). All ventilators require the patient to lower airway pressure below external PEEP and then some more by an amount that produces the change in airway pressure or flow required for triggering (trigger sensitivity). In such cases, a higher external PEEP reduces the difference between end-expiratory alveolar pressure and external PEEP and facilitates triggering. Regardless of DH, low trigger sensitivity requires more effort to trigger a breath. Particularly when efforts are weak (muscle weakness or overassist), some efforts fail to trigger the ventilator (expiratory ineffective efforts [IEs]). On the other hand, high trigger sensitivity promotes false triggering by circuit noise or cardiac oscillations, which may result in overventilation. Adjustments to these settings may be quite effective in mitigating poor interactions and the direction of adjustment depends on the nature of poor interaction (eg, increase trigger sensitivity with IEs and decrease it with false triggering).

Mode-specific settings The mode-specific settings most relevant to control of breathing on MV are those that determine V_T and duration of inflation (T_I):

Volume-cycled and pressure-control ventilation In the volume-cycled mode, both V_T and T_I are preset. In the pressure-control mode, T_I is preset, whereas the set pressure determines a minimum V_T that, similar to volume-cycled mode, will not decrease if efforts become weak. Considering that patient's RR does not decrease in response to hypocapnia (see Determinants of desired breathing pattern section), there is no way in either case for hypocapnia to be mitigated unless efforts cease completely (central apnea). At this point, however, the backup ventilator rate is activated. Whether breathing efforts resume depends on the set V_T or pressure (minimum V_T) and the backup rate. If the backup rate is sufficiently high, central apnea continues and the patient is then in totally controlled ventilation with all its complications. If efforts resume, $Paco_2$ decreases again below the apneic threshold and the patient alternates between triggered and automatic breaths with continued overventilation. The tendency for these modes to cause overventilation is compounded because, in alert patients, constant V_T is not tolerated unless ventilation is higher than what is required to maintain normocapnia (see Determinants of desired breathing pattern section). Thus, among the main disadvantages of these modes is the tendency to result in overassistance and respiratory muscle dysfunction.

V_T and T_I determine the mean inspiratory flow. The setting of peak-flow in assist-control ventilation has a specific influence on the respiratory drive and the patient's effort. An insufficient peak-flow compared with the needs of the patient is very uncomfortable and leads to increased effort. When this parameter is not directly set or displayed, a low peak flow will create air hunger or flow starvation. If misdiagnosed by the clinician, it will prompt the administration of sedation, whereas a readjustment of the setting will quickly improve the clinical tolerance. A drawback of high flow in the era of low tidal ventilation is that it may result in a very short insufflation phase. The latter may facilitate the occurrence of double triggering when neural inspiratory time is prolonged beyond the end of the insufflation.

Other types of poor interactions with these modes are related to the set T_I. The ventilator has no way of knowing when the patient's effort ends. Furthermore, the patient's T_I varies over a wide range (0.4–2.0 seconds). Thus, it is difficult to set a T_I that matches the patient's T_I. To compound matters, inspiratory pressure must increase a finite amount before triggering occurs (see Settings common to all modes section). Thus, a substantial portion of the patient's inspiratory phase can elapse before triggering (trigger delay). In most patients, the end of inflation is well beyond the end of patient's effort. Little time is then available for lung volume to return to FRC before the next effort. What happens then depends on the speed of lung emptying (the time constant; see Mechanical properties of the thorax), how strong the inspiratory efforts are, and how much time is available before the next effort. In one extreme (a long time constant and/or weak efforts and/or little available time) the next effort begins at a time when DH is high and fails to trigger (IE; **Fig. 2**). On the other extreme (a short time constant), lung volume can return to close to FRC. A new breath is triggered with every effort. With a high undistressed RR, the ventilator is triggered at a high rate, resulting in overventilation.

Other types of timing abnormalities can occur with these modes. If ventilator T_I is set too short relative to the patient's T_I, the patient's effort continues after airway pressure is reset to PEEP. A second breath can be triggered from the same initial effort, resulting in double triggering and breath-stacking. Finally, a ventilator-triggered breath can trigger a patient's inspiratory effort that would not have occurred otherwise, a phenomenon called entrainment or reverse triggering. Timing of the entrained breath can vary. Regular and repeated activation of respiratory muscles after time-initiated ventilator cycles during controlled MV is

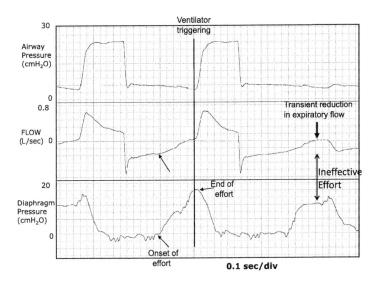

Fig. 2. Impact of long time constant on synchrony. A patient with severe COPD. Note that the onset of effort in diaphragm pressure began when expiratory flow was well above 0, indicating DH. Much of patient's inspiratory time was spent simply reducing the expiratory flow to 0 (note the change in trajectory of expiratory flow at the onset of diaphragm activity). This effort just managed to trigger the ventilator. The ventilator's inhalation phase is completely out of phase with patient's cycle. The next inspiratory effort fails to trigger the ventilator (Ineffective Effort at *arrows*), identified by transient reduction in expiratory flow.

referred to as respiratory entrainment or phase-locking phenomenon. Regular entrainment is not always present, and the pattern can be irregular or modified by the reverse breaths, such as incomplete expiration, air trapping, or double cycling. Reverse triggering has been described in ICUs in sedated mechanically ventilated patients with acute respiratory distress syndrome (ARDS) but also in brain dead patients, suggesting that different mechanisms may explain its occurrence. Should the entrained breath occur during the ventilator's exhalation phase it can result in an IE or trigger an extra breath (resulting in overventilation), depending on how strong the entrained effort is. If it occurs during inhalation, it may result in double triggering and breath-stacking.

> *Overassistance leading to hyperventilation and respiratory muscle dysfunction, insufficient peak-flow, and entrainment or reverse triggering are some of the drawbacks of volume-cycled and pressure-control ventilation.*

Pressure Support Ventilation As with pressure control ventilation, the set pressure in pressure support ventilation (PSV) dictates a minimum V_T that does not decease no matter how weak the efforts are. Unlike pressure control, however, ventilator T_I is not fixed, and there is no backup rate. These differences result in substantial differences from the control of breathing during controlled modes.

In PSV inhalation ends when the inspiratory flow, which peaks early in the inflation phase, decreases to a preset level or percent of the peak flow. Similar to the lung emptying during exhalation, the rate at which the volume increases and the inspiratory flow declines during inspiration is exponential, as determined by the time constant. With a long time constant (eg, chronic obstructive pulmonary disease [COPD]), the inhalation phase may continue for several seconds, pending the decline of flow to the threshold level. During this long inhalation, one or more inspiratory efforts may occur. Because the ventilator is already triggered, they present as transient increases in flow above the background exponential decline (inspiratory IEs; **Figs. 3** and **4**). For the same reason, (a long time constant) flow rate declines slowly during exhalation, which can result in expiratory IEs (see **Figs. 2–4**). Several breathing cycles may occur within one ventilator cycle (**see Fig. 4**).

Clearly, such a state would be poorly tolerated in alert patients. Alert patients are capable of establishing synchrony because of their higher respiratory drive or through operation of high-level reflexes that require wakefulness. However, once the patient falls asleep, respiratory efforts decrease and consciousness-dependent reflexes no longer operate. Slow deep breathing with IEs may suddenly develop on falling asleep or after sedation. Here, the change in breathing pattern with sleep onset is simply unmasking the presence of a long time constant.

The solution to excessive IEs is to reduce the pressure support level so that respiratory efforts become stronger and more able to overcome the DH that results from the long time constant. When the pressure level is reduced in such cases, the breathing pattern may rapidly change from slow deep breathing (with IEs) to rapid shallow breathing (see **Fig. 4**). This is often interpreted as respiratory distress even though it simply reflects the

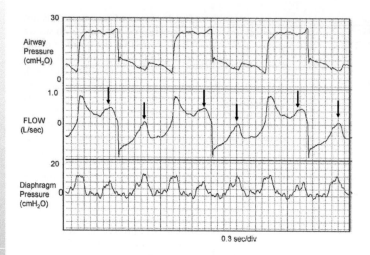

Fig. 3. A more severe case of nonsynchrony with IEs occurring both during the inhalation and exhalation phases of the ventilator (*arrows*), resulting in 3:1 rhythm (the patient's RR is 3 times that of the ventilator).

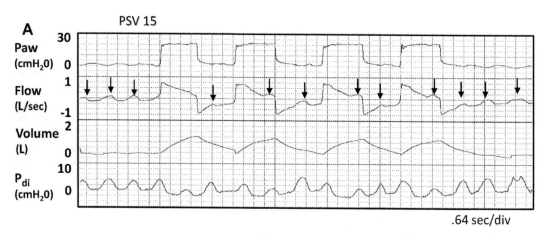

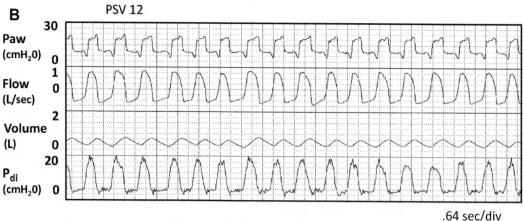

Fig. 4. Thirty-second tracings before (*A*) and after (*B*) reducing pressure support from 15 to 12 cmH$_2$O. Note the marked change in breathing pattern from slow deep breathing to rapid shallow breathing. However, the patient's RR remained the same (35/min). The amplitude of inspiratory efforts increased following reduction of pressure assist, resulting in the patient being able to trigger the ventilator with every effort. V$_T$ decreased in part because of the lower PSV pressure but mostly because inspiratory duration is now much shorter, which, in the presence of a long time constant, results in incomplete filling of the lungs at the end of the short inhalation phase. Arrows in A indicate IEs. Paw: airway pressure; Pdi, diaphragm pressure. (*Reprinted* by permission from Springer Nature: Springer Control of Breathing During Mechanical Ventilation by M. Younes Copyright 2005.)

unmasking of the patient's true RR. Pressure is increased again, perpetuating the overassist and associated nonsynchrony. Lack of awareness of this phenomenon can result in unnecessary delays in extubation. An increase in the RR on reduction of PSV pressure should not be considered a sign of distress unless accompanied by other indications of distress (eg, accessory muscle use, tachycardia).

By contrast, in patients with a short time constant (eg, stiff respiratory system) lung filling during inhalation is fast so that the patient receives the minimum V_T (which could be large) with every triggered breath. Furthermore, the flow threshold for terminating inhalation is reached quickly. There is, accordingly, no encroachment on exhalation time. This and the fast emptying during exhalation preclude DH and IEs. Thus, the ventilator is triggered with every inspiratory effort. Patients with fast undistressed RR will receive relatively large V_T at a fast rate. $Paco_2$ declines rapidly, resulting in central apnea. Without a backup rate, apnea persists until $Paco_2$ increases to above the apneic threshold. Rapid breathing with large V_T resumes and the cycle repeats. Development of recurrent central apneas on PSV should be attributed to high PSV pressure unless there are other signs of respiratory depression (hypercapnia, acidemia).

An advantage of PSV is that marked overventilation cannot develop. In patients with a long time constant, reduction in inspiratory efforts associated with mild hypocapnia will result in some efforts failing to trigger so that ventilator rate decreases. In patients with a short time constant, delivered ventilation will be reduced by intermittent central apnea. In either case, $Paco_2$ is constrained to be near the apneic threshold but not much below it.

Although PSV has the advantage of not being associated with marked hyperventilation, the inhalation phase may continue for several seconds, depending on the decline of flow to the threshold level in patients with a long time constant (eg, COPD). During this long inhalation, one or more inspiratory efforts may occur. Because the ventilator is already triggered, they present as transient increases in flow above the background exponential decline. Due to a long time constant, the flow rate declines slowly during exhalation, which can result in expiratory IEs. Thus, several breathing cycles may occur within one ventilator cycle.

Proportional assist ventilation and neurally adjusted ventilatory assist Proportional assist ventilation (PAV) and neurally adjusted ventilatory assist (NAVA) are radically different from

conventional modes in that there is no set V_T, airway pressure, or inspiratory time. The pressure assist is simply made proportional to the instantaneous inspiratory effort of the patient. What is adjusted is the proportionality between the instantaneous effort and the pressure generated by the ventilator. The ventilator simply amplifies the effort of the patient and the control of breathing is relegated back to the patient's control system.

When working properly, these modes are well synchronized with patient efforts so that comfort is enhanced and there are few, if any, IEs or central apneas. Because there is no minimum V_T, the risk of overventilation is minimal, thereby protecting against respiratory muscle dysfunction.

The 2 modes differ in the way the instantaneous inspiratory effort is detected. In PAV, it is calculated noninvasively from the pressure and flow signals. With NAVA, instantaneous inspiratory activity is measured using a specialized esophageal catheter that measures diaphragm activity. The main disadvantage of PAV is that triggering is still conventional; therefore, the effort must first increase to overcome any DH and the triggering threshold before the ventilator begins responding to the effort. In patients with DH and brief inspiratory effort (fast undistressed rate), this leaves little time for the ventilator to provide assist (note that ventilator cycles off when inspiratory effort ends). Patients may then develop distress despite high levels of assist. This can be obviated by using the initial increase in calculated inspiratory pressure to trigger. However, this is not yet available. NAVA is not subject as much to this problem because triggering occurs when inspiratory activity begins regardless of the presence of DH. Nonetheless, to avoid false triggering, diaphragm activity must still increase above a set threshold before triggering occurs; therefore, the same problem can occur if there is important baseline noise in the diaphragm activity signal. This mode also entails insertion of an esophageal catheter and requires the diaphragm signal to be stable over extended periods (days).

In the event that the patient's undistressed rate is high, and in the presence of many IEs before switching from another mode, switching to either of these modes will be associated with a sudden, often marked, change in the breathing pattern to a rapid shallow breathing. As in the case of reducing PSV pressure in patients with excessive IEs (see Pressure Support Ventilation), such a change simply unmasks the high undistressed RR of the patient and should not be considered as reflecting respiratory distress in the absence of other signs of distress. Particularly if the change occurs suddenly (eg, within 15 seconds after switching) it is almost certain that it is not distress related. Distress due to underassist takes a minute or more to develop.

In PAV, the instantaneous inspiratory effort is detected and calculated noninvasively from the pressure and flow signals. With NAVA, instantaneous inspiratory activity is measured using a specialized esophageal catheter that measures diaphragm activity. The main disadvantage of PAV is that the effort must first increase to overcome any DH and the triggering threshold before the ventilator begins responding to the effort. NAVA is not subject as much to this problem because triggering occurs when inspiratory activity begins regardless of the presence of DH. Nonetheless, to avoid false triggering, diaphragm activity must still increase above a set threshold before triggering occurs, so that the same problem can occur if there is important baseline noise in the diaphragm activity signal.

CLINICAL CONSEQUENCES OF POOR PATIENT–VENTILATOR INTERACTIONS

Patient–ventilator dyssynchrony is associated with poor outcomes, including higher mortality and longer durations of ventilation. Although an association is not a synonym of causality, these observations could be explained by several factors. Mechanisms of lung or diaphragm injury may coexist. It is possible that spontaneously breathing patients develop self-inflicted lung injury and dyssynchronies can contribute to this result. Repeated ultrasound examination of diaphragm thickness have shown that almost 60% of patients exhibit changes in thickness over time under MV; mostly decreased thickness but also increased thickness, suggesting muscle injury.

In cases of a high respiratory drive with volume control ventilation, high inspiratory efforts, presenting as flow starvation, can result in both diaphragm (excessive effort) and lung injury, through the generation of high regional forces generating pendelluft. When the respiratory drive is high and/or in the concomitant presence of inspiratory threshold loading by auto-PEEP and high airway resistance, load-induced diaphragm injury may develop. In both volume and pressure control, these efforts can also induce double cycles and breath-stacking. Then, increased V_T can lead to failure of lung protective ventilation, resulting in a worse outcome.

In sedated patients with a low respiratory drive, respiratory entrainment and reverse triggering can also generate double cycling with similar deleterious consequences due to a high delivered ventilation. In addition, because diaphragm contractions start late during the insufflation phase, peak activity occurs during the expiration, at a time when the lung volume is decreasing and the muscle is lengthening. This creates conditions of eccentric or plyometric contraction, which can be injurious for the diaphragm. In patients with ARDS, paralysis in the first 2 days of MV suppresses all these dyssynchronies, which may explain an observed reduction in mortality.

Finally, in patients with ineffective triggering, the same mechanisms may exist. In addition, the reduction in pressure support unmasks these non-triggered respiratory efforts, and this apparent increase in RR is often misinterpreted as a sign of distress. The patient is kept with excessive levels of support that result in delayed weaning from the ventilator. Also, as previously explained, repeated apneas during sleep result in multiple arousals and awakenings and a very poor sleep quality, with the potentially important consequence of sleep deprivation. IEs are most often related to overassistance. As previously explained, overassistance is very frequent with assisted ventilation and it can lead to disuse atrophy of the respiratory muscles, diaphragmatic weakness, and subsequent difficulties in weaning. If overassistance is avoided during MV or the diaphragm is activated by phrenic nerve stimulation, disuse atrophy is attenuated. Therefore, it is important to suspect it and the presence of IEs and low RR (below 20 per minute) is a simple clinical way to detect it.

Different studies have shown that IEs were associated with increased duration of MV and a lower rate of weaning success. Using the ratio of the number of dyssynchronous breaths to the total number of breaths, it was shown that having an asynchrony index higher than 10%, which existed in 26% of the patients, was associated with a longer duration of MV and a higher rate of tracheostomy. These results were confirmed using multivariate analysis to demonstrate that a high level of asynchrony was an independent predictor of a prolonged stay. The development of automatized techniques made the analysis of longer recordings feasible and not limited by the time to visually review recordings. Using such techniques over prolonged duration, it was shown than a high level of mortality was associated with higher ICU and hospital mortality. Finally, it has been observed that patients often present clusters of dyssynchrony; for example, more than 30 dyssynchronies in a 3-minute period. These events were very strongly associated with poor outcomes.

> *Patient–ventilator dyssynchrony is associated with higher mortality and longer durations of ventilation. Although it remains uncertain whether this reflects a cause-and-effect relationship, lung and/or diaphragm injury may coexist, leading to a poorer outcome.*

REFERENCES

1. Younes M. Patient-ventilator interaction with pressure-assisted modalities of ventilatory support. Semin Respir Crit Care Med 1993;14:299–322.
2. Akoumianaki E, Vaporidi K, Georgopoulos D. The injurious effects of elevated or nonelevated respiratory rate during mechanical ventilation. Am J Respir Crit Care Med 2019;199:149–57.
3. Younes M. Proportional assist ventilation. In: Tobin M, editor. Principles and practice of mechanical ventilation. 3rd edition. New York: McGraw Hill; 2013. p. 315–49 [Chapter 12].
4. Georgopoulos D. Effects of mechanical ventilation on control of breathing. In: Tobin M, editor. Principles and practice of mechanical ventilation. 3rd edition. New York: McGraw Hill; 2013. p. 805–20 [Chapter 35].
5. Younes M, Georgopoulos D. Control of breathing relevant to mechanical ventilation. In: Marini J, Slutsky A, editors. Physiological basis of ventilatory supportvol. 118. New York: Dekker; 1998. p. 1–74. Lung Biol In Health and Dis. [Chapter 1].
6. Pham T, Telias I, Piraino T, et al. Asynchrony consequences and management. Crit Care Clin 2018;34: 325–41.
7. Dres M, Rittayamai N, Brochard L. Monitoring patient-ventilator asynchrony. Curr Opin Crit Care 2016;22:246–53.
8. Sinderby C, Beck JC. Neurally adjusted ventilatory assist. In: Tobin M, editor. Principles and practice of mechanical ventilation. 3rd edition. New York: McGraw Hill; 2013. p. 351–76 [Chapter 13].
9. Pham T, Brochard LJ, Slutsky AS. Mechanical ventilation: state of the art. Mayo Clin Proc 2017;92: 1382–400.
10. Goligher E, Brochard LJ, Ried D, et al. Diaphragmatic myotrauma: a mediator of prolonged ventilation and poor patient outcomes in acute respiratory failure. Lancet Respir Med 2019;7:90–8.
11. Brochard L, Slutsky A, Pesenti A. Mechanical ventilation to minimize progression of lung injury in acute respiratory failure. Am J Respir Crit Care Med 2017; 195:438–42.
12. Tobin MJ, Jubran A, Laghi F. Patient-ventilator interaction. Am J Respir Crit Care Med 2001;163: 1059–63.
13. Yoshida T, Fujino Y, Amato MBP, et al. Fifty years of research in ARDS. Spontaneous breathing during mechanical ventilation. Risks, mechanisms, and management. Am J Respir Crit Care Med 2017; 195:985–92.

Update on Chemoreception
Influence on Cardiorespiratory Regulation and Pathophysiology

Jerome A. Dempsey, PhD*, Curtis A. Smith, PhD

KEYWORDS

- Sensory hyperreflexia in chronic diseases • Carotid-medullary chemoreceptor interdependence
- Hypersensitization of chemoreception

KEY POINTS

- Peripheral chemoreceptor stimulation has marked hyperadditive influences on central chemoreceptor responsiveness and central nervous system hypoxia is stimulatory to ventilation in physiologic preparations.
- Peripheral and central chemoreceptors and their interdependence as well as muscle metaboreceptors exert tonic influences on ventilatory drive and sympathetic vasomotor activity in health at rest and/or exercise.
- States of hyperreflexia occur in obstructive sleep apnea, chronic obstructive pulmonary disease, congestive heart failure, and hypertension and effective treatment of the resultant hyperadrenergic state, sleep apnea, and exertional dyspnea should require targeting of these hypersensitivities.

INTRODUCTION

The past decade has provided major advances in our understanding of chemoreception: its basic mechanisms of transduction; its role in cardiorespiratory regulation in wakefulness, sleep, and exercise; and its contributions to the "sensory hyperreflexia" and aberrant afferent tonicity[1] known to exist in such chronic diseases as hypertension, heart failure, chronic obstructive pulmonary disease (COPD), and sleep apnea. Our brief essay updates these topics with emphasis on key feedback influences on cardiorespiratory control emanating from carotid and medullary chemoreceptors and their interdependence, as well as from group III-IV metaboreceptors and mechanoreceptors in skeletal muscle.

PERIPHERAL/CENTRAL CHEMORECEPTION
Peripheral Chemoreception

The location and function of 2 distinct sets of chemoreceptors have been identified that play key roles in regulating both ventilation and sympathetic nerve activity. The primary oxygen sensors, the carotid body (CB) chemoreceptors, have the primary function of sensing P_{O_2}, $CO_2/H+$ in arterial blood. They are polymodal receptors that also sense many factors including but not limited to K+, temperature, osmolarity, glucose, and insulin.[2] Hypoxia is thought to be transduced by CO-modulated production of H_2S, which in turn promotes Ca_2+ release via mitochondrial and membrane pathways resulting in neurotransmitter release and increased neural activity in the carotid sinus nerve, which is

Disclosure Statement: No disclosures.
Department Population Health Sciences, University of Wisconsin-Madison, 707 WARF Building, 610 N. Walnut Street, WI 53726, USA
* Corresponding author.
E-mail address: jdempsey@wisc.edu

then transmitted to the central nervous system via the nucleus tractus solitarius (NTS) (**Fig. 1**). Transduction of $CO_2/H+$ at the carotid chemoreceptor occurs via a fall in glomus cell intracellular pH, which inhibits K+ channels, leading to membrane depolarization and a voltage-gated increase in intracellular $[Ca^{2+}]$, which triggers neurotransmitter release and increased neural activity in the carotid sinus nerve.[3] The carotid sinus nerve and ventilatory and sympathetic responses to hypoxia/hypercapneic combinations (ie, asphyxia) are powerful and hyperadditive, with the site of this hyperaddition occurring almost exclusively at the level of the carotid chemoreceptor.[4] The carotid chemoreceptor

response to hypoxia, per se, is curvilinear with respect to a falling Pao_2 and, owing to the Hbo_2 dissociation curve sigmoid shape, fairly linear with respect to arterial Hbo_2 percent saturation.

The ventilatory response to carotid chemoreceptor CO_2, in the absence of concomitant changes in PaO_2, appears to be relatively sluggish, as best demonstrated in awake goats and awake or sleeping dogs using extracorporeal perfusion of the isolated carotid chemoreceptor. In these animals, the raising of the isolated carotid chemoreceptor Pco_2 more than 15 to 20 mm Hg above eupneic air-breathing levels was required to elicit a significant hyperventilatory response.[5,6] The

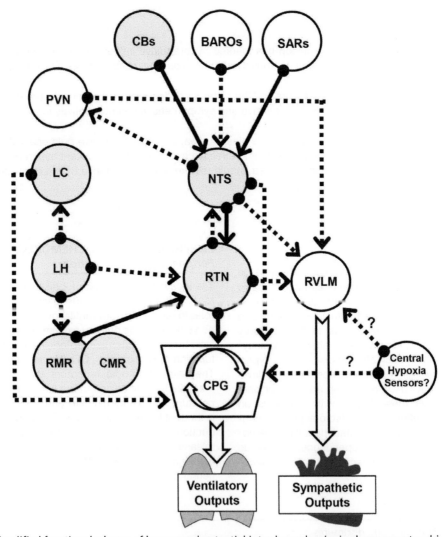

Fig. 1. Simplified functional schema of known and potential interdependencies in chemoreceptor-driven cardiorespiratory control systems. Yellow shading indicates structures known to be chemosensitive. Arrows indicate reported pathways; solid arrows indicate pathways known to show interdependence. See text for details. BAROs, baroreceptors; CMR, caudal medullary raphé; CPG, central respiratory pattern generator; LC, locus ceruleus; LH, lateral hypothalamus; NTS, nucleus tractus solitarius; PVN, paraventricular nucleus; RMR, rostral medullary raphé; RTN, retrotrapezoid nucleus; RVLM, rostral ventrolateral medulla; SAR, lung slowly adapting receptors.

hypoventilatory response to hypocapnic blood delivered to the isolated carotid chemoreceptor was more sensitive , as transient reductions in $P_{CB}CO_2$ during NREM sleep over the 3-14 mmHg range elicited immediate, dose-dependent reductions in Vt and mean inspiratory flow - but no alteration in breath timing.[7]

Central Chemoreception

Sufficient evidence now exists to support the medullary retrotrapezoid nucleus (RTN) as the primary and most sensitive site of "central" chemoreception of $CO_2/H+$ in its environment of the brain extracellular fluid. Several unique features distinguish the RTN from the surrounding glia and remainder of the lower brain stem respiratory network, including glutaminergic neurons characterized by expression of Phox2b and NK1 receptors.[8] Recent findings have shown that in contrast to the highly sensitive vascular reactivity of most of the cerebral vasculature to hypercapnic-induced vasodilation and hypocapnic-induced vasoconstriction, the RTN vasculature appears to be nonresponsive to changes in P_{CO_2} in its local environment.[9] Given that the vascular reactivity is intended to minimize changes in brain extracellular fluid (ECF) CO_2/H^+ for any given change in arterial P_{CO_2},[10] this lack of RTN CO_2 vasoreactivity means that RTN H^+ homeostasis would be sacrificed while preserving a hypersensitive RTN chemoresponsiveness.

Central Nervous System Hypoxia

Contrary to what has been commonly assumed from the results of studies in anesthetized animals, in the unanesthetized state central nervous system (CNS) hypoxia is stimulatory, rather than inhibitory, to ventilatory drive and sympathetic nerve activity. This stimulatory effect of CNS hypoxia is not always evident following CB denervation but is consistent in awake or sleeping animals when selective CNS hypoxia is produced (via inhalation of hypoxic concentrations) simultaneous with preserving tonic input from the isolated carotid chemoreceptor perfused with normoxic normocapnic blood (**Fig. 2**).[11,12] The CNS hypoxic ventilatory response is dose-dependent and approximately one-third the magnitude of that obtained when both CB and CNS are exposed to hypoxia, as in the intact animal. This ventilatory response is entirely driven by an increase in breathing frequency as opposed to increases in both tidal volume and frequency in the intact animal. Hyperventilation with CNS hypoxia first appears within 15 to 20 seconds following the onset of alveolar hypoxia, that is, in close proximity to the response time in the intact animal. CNS hypoxia, per se, also elicits a sympatho-excitatory response, although this response required quite severe levels of hypoxia, at least in the anesthetized animal.[13]

Although some medullary respiratory neurons have been shown to be directly stimulated via hypoxia in their immediate environment, recent evidence suggests a "non-neural" mechanism.[14] First, brain astrocytes are capable of sensing even small reductions in P_{O_2} via inhibition of mitochondrial respiration and subsequent release of ATP in close proximity to the brain stem respiratory network. Secondly, given that specific CNS hyperoxia, with maintained tonic input from the isolated carotid body or following carotid body resection (CBX), also stimulates ventilation, then increased reactive oxygen species are also likely to be a significant mechanism in this signaling cascade[15] (see **Fig. 2**). Thus, although carotid chemoreceptor tonic input appears to be required for a stimulatory response to CNS hypoxia, in the intact hypoxic animal both the CB (primarily) and the CNS (to a lesser extent) would be expected to contribute to the total cardiorespiratory response.

HYPERADDITIVE INTERDEPENDENCE IN THE EXPANDED CHEMORECEPTOR PATHWAY

Phox2b, a key gene product proliferating in early embryonic development of the autonomic nervous system, is strongly expressed in neurons that are part of an uninterrupted chain in a circuit that includes the CB and their afferents as well as the NTS projection to the RTN. Carotid chemoreceptor input also has a direct pathway from NTS to the central respiratory pattern generator (CPG) and even higher to the paraventricular nucleus (PVN) in the hypothalamus[8] (see **Fig. 1**). As outlined later, this entire "expanded" interdependent chemoreceptor pathway comes into play to explain the ventilatory and sympathetic vasomotor responses when carotid bodies are stimulated or inhibited via changes in arterial P_{O_2} or CO_2, or even when "tonic" carotid chemoreceptor activity is withdrawn under normoxic conditions during eupneic air breathing.

Fig. 3 reveals in the awake canine the importance of these interdependencies throughout the chemoreceptor pathway and especially the influence of carotid chemoreceptor input on "central" CO_2 chemosensitivity. Note in **Fig. 3**A that with CB inhibition achieved via perfusion of the isolated CB with hyperoxic hypocapnic blood, eupneic air-breathing ventilation falls immediately and reaches a nadir of approximately 60% below control after approximately 30 seconds of exposure on average. Beyond 30 seconds of continued CB inhibition, ventilation ($\dot{V}_E$) rises to approximately

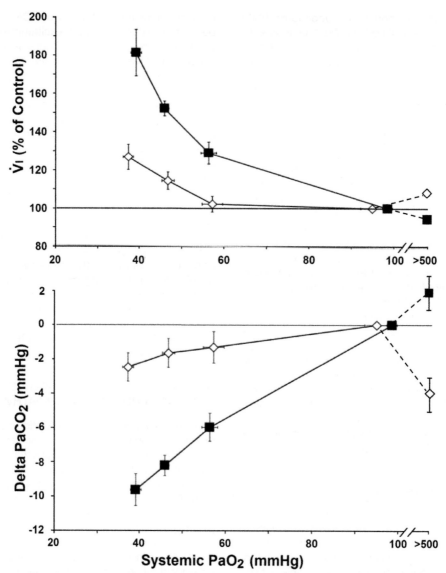

Fig. 2. Steady-state ventilatory responses to CNS hypoxia/hyperoxia alone (*open diamonds*) versus CNS plus CB hypoxia/hyperoxia (*filled squares*) in awake canines. The CNS hypoxic data were obtained using a perfused carotid body canine preparation to isolate the CNS from the CB with the CB held at normoxic and normocapnic levels via perfusion during inhalation of hypoxic gases (n = 11). The CNS hyperoxia data were obtained in bilaterally CB denervated dogs (n = 5). Note that when the CNS was exposed to hypoxia with CB held normoxic, dose-dependent hyperventilatory responses occurred that were approximately one-third of the response obtained in the intact animal when both CB and CNS were hypoxic. With CNS hyperoxia, a moderate hyperventilation occurred. The hyperventilation with CNS hypoxia was due entirely to a progressive increase in breathing frequency, whereas the hyperventilation in CNS hyperoxia was due primarily to an increase in VT. (*Data from* Curran AK, Rodman JR, Eastwood PR, et al. Ventilatory responses to specific CNS hypoxia in sleeping dogs. J Appl Physiol (1985) 2000;88(5):1840–52; and Rodman JR, Curran AK, Henderson KS, et al. Carotid body denervation in dogs: eupnea and the ventilatory response to hyperoxic hypercapnia. J Appl Physiol (1985) 2001;91(1):328–35.)

35% below control and remains at this level for 25 + minutes despite the substantial sustained systemic and CNS hypercapnic acidosis. That CB inhibition was markedly suppressing the central CO_2 chemosensitivity is further evidenced in the 30% ventilatory overshoot apparent immediately on termination of the CB hyperoxic hypocapnia.[16] This critical dependence of CB input on responses to central CO_2 accumulation was also shown via the hyperadditive effects of CB stimulation/inhibition on the ventilatory response slope to "central" CO_2, as illustrated in

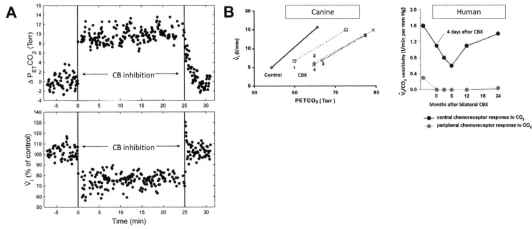

Fig. 3. (*A*) Effects of carotid chemoreceptor inhibition on breath-by-breath $\dot{V}_E$ and end-tidal CO_2 (PETCO$_2$) in normoxia in the awake canine. At time zero, the isolated and perfused CB was inhibited by suddenly reducing perfusate Pco$_2$ from 40 to 20 mm Hg and increasing perfusate Po$_2$ from 90 to ∼500 mm Hg. Normal CB blood gases were abruptly restored at the +25 minute mark. The persistent hypoventilatory response to CB inhibition despite the continued systemic and CNS hypercapnic acidosis consisted of a reduced VT, fb, VT/TI and EMG$_{di}$ and prolonged TE. (*B*) Thirty-five percent to 70% reduction in the slope of the hyperoxic CO_2 ventilatory response in the awake canine (left) and human (right) resulting from bilateral CB denervation. In canines, the response slopes are shown pre-CBX and at 1 to 4 days post-CBX (adapted with permission from Rodman and colleagues, 2001[18]). In the human, the plotted ventilatory response slope values represent those obtained early (less than 15 seconds) ("peripheral chemoreceptor") and later ("central chemoreceptor") in the CO_2 exposure period. The gradual rise in the "central chemoreceptor" CO_2 response slope at 6 months post-CBX shows the long-term plasticity of the CO_2 response following CBX. (*Adapted from* [A] Blain GM, Smith CA, Henderson KS, et al. Contribution of the carotid body chemoreceptors to eupneic ventilation in the intact, unanesthetized dog. J Appl Physiol (1985) 2009;106(5):1564–73; with permission; and [B] Dahan A, Nieuwenhuijs D, Teppema L. Plasticity of central chemoreceptors: effect of bilateral carotid body resection on central CO2 sensitivity. PLoS Med 2007;4(7):e239.)

the awake canine with extracorporeal perfusion of the carotid chemoreceptor. These hyperadditive effects occurred whether CB excitation/inhibition was accomplished via changes in oxygen, CO_2, or their combination.[6] These hyperadditive influences are also consistent with the effects of bilateral CB denervation in several species, including humans,[17,18] which resulted in a 40% to 70% reduction in the steady-state ventilatory response to hyperoxic hypercapnia (see **Fig. 3**B) and in a reduced response to focal cerebral acidosis.[19]

Souza, Guyenet and colleagues[20,21] questioned whether the marked hypoventilation/CO_2 retention accompanying CBX could be interpreted to mean that carotid body afferents contribute significantly to the drive to breathe under control (normoxic) conditions. These investigators critiqued use of the CBX approach to this question by raising the possibility that the surgical deafferentation procedure, with accompanying potential collateral damage to baroreceptors and sympathetic innervation, along with inflammation and synaptic rearrangement, was *not* equivalent to merely silencing the CBs. To the contrary, we argue that CB inhibition using the isolated perfused chemoreceptor preparation (see **Fig. 3**A) provides clear evidence that carotid chemoreceptors do indeed provide a substantial tonic

input to the eupneic drive to breathe. Based on the substantial, sustained depressive effect of carotid chemoreceptor inhibition on ventilation shown in **Fig. 3**A, together with evidence of a marked reduction in the central CO2 response slope in the face of carotid chemoreceptor inhibition,[6] the sources of this topic input would appear to include both the direct afferent input to the CPG plus the interdependence of central chemosensitivity on the level of peripheral chemoreceptor activity.

The chemoreceptor pathway involves integrative regulation of cardiorespiratory control extending from the carotid chemoreceptor to the hypothalamus.

The carotid chemoreceptor exerts a marked tonic input on the normal, eupneic drive to breathe even in health through its "direct" effect on the medullary respiratory pattern generator plus its significant hyperadditive influence on the central chemoreceptor sensitivity to CO_2.

This interdependence of chemoreceptor function also means that the common practice of assessing "central" chemosensitivity, per se, in intact humans and animals via the use of hyperoxic/hypercapnic inhalation is not justified.

To what extent tonic CB input in normoxia also influences sympathetic nerve activity is less clear. For example, transient inhibition of CBs in the healthy dog (using close carotid body injection of dopamine or hyperoxic saline) or in healthy humans with transient hyperoxia has no discernible effect on limb vascular conductance or on muscle sympathetic nerve activity (MSNA) at rest, but does cause significant MSNA inhibition and enhanced limb vascular conductance and blood flow during even mild-intensity exercise.[22,23] These sympathetic vasomotor responses were prevented via sympathetic blockade in the canine.[23] In many disease states (see later in this article) excessive chemosensitivity is manifested in chronically elevated sympathetic vasomotor activity.

Is the Rodent Model Exceptional/Appropriate?

Like other species, the rodent expresses a substantial and sustained hypoventilation and CO_2 retention following CB denervation, but unlike other mammals shows no reduction in the slope of the ventilatory response to CO_2.[24–26] We have no explanation for this puzzling dissociation between the marked effects of CBX on eupneic air-breathing ventilation and CO_2 retention in the absence of coincident changes in (superimposed) CO_2 sensitivity, other than they suggest an absence of any hyperadditive effects of CB input on the "central" CO_2 response sensitivity in this species. Despite these puzzling species differences, the anesthetized rodent does show a significant effect of systemic hypoxemia on the activity of CO_2 sensitive RTN neurons, which is prevented via CBX,[26] that is, a CB-RTN functional link does exist. Further, the rodent has provided all of the evidence thus far supporting CO_2-sensitive neurons in the RTN as an integrative site in the medulla whose output and cardiorespiratory effects are influenced by inputs from the vagally mediated stretch receptors from the lung as well as from locomotor areas of the hypothalamus[8] (see **Fig. 1**). Finally, recent studies in the awake rodent showed that obliteration of almost all neurons in the RTN will cause acute alveolar hypoventilation and CO_2 retention, similar to that achieved via CBX, but the alveolar hypoventilation was caused by an increase in breathing frequency and dead space ventilation with a reduced tidal volume (VT) and no change in overall ventilation ($\dot{V}_E$).[20] Given the almost exclusive use of the rodent currently for mechanistic studies of chemoreceptor-driven cardiorespiratory regulation, these differences between species limit generalization of findings. Similar concerns in assessing chemoreceptor

characteristics in the rodent and other small mammals stem from the marked reductions in their metabolic rate elicited on acute exposure to hypoxia. (Hypoxic stimulation of arterial chemoreceptor afferents coincides with a reduction in sympathetic outflow to brown adipose tissue, which in turn inhibits nonshivering thermogenesis, thereby contributing to hypoxia-induced reductions in body temperature and metabolic rate.[27]) Because CO_2 production (and/or pulmonary exchange of CO_2) is an important drive to breathe, it must always be measured and accounted for in quantifying hypoxic cardiorespiratory responsiveness.[28]

> The rodent is the mammal currently used almost exclusively for the study of mechanisms underlying chemoreception in health and disease. However, there are several fundamental differences between rodents and larger mammals in such factors as chemoreceptor interdependence and metabolic plasticity that need clarification before generalizations from rodents to humans are accepted.

HYPERSENSITIZATION OF CHEMORECEPTION/MUSCLE AFFERENT FEEDBACK EFFECTS ON BREATHING AND SYMPATHETIC NERVE ACTIVITY

Substantial evidence now exists to support a susceptibility to sensitization of such key autonomic afferent regulators as chemoreception and metaboreceptor and mechanoreceptor muscle afferents. For chemoreceptors, variations in the amount and "pattern" of O_2 supply are critical regulators of chemosensitivity, as shown in the following examples:

- On exposure to even moderate levels of constant hypoxia, carotid chemoreceptors begin to increase sensitivity within a few hours and continue to increase for several days, eliciting time-dependent hyperventilation, increased MSNA, and systemic hypertension, all of which persist for some days on return to normoxic environments following cessation of hypoxia. These time-dependent ventilatory changes occur even in the presence of a persistent hypocapnia and alkalosis. Proliferation of type 1, hypoxic-sensing glomus cells in the CB begins to appear early in the hypoxic exposure.[29]
- The intermittent hypoxemia (IH) attending sleep apnea is especially sensitizing to the entire chemoreceptor pathway, as the pro-oxidant transcriptional regulator HIF1 (HIF-1α) is fully

expressed without the accompanying upregulation of the opposing antioxidant HIF-2α[30] (**Fig. 4**). This results in sustained oxidative stress and proinflammatory molecules distributed to neuronal structures throughout the chemoreceptor pathway and to the systemic resistance vessels. The very fast reoxygenation phase following each apnea in the patient with obstructive sleep apnea (OSA) is a key element in the deleterious widespread, excessive inflammatory response triggered by IH.[31]

- Chronic heart failure (CHF) in animal models and humans is characterized by increased chemosensitivity with accompanying autonomic imbalance in the form of increased sympathetic nerve activation (SNA), renal vasoconstriction, cardiac arrhythmias, and unstable breathing. The enhanced chemosensitivity usually occurs in the absence of arterial hypoxemia. Rather, it has been attributed to a reduced CB blood flow leading to a reduced expression of a sheer-stress–induced mechano-sensitive transcription of target genes, which in turn determine NO availability, and antioxidant defenses in the CB.[32]
- Carotid bodies are sensitized and tonically active in the spontaneously hypertensive rat, accounting for excessive levels of renal SNA and high vascular resistance. The precise

source of CB sensitization in this hypertensive model has not been completely elucidated, although reduced carotid body flow and sheer stress could occur via excessive sympathetic vasoconstriction of the carotid body vasculature.[1] Increased renal afferent activity has also been identified as another source of excessive SNA in chronic hypertension.

> Hypersensitization of carotid chemoreception occurs via exposure to hypoxia and especially to IH with its rapid restoration to normoxia attending cyclical sleep apneas, and also to the reduced CB blood flow and sheer stress attending CHF and chronic hypertension.
>
> This hypersensitivity is manifested as chronically high levels of sympathetic vasomotor activity as well as breathing instability and periodic breathing.

- A coupling of high central respiratory drive to sympathetic output has been shown in reduced rodent preparations and suggested as an important source for excessive SNA in chronic hypertension.[33] Whether this link is an important source of excessive SNA in

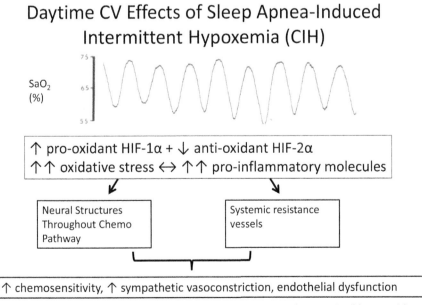

Fig. 4. Summary of effects of chronic IH induced via cyclical sleep apnea characterized by a rapid reoxygenation phase at apnea termination following each O_2 desaturation. up and down arrows indicate increases and decreases. (*Data from* Semenza GL, Prabhakar NR. Neural regulation of hypoxia-inducible factors and redox state drives the pathogenesis of hypertension in a rodent model of sleep apnea. J Appl Physiol (1985) 2015;119(10):1152–56; and Lim DC, Brady DC, Soans R, et al. Different cyclical intermittent hypoxia severities have different effects on hippocampal microvasculature. J Appl Physiol (1985) 2016;121(1):78–88.)

intact humans is confounded by the following evidence: (1) MSNA is *inhibited* during most of inspiration and the onset of inhibition during inspiration is dependent on the absolute level of lung inflation and in part mediated by lung afferents[34]; (2) changing central respiratory motor output, per se (either increased via voluntary efforts or reduced via mechanical ventilation), was without significant effect on MSNA[35] (**Fig. 5**); and (3) steady-state, as opposed to within-breath, MSNA levels are not influenced by substantial voluntary increases or decreases in breathing frequency, tidal volume, and $\dot{V}_E$.[36,37] Guyenet and colleagues[21] emphasized the importance of chemoreceptor-mediated "direct" activation of presympathetic medullary neurons that operate via a pathway from the NTS independently of the CPG.

- Thinly myelinated and unmyelinated skeletal muscle afferents are also highly sensitized in animal models of CHF and hypertension, leading to excessive sympatho-excitation and vasoconstriction and exaggerated

pressor and ventilatory responses to exercise[38,39] (also see later in this article).

VENTILATORY VERSUS SYMPATHETIC REGULATION VIA CHEMOSENSITIZATION

Although chemorecepter activation certainly stimulates both phrenic nerve activity and ventilation as well as SNA with accompanying vasoconstriction, there are important instances in which chemoreceptor stimulation might elicit quite different outcomes. For example, following several minutes of IH or intermittent asphyxia in humans, SNA stays elevated for up to 2 hours or more on return to room air, whereas ventilation returns immediately to control values.[40] It has also been suggested that the carotid chemoreceptor sensitization accompanying chronic intermittent hypoxemia or CHF is sufficient to increase SNA and its cardiovascular sequelae in the resting air-breathing state but has little effect on ventilation. Apparently this dichotomy may occur because the barroreflex countervailing influence on SNA is reduced with

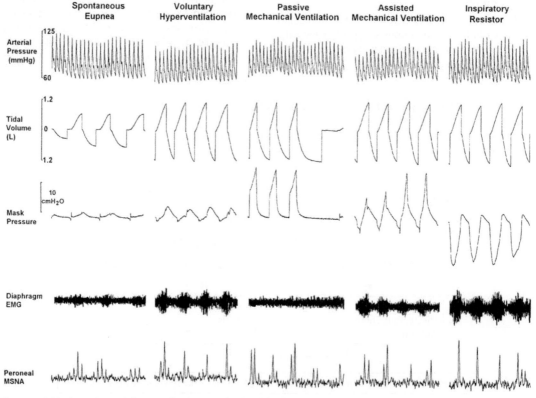

Fig. 5. Within-breath modulation of MSNA in the healthy human. Note the increase in MSNA modulation with increased VT above spontaneous eupnea (PETCO₂ maintained normocapnic), but with no further modulating effect of increases or decreases in central respiratory motor output. For example, contrast high central drive (voluntary hyperventilation and inspiration against high resistance) versus no or reduced central drive (passive or assisted mechanical ventilation). (*From* St Croix CM, Satoh M, Morgan BJ, et al. Role of respiratory motor output in within-breath modulation of muscle sympathetic nerve activity in humans. Circ Res 1999;85(5):457–69; with permission.)

increasing chemoreceptor activity and therefore will not oppose the increased SNA, whereas the RTN countervailing influence on ventilatory control will be "silenced" by the cerebral alkalosis accompanying carotid chemoreceptor stimulation.[41] However, not to be overlooked is the substantial evidence that chemosensitization in chronic states has significant effects on ventilatory control. Consider in CHF the periodic breathing during wakefulness and sleep, the failure of $\dot{V}_E$ to decrease and $Paco_2$ to increase on transition from rest to sleep, thereby sensitizing the hypocapnic-induced apneic threshold[42] and the tachypneic hyperventilatory response to even mild-intensity exercise in CHF.[43] Even the supposed silencing of the RTN CO_2-sensitive neurons with CB stimulation[41] must derive from some significant degree of respiratory alkalosis and in turn this must stem from hyperventilation-induced hypocapnia, even of a mild degree. Further, in the face of marked carotid chemoreceptor stimulation and systemic alkalosis, the central chemoreceptors remain highly sensitive to small changes in the CO_2 in their environment (see also Exertional Periodic Breathing in Heart Failure: Mechanisms and Clinical Implications).[6]

ROLE OF HYPERSENSITIZED CHEMORECEPTOR AND MUSCLE AFFERENTS IN CYCLICAL SLEEP APNEA PATHOGENESIS, DYSPNEA, AND HYPERTENSION
Obstructive Sleep Apnea

A case has been made for an important role for instability of central motor output in cyclical sleep apnea, both central sleep apnea (CSA) and OSA.[44,45] The link of central instability to obstructive apnea occurs at the nadir of the oscillatory central drive to breathe in patients with a collapsible upper airway.[44] In turn the causes of ventilatory undershoot and overshoot with central respiratory instability are deeply rooted in the excessive chemosensitivity underlying increases in "loop gain" (**Fig. 6**).[46] In brief, sleep unmasks a critical dependence of ventilatory control on CO_2 and in particular an apneic threshold, which occurs just a few mm Hg $Paco_2$ below eupnea. CB denervation studies in rats and dogs show that carotid chemoreceptors are required for apneas to occur following a brief ventilatory overshoot, but use of the isolated carotid chemoreceptor perfusion preparation in sleeping dogs shows that transient hypocapnia at *both* the level of the carotid chemoreceptor as well as the level of the medullary chemoreceptors is required to cause apnea, again demonstrating the functional importance of peripheral central chemoreceptor interdependence.[44,47] In addition, use of a sleeping canine preparation with reversible

vagal blockade showed that vagal inhibitory feedback influences via lung stretch during the ventilatory overshoot phase were also important contributors to subsequent apneas.[48] Another key element underlying repeated ventilatory overshoots and undershoots is the patient's arousal threshold in response to chemoreceptor-driven sensory input during an apnea.[45] Transient arousals will augment the accompanying transient ventilatory overshoot at apnea termination, thereby enhancing the hypocapnia and tidal volume achieved before returning to sleep and perpetuating repeated apneas (further discussion on this topic is provided in Pathogenesis of Obstructive Sleep Apnea).

Congestive Heart Failure

Many patients with CHF present a "perfect storm" for high loop gain and periodic breathing in sleep, as their high chemosensitivity sensitizes both their ventilatory overshoot and apneic threshold (see **Fig. 6**). In addition, their high pulmonary vascular pressures lead to sensitization of the apneic threshold and the high drive to breathe emanating from both chemoreceptor and pulmonary vascular receptor stimulation constrains the hypoventilation normally accompanying sleep onset and reduces the CO_2 "reserve," that is, the differences in $Paco_2$ between eupnea and the apneic threshold.[42] Further, the blunted CO_2 cerebrovascular responsiveness commonly accompanying CHF means that cerebral ECF Pco_2 is less well "protected" from accompanying changes in arterial PCO_2, again leading to a reduced CO_2 reserve and sensitized apneic threshold. Finally, the prolonged circulation time means longer apneas and cycle times and more blood gas disturbances accompanying each apnea, thereby exacerbating the ventilatory overshoot (further discussion on this topic is provided in Pulmonary Limitations in Heart Failure and Exertional Periodic Breathing in Heart Failure: Mechanisms and Clinical Implications).

Periodic breathing with cyclical central apneas occurs primarily because of increased "loop gain," wherein transient perturbations in breathing result in exaggerated hyperventilatory and/or hypoventilatory responses and continued instability. Chemosensitivity is a major source of loop gain and is one of several key contributors to the periodic breathing of heart failure. Cyclical OSAs are often dependent on the presence of a collapsible airway, excessive chemosensitivity, and a sensitized arousal threshold, leading to sustained oscillations in central respiratory motor output, with obstructions occurring at the nadir of the central motor drive.

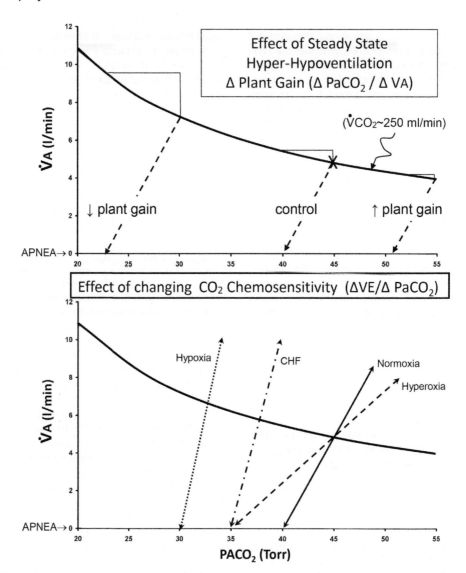

Fig. 6. Diagramatic representation of the relationships in the alveolar gas equation ($PACO_2 = \dot{V}CO_2/\dot{V}A \times K$) at an isometabolic $\dot{V}CO_2$ of 250 mL/min, illustrating the effects of changes in plant gain (top) and controller gain (or chemosensitivity: bottom) on susceptibility to apnea/instability. Note: Owing to the hyperbolic $\dot{V}$ E:$PACO_2$ relationship, as $Paco_2$ is reduced via steady-state hyperventilation (eg, acetazolamide therapy), the reduced plant gain means that a transient ventilatory overshoot much larger than that under control conditions is required to reach the apneic threshold. Conversely with steady-state hypoventilation (eg, metabolic alkalosis or non–rapid eye movement sleep) a much smaller ventilatory overshoot is required to reduce $Paco_2$ to the apneic threshold. In bottom panel, note increased propensity for apnea and destabilization of breathing with increases in CO_2 sensitivity (eg, hypoxia, CHF), because the hypocapnic-induced apneic threshold resides much closer to eupneic $Paco_2$ than in control conditions plus the ventilatory overshoot response to increases in chemical stimuli is exaggerated. Stabilization of breathing occurs with reduced chemosensitivity (eg, hyperoxia) because ventilatory overshoots are reduced and reaching the apneic threshold $Paco_2$ requires a much greater increase in ventilation and reduction in $Paco_2$. (*Data from* Khoo MC, Kronauer RE, Strohl KP, et al. Factors inducing periodic breathing in humans: a general model. J Appl Physiol Respir Environ Exerc Physiol 1982;53(3):644–59; Dempsey JA, Veasey SC, Morgan BJ, et al. Pathophysiology of Sleep Apnea. Physiol Rev 2010;90:47–112.)

Muscle Afferents

Hypersensitized muscle metaboreceptor/mechanoreceptor afferents also play a significant role in the cardiorespiratory response to exercise and to exercise limitation. This was best demonstrated by the effect of locomotor muscle afferent partial blockade during exercise in CHF, COPD, and hypertensive patients achieved via intrathecal administration of the opiate agonist Fentanyl.[49] In all of these cases, major effects of blockade on cardiorespiratory responses to exercise occurred as follows: (1) breathing frequency, dead space ventilation, and dyspnea were markedly reduced and exercise performance prolonged in COPD[50]; (2) in CHF, marked hypoventilation occurred and limb muscle vascular conductance blood flow and cardiac output increased[23,51]; and (3) in chronically hypertensive patients, the excessive pressor response to exercise was normalized.[52] These cardiorespiratory effects of muscle afferent blockade were also reported in young healthy exercising subjects,[49] but appear to be significantly greater in patients with CHF or COPD and hypertensive patients in whom sympathetic vasomotor activity and the drive to breathe during exercise are excessive.

Excessive feedback from sensitized muscle afferent group III-IV mechanoreceptors and metaboreceptors during exercise precipitates excessive ventilatory drive, hyperinflation, and dyspnea in COPD, high cardiac output, muscle vasoconstriction, and hyperventilation in CHF and excessive pressor responses in chronic hypertension, all of which negatively impact locomotor muscle O_2 transport and fatigue, dyspnea, exercise performance, and quality of life.

TREATMENT IMPLICATIONS OF "SENSORY HYPERREFLEXIA"

There are some limited but promising findings recently in both animal models and in humans in support of attempts to modify excessive sensitivities of feedback pathways in treating/rehabilitating patients with OSA, CHF, COPD, and hypertension.

Obstructive Sleep Apnea

Continuous positive airway pressure (CPAP) is clearly the preferred, effective treatment of sleep-induced cyclical obstruction and its accompanying IH. The problem is that many patients with OSA either refuse CPAP treatment or use it for less than 4 hours per night, a level of usage that is inadequate for effectively treating the cardiovascular sequelae attending OSA.[53] Alternatively, reductions in loop gain can be achieved through the use of supplemental O_2 (to reduce chemoreceptor gain) or ventilatory stimulation (acetazolamide, to reduce plant gain) (see **Fig. 6**). If these

approaches are applied to those patients with high loop gain and moderate degrees of airway collapsibility, they may often be effective in significantly reducing sleep-disordered breathing.[44,54] Any residual apneas are commonly prolonged with supplemental O_2 but hypoxemia does not occur. Combination therapies of supplemental O_2 plus hypnotics used to reduce the arousal threshold have also shown promise, again in selected patients with OSA.[55] Phenotyping the patient for high loop gain is important in determining the feasibility of these approaches and this might be accomplished by examining patterns of ventilatory overshoot or a high prevalence of "mixed" apneas in the routine polysomnogram or even by simple breath hold or CO_2 chemosensitivity tests in wakefulness.[56] Some claims that CPAP effects on selected cardiovascular outcomes in patients with OSA exceeded those of supplemental O_2 were based on studies that applied these treatments for <5 hours per night and in patients with OSA with very minimal sleep time spent below 90% HbO_2 saturation.[57] Again there is a need to tailor treatment to individual patient characteristics.[54]

Cyclical Central Sleep Apnea

CSA is common in heart failure, with its accompanying IH and resulting hyperadrenergic state.[53] CPAP is usually not effective or only partially effective in treating central apneas and therefore may even be harmful to those whose CSA is not suppressed.[58] In animal models of CHF, CBX or pharmacologic blockade of carotid body excitatory neurotransmitters effectively prevents unstable breathing.[44] Systematic studies in humans using nocturnal supplemental oxygen show substantial improvement in CSA, reduced sympathetic activity and arrhythmias, and improved cardiac function.[53] Importantly, only supplemental O_2 in quantities sufficient to prevent HbO_2 desaturation and CSA should be used, as determined via titration during sleep. Inducing hyperoxia for sustained periods has been shown to increase vasoconstriction and impair ventricular function. A strong case has been made for clinical trials to determine the role of supplemental O_2 in treating CSA in CHF.[53]

Attention also should be paid to the use of acetazolamide to reduce plant and loop gain via moderate reductions in $Paco_2$.[53] Clearly, lowering steady-state $Paco_2$ and plant gain moves the apneic threshold Pco_2 farther away, not closer, to the eupneic $Paco_2$ (see **Fig. 6**). In patients with CHF who develop obstructive as well as central apneas secondary to excess fluid accumulation around the upper airway, a diuretic therapy might be combined with these measures to lower loop gain. Finally, there may even be ways to address the underlying mechanism of CB sensitization in CHF by enhancing carotid body blood flow: (1) statin use in a postinfarction CHF rodent model upregulated CB blood flow, enhanced endothelial NO synthase within the CB, and reduced chemosensitivity, resulting in less ventilatory instability and fewer cardiac arrhythmias[59]; and (2) exercise training in CHF rodents and human patients augmented cardiac output and blood flow in moderate amounts, apparently sufficient to reduce CB hypersensitivity.[60,61]

Chemosensitivity and Systemic Hypertension

In the rodent chronic hypertensive model, the hypersensitized CB is tonically active during normoxic, air-breathing conditions. CBX lowers blood pressure (BP) and renal SNA and improves baroreflex and renal function.[62] How might this be accomplished in humans who are resistant to antihypertensive medications and show enhanced chemosensitivity? Limited numbers of hypertensive patients have undergone single or even bilateral CB denervation with a number of the "responders" showing significant reductions in BP, but such approaches are nonreversible and could elicit serious consequences in circumstances of sleep apnea or exposure to hypoxic environments. Other approaches to reduce CB hypersensitivity include exercise training and statin use (see earlier in this article). Another exciting recent idea identifies a pure adrenergic receptor P_2X3 messenger RNA expression in chemoreceptive petrosal sensory neurons as a source of enhanced CB tonic drive and hyperreflexia in the CHF rodent model. Specific pharmacologic antagonists of these neurons might provide a means of reducing high tonic activity from the CB while preserving its emergency function.[63] Stay tuned!

Exertional Dyspnea/Increased Respiratory Drive

An abnormally high drive to breathe during exercise is commonly encountered in patients with COPD or CHF, leading to flow limitation, hyperinflation, dyspnea, limb fatigue, and exercise limitation (further discussion on thsi topic ia also provided in The Pathophysiology of Dyspnea and Exercise Intolerance in COPD). Significant sources of these high drives are to be found in sensitized afferents in both the CBs and muscle group III-IV afferents (see earlier in this article). Accordingly, rehabilitation efforts that target

these muscle afferent hypersensitivities will allow these patients to train at higher intensities and experience more beneficial training effects in their markedly fatigueable locomotor muscles and improve exercise performance and quality of life. These approaches would include the following: (1) the use of O_2 supplementation during training sessions to enhance O_2 transport and reduce the ventilatory response and dyspnea, thereby raising work output (see also Physiologic Effects of O_2 Supplementation During Exercise in Chronic Obstructive Pulmonary Disease); and (2) exercise training of single limbs, which will upregulate the low aerobic capacity in limb muscles via increased mitochondrial volume and capillarization, thereby reducing metabolite accumulation and sensory input from muscle metaboreceptors and

---

Box 1
Treatment implications targeting hypersensitive chemoreceptors and/or muscle afferents

Treatment implications targeting hypersensitive chemoreceptors and/or muscle afferents, include reducing their sensitivity via

a. Use of supplemental O_2 during sleep to treat central apnea and even obstructive apneas in some patients with obstructive sleep apnea with high chemosensitivity and moderately collapsible airways (see also Pathogenesis of Obstructive Sleep Apnea)

b. Exercise training of single limbs plus supplemental O_2 to increase training intensity, thereby leading to improved aerobic capacity of locomotor muscles and reduced muscle metabolite accumulation and afferent stimulation in chronic obstructive pulmonary disease (see also Physiologic Effects of O_2 Supplementation during Exercise in Chronic Obstructive Pulmonary Disease and The Relevance of Limb Muscle Dysfunction In COPD: A Review for Clinicians)

c. Specific training of respiratory muscles to reduce the metabolite accumulation during exercise, thereby preventing/delaying sympathetic -induced vasoconstriction in locomotor muscles.

d. Use of physical training and statin therapy in chronic heart failure to enhance chemoreceptor blood flow

e. Ongoing research to selectively reduce excessive *tonic* carotid chemoreceptor activity in drug-resistant hypertension without sacrificing chemoreceptor emergency function.

reducing the ventilatory drive and its negative sequelae during exercise (see also The Relevance of Limb Muscle Dysfunction In COPD: A Review for Clinicians).[50] Respiratory muscle unloading studies have also revealed the high sensitivity of respiratory muscle metaboreceptors in patients with CHF or COPD causing sympathoexcitation, redistribution of blood flow, and exacerbating limb fatigue during exercise.[64] Accordingly, specific respiratory muscle training studies have been shown to delay the onset of diaphragm fatigue and metabolite accumulation during exercise, thereby delaying the metaboreflex-induced sympathoexcitation, improving blood flow distribution, and reducing locomotor muscle fatigue[64] (**Box 1**).

SUMMARY

Recent research has unraveled many of the mechanisms underlying central and peripheral chemoreception and revealed a highly interdependent chemoreceptor pathway extending from carotid chemoreceptors to the hypothalamus. Thus, in physiologic preparations, input from the carotid chemoreceptor exerts hyperadditive effects on central CO_2 ventilatory responsiveness, and central chemoreceptor CO_2-sensitive neurons are also influenced by input from both the hypothalamus and lung stretch. Hyperchemosensitivity results from sustained hypoxic exposure, IH, and reduced blood flow, resulting in unstable breathing and enhanced tonic vasomotor sympathetic activity and its cardiovascular sequalae. Hypersensitivity of group III-IV muscle afferents have also been documented, especially in sedentary, deconditioned patient populations, resulting in excessive pressor, ventilatory, and dyspneic responses to exercise and exercise limitation. These states of "hyperreflexia" occur in OSA, CHF, COPD, and chronic hypertension. Specific targeting of the sensitized reflexes may provide effective alternate treatments in selected patient populations.

ACKNOWLEDGMENTS

The authors are grateful to Ben Dempsey for his excellent article preparation and to Barbara Morgan who served as a technical consultant. Original research reported here was supported by the National Heart, Lung, and Blood Institute and American Heart Association.

REFERENCES

1. Koeners MP, Lewis KE, Ford AP, et al. Hypertension: a problem of organ blood flow supply-demand mismatch. Future Cardiol 2016;12(3):339–49.

2. Kumar P, Bin-Jaliah I. Adequate stimuli of the carotid body: more than an oxygen sensor? Respir Physiol Neurobiol 2007;157(1):12–21.

3. Prabhakar NR, Semenza GL. Oxygen sensing and homeostasis. Physiology (Bethesda) 2015;30(5): 340–8.

4. Daristotle L, Bisgard GE. Central-peripheral chemoreceptor ventilatory interaction in awake goats. Respir Physiol 1989;76(3):383–91.

5. Bisgard GE, Busch MA, Daristotle L, et al. Carotid body hypercapnia does not elicit ventilatory acclimatization in goats. Respir Physiol 1986;65(1): 113–25.

6. Smith CA, Blain GM, Henderson KS, et al. Peripheral chemoreceptors determine the respiratory sensitivity of central chemoreceptors to CO2 : role of carotid body CO2. J Physiol 2015;593(18): 4225–43.

7. Smith CA, Saupe KW, Henderson KS, et al. Ventilatory effects of specific carotid body hypocapnia in dogs during wakefulness and sleep. J Appl Physiol (1985) 1995;79(3):689–99.

8. Guyenet PG, Bayliss DA, Stornetta RL, et al. Proton detection and breathing regulation by the retrotrapezoid nucleus. J Physiol 2016;594(6):1529–51.

9. Hawkins VE, Takakura AC, Trinh A, et al. Purinergic regulation of vascular tone in the retrotrapezoid nucleus is specialized to support the drive to breathe. Elife 2017;6 [pii:e25232].

10. Xie A, Skatrud JB, Morgan B, et al. Influence of cerebrovascular function on the hypercapnic ventilatory response in healthy humans. J Physiol 2006; 577(Pt 1):319–29.

11. Daristotle L, Engwall MJ, Niu WZ, et al. Ventilatory effects and interactions with change in PaO2 in awake goats. J Appl Physiol (1985) 1991;71(4):1254–60.

12. Curran AK, Rodman JR, Eastwood PR, et al. Ventilatory responses to specific CNS hypoxia in sleeping dogs. J Appl Physiol (1985) 2000;88(5):1840–52.

13. Sun MK, Reis DJ. Hypoxia selectively excites vasomotor neurons of rostral ventrolateral medulla in rats. Am J Physiol 1994;266(1 Pt 2):R245–56.

14. Gourine AV, Funk GD. On the existence of a central respiratory oxygen sensor. J Appl Physiol (1985) 2017;123(5):1344–9.

15. Dean JB, Mulkey DK, Henderson RA, et al. Hyperoxia, reactive oxygen species, and hyperventilation: oxygen sensitivity of brain stem neurons. J Appl Physiol (1985) 2004;96(2):784–91.

16. Blain GM, Smith CA, Henderson KS, et al. Contribution of the carotid body chemoreceptors to eupneic ventilation in the intact, unanesthetized dog. J Appl Physiol (1985) 2009;106(5):1564–73.

17. Dahan A, Nieuwenhuijs D, Teppema L. Plasticity of central chemoreceptors: effect of bilateral carotid body resection on central CO2 sensitivity. PLoS Med 2007;4(7):e239.

18. Rodman JR, Curran AK, Henderson KS, et al. Carotid body denervation in dogs: eupnea and the ventilatory response to hyperoxic hypercapnia. J Appl Physiol (1985) 2001;91(1):328–35.

19. Hodges MR, Opansky C, Qian B, et al. Carotid body denervation alters ventilatory responses to ibotenic acid injections or focal acidosis in the medullary raphe. J Appl Physiol (1985) 2005;98(4):1234–42.

20. Souza GMPR, Kanbar R, Stornetta DS, et al. Breathing regulation and blood gas homeostasis after near complete lesions of the retrotrapezoid nucleus in adult rats. J Physiol 2018;596(13):2521–45.

21. Guyenet PG, Bayliss DA, Stornetta RL, et al. Interdependent feedback regulation of breathing by the carotid bodies and the retrotrapezoid nucleus. J Physiol 2018;596(15):3029–42.

22. Stickland MK, Morgan BJ, Dempsey JA. Carotid chemoreceptor modulation of sympathetic vasoconstrictor outflow during exercise in healthy humans. J Physiol 2008;586(6):1743–54.

23. Stickland MK, Miller JD, Smith CA, et al. Carotid chemoreceptor modulation of regional blood flow distribution during exercise in health and chronic heart failure. Circ Res 2007;100(9):1371–8.

24. Mouradian GC, Forster HV, Hodges MR. Acute and chronic effects of carotid body denervation on ventilation and chemoreflexes in three rat strains. J Physiol 2012;590(14):3335–47.

25. da Silva GS, Giusti H, Benedetti M, et al. Serotonergic neurons in the nucleus raphe obscurus contribute to interaction between central and peripheral ventilatory responses to hypercapnia. Pflugers Arch 2011;462(3):407–18.

26. Takakura AC, Moreira TS, Colombari E, et al. Peripheral chemoreceptor inputs to retrotrapezoid nucleus (RTN) CO2-sensitive neurons in rats. J Physiol 2006;572(Pt 2):503–23.

27. Morrison SF. 2010 Carl Ludwig distinguished lectureship of the APS neural control and autonomic regulation section: central neural pathways for thermoregulatory cold defense. J Appl Physiol (1985) 2011;110(5):1137–49.

28. Morgan BJ, Adrian R, Bates ML, et al. Quantifying hypoxia-induced chemoreceptor sensitivity in the awake rodent. J Appl Physiol (1985) 2014;117(7):816–24.

29. Wang ZY, Olson EB, Bjorling DE, et al. Sustained hypoxia-induced proliferation of carotid body type I cells in rats. J Appl Physiol (1985) 2008;104(3):803–8.

30. Semenza GL, Prabhakar NR. Neural regulation of hypoxia-inducible factors and redox state drives the pathogenesis of hypertension in a rodent model of sleep apnea. J Appl Physiol (1985) 2015;119(10):1152–6.

31. Lim DC, Brady DC, Soans R, et al. Different cyclical intermittent hypoxia severities have different effects on hippocampal microvasculature. J Appl Physiol (1985) 2016;121(1):78–88.

32. Marcus NJ, Del Rio R, Ding Y, et al. KLF2 mediates enhanced chemoreflex sensitivity, disordered breathing and autonomic dysregulation in heart failure. J Physiol 2018;596(15):3171–85.

33. Simms AE, Paton JF, Pickering AE, et al. Amplified respiratory-sympathetic coupling in the spontaneously hypertensive rat: does it contribute to hypertension? J Physiol 2009;587(3):597–610.

34. Seals DR, Suwarno NO, Joyner MJ, et al. Respiratory modulation of muscle sympathetic nerve activity in intact and lung denervated humans. Circ Res 1993;72(2):440–54.

35. St Croix CM, Satoh M, Morgan BJ, et al. Role of respiratory motor output in within-breath modulation of muscle sympathetic nerve activity in humans. Circ Res 1999;85(5):457–69.

36. Fatouleh R, Macefield VG. Respiratory modulation of muscle sympathetic nerve activity is not increased in essential hypertension or chronic obstructive pulmonary disease. J Physiol 2011;589(Pt 20):4997–5006.

37. Limberg JK, Morgan BJ, Schrage WG, et al. Respiratory influences on muscle sympathetic nerve activity and vascular conductance in the steady state. Am J Physiol Heart Circ Physiol 2013;304(12):H1615–23.

38. Vongpatanasin W, Wang Z, Arbique D, et al. Functional sympatholysis is impaired in hypertensive humans. J Physiol 2011;589(Pt 5):1209–20.

39. Wang HJ, Li YL, Gao L, et al. Alteration in skeletal muscle afferents in rats with chronic heart failure. J Physiol 2010;588(Pt 24):5033–47.

40. Xie A, Skatrud JB, Puleo DS, et al. Exposure to hypoxia produces long-lasting sympathetic activation in humans. J Appl Physiol (1985) 2001;91(4):1555–62.

41. Basting TM, Burke PG, Kanbar R, et al. Hypoxia silences retrotrapezoid nucleus respiratory chemoreceptors via alkalosis. J Neurosci 2015;35(2):527–43.

42. Xie A, Skatrud JB, Puleo DS, et al. Apnea-hypopnea threshold for CO2 in patients with congestive heart failure. Am J Respir Crit Care Med 2002;165(9):1245–50.

43. Woods PR, Olson TP, Frantz RP, et al. Causes of breathing inefficiency during exercise in heart failure. J Card Fail 2010;16(10):835–42.

44. Dempsey JA, Xie A, Patz DS, et al. Physiology in medicine: obstructive sleep apnea pathogenesis and treatment–considerations beyond airway anatomy. J Appl Physiol (1985) 2014;116(1):3–12.

45. Younes M, Ostrowski M, Atkar R, et al. Mechanisms of breathing instability in patients with obstructive sleep apnea. J Appl Physiol (1985) 2007;103(6):1929–41.

46. Khoo MC, Kronauer RE, Strohl KP, et al. Factors inducing periodic breathing in humans: a general model. J Appl Physiol Respir Environ Exerc Physiol 1982;53(3):644–59.

47. Smith CA, Chenuel BJ, Henderson KS, et al. The apneic threshold during non-REM sleep in dogs: sensitivity of carotid body vs. central chemoreceptors. J Appl Physiol (1985) 2007;103(2):578–86.

48. Chow CM, Xi L, Smith CA, et al. A volume-dependent apneic threshold during NREM sleep in the dog. J Appl Physiol (1985) 1994;76(6):2315–25.

49. Amann M, Blain GM, Proctor LT, et al. Group III and IV muscle afferents contribute to ventilatory and cardiovascular response to rhythmic exercise in humans. J Appl Physiol (1985) 2010;109(4):966–76.

50. Gagnon P, Bussières JS, Ribeiro F, et al. Influences of spinal anesthesia on exercise tolerance in patients with chronic obstructive pulmonary disease. Am J Respir Crit Care Med 2012;186(7):606–15.

51. Olson TP, Joyner MJ, Eisenach JH, et al. Influence of locomotor muscle afferent inhibition on the ventilatory response to exercise in heart failure. Exp Physiol 2014;99(2):414–26.

52. Barbosa TC, Vianna LC, Fernandes IA, et al. Intrathecal fentanyl abolishes the exaggerated blood pressure response to cycling in hypertensive men. J Physiol 2016;594(3):715–25.

53. Javaheri S, Barbe F, Campos-Rodriguez F, et al. Sleep apnea: types, mechanisms, and clinical cardiovascular consequences. J Am Coll Cardiol 2017;69(7):841–58.

54. Sands SA, Edwards BA, Terrill PI, et al. Identifying obstructive sleep apnoea patients responsive to supplemental oxygen therapy. Eur Respir J 2018;52(3) [pii:1800674].

55. Edwards BA, Sands SA, Owens RL, et al. The combination of supplemental oxygen and a hypnotic markedly improves obstructive sleep apnea in patients with a mild to moderate upper airway collapsibility. Sleep 2016;39(11):1973–83.

56. Messineo L, Taranto-Montemurro L, Azarbarzin A, et al. Breath-holding as a means to estimate the loop gain contribution to obstructive sleep apnoea. J Physiol 2018;596(17):4043–56.

57. Gottlieb DJ, Punjabi NM, Mehra R, et al. CPAP versus oxygen in obstructive sleep apnea. N Engl J Med 2014;370(24):2276–85.

58. Javaheri S. CPAP should not be used for central sleep apnea in congestive heart failure patients. J Clin Sleep Med 2006;2(4):399–402.

59. Haack KK, Marcus NJ, Del Rio R, et al. Simvastatin treatment attenuates increased respiratory variability and apnea/hypopnea index in rats with chronic heart failure. Hypertension 2014;63(5):1041–9.

60. Marcus NJ, Pügge C, Mediratta J, et al. Exercise training attenuates chemoreflex-mediated reductions of renal blood flow in heart failure. Am J Physiol Heart Circ Physiol 2015;309(2):H259–66.

61. Zurek M, Corrà U, Piepoli MF, et al. Exercise training reverses exertional oscillatory ventilation in heart failure patients. Eur Respir J 2012;40(5):1238–44.

62. Niewinski P, Janczak D, Rucinski A, et al. Carotid body resection for sympathetic modulation in systolic heart failure: results from first-in-man study. Eur J Heart Fail 2017;19(3):391–400.

63. Pijacka W, Moraes DJ, Ratcliffe LE, et al. Purinergic receptors in the carotid body as a new drug target for controlling hypertension. Nat Med 2016;22(10):1151–9.

64. Sheel AW, Boushel R, Dempsey JA. Competition for blood flow distribution between respiratory and locomotor muscles: implications for muscle fatigue. J Appl Physiol (1985) 2018;125(3):820–31.

Incorporating Lung Diffusing Capacity for Carbon Monoxide in Clinical Decision Making in Chest Medicine

J. Alberto Neder, MD, PhD, FRCPC, FERS[a],*,
Danilo C. Berton, MD, PhD[b], Paulo T. Muller, MD, PhD[c],
Denis E. O'Donnell, MD, FRCPI, FRCPC, FERS[d]

KEYWORDS

- Lung function • Lung diffusing capacity • Gas exchange • Dyspnea • Hypoxia

KEY POINTS

- Measurements of single-breath lung diffusing capacity for carbon monoxide (DLCO) provide an integrated picture of the complex mechanisms involved in the transfer of oxygen from atmospheric air to lung capillaries.
- To maximize the clinical information derived from those measurements, DLCO should be analyzed taking into consideration the ratio between total lung capacity and the accessible alveolar volume (TLC/VA ratio), VA, and the diffusion coefficient for carbon monoxide (KCO).
- Clinical scenarios in which DLCO is more likely to provide relevant information include dyspnea of unknown origin or out-of-proportion dyspnea, investigation of the mechanisms of dyspnea and exercise intolerance in chronic obstructive pulmonary disease (COPD), differential diagnosis between asthma and COPD, investigation of the causes underlying a restrictive ventilatory defect, management of patients with pulmonary vascular disease and interstitial lung disease, and preoperative assessment.

INTRODUCTION

The transfer of oxygen (O_2) from atmospheric air to pulmonary capillaries, and carbon dioxide (CO_2) in the opposite direction, is the key task of the lungs in terrestrial animals. Because most respiratory diseases in humans impair the efficiency of the lungs as gas exchangers, there is a strong rationale for pulmonary function tests (PFTs) aimed at exploring the integrity of such a crucial endeavor.[1]

Clinically, this is more commonly carried out by tests of lung diffusing capacity (DL)[2] using a highly diffusible gas such as carbon monoxide (CO).[3] More than 100 years ago,[4] Marie Krogh used the

Disclosure Statement: No author has any relationship with a commercial company that has a direct financial interest in the subject matter or materials discussed in this article or with a company making a competing product.
a Laboratory of Clinical Exercise Physiology, Division of Respirology and Sleep Medicine, Department of Medicine, Kingston Health Science Center, Queen's University, Richardson House, 102 Stuart Street, Kingston, Ontario K7L 2V6, Canada; b Division of Respirology, Federal University of Rio Grande do Sul, Porto Alegre, Brazil; c Division of Respirology, Federal University of Mato Grosso do Sul, Campo Grande, Brazil; d Respiratory Investigation Unit, Division of Respirology and Sleep Medicine, Kingston Health Science Center & Queen's University, Kingston, Ontario, Canada
* Corresponding author.
E-mail address: alberto.neder@queensu.ca

Clin Chest Med 40 (2019) 285–305
https://doi.org/10.1016/j.ccm.2019.02.005
0272-5231/19/© 2019 Elsevier Inc. All rights reserved.

exquisite affinity of hemoglobin for CO (230 times greater than its affinity for O_2) to show that, even at the extremes of exercise and altitude,[5] passive diffusion alone is sufficient to explain how O_2 is transferred from alveolar air to capillary blood.[6] A standardized technique to measure D_L after a single inhalation of a small fraction of CO was subsequently developed by Ogilvie and colleagues[3] in 1957. Using a tracer gas, these investigators also proposed a method to estimate the volume of the gas exchanging areas that received the inhaled mixture (the accessible alveolar volume, V_A).[3] With only some few modifications, 6 decades later this remains the standard approach to measure the diffusion factor for CO (D_{LCO}), V_A, and the diffusion coefficient for CO (D_{LCO}/V_A, K_{CO}) in most clinical laboratories worldwide.[7]

Tests of lung diffusing capacity (D_L) are wrongly named; these tests do not only assess the diffusion process across the alveolar–capillary membrane and they do not provide a metric of capacity (the maximal ability of the lungs to transfer the respiratory gases from atmosphere to blood).

Despite its widespread availability, there remains substantial misunderstanding of the physiologic meaning of D_{LCO} and its derived measurements. This is further complicated by some complex interpretative considerations,[8–10] which have not been extensively tested in prospective studies.[11,12] The poor specificity of a low D_{LCO}, particularly when used in isolation,[7] has also contributed to a somewhat negative view of D_{LCO} in modern day pulmonology. Nevertheless, D_{LCO} is to date the only noninvasive PFT to provide an integrated picture of gas exchange efficiency in the human lungs.[13]

The current chapter aims to provide a comprehensive and updated overview of the clinical value of D_{LCO}, V_A, and K_{CO} in providing relevant information. The authors initially present the physiologic and methodologic bases of these measurements. After detailing the key pitfalls that commonly bring challenges to interpretation, the authors outline a clinically friendly approach for D_{LCO} interpretation that takes those caveats into consideration. The authors conclude by describing the different clinical scenarios in which D_{LCO} can effectively assist the chest physician in the management of patients with cardiorespiratory diseases. Illustrative clinical cases are presented in this section to highlight the advantages of the above-mentioned interpretative approach. Because of space constraints, the authors focus on the single-breath technique, used most commonly in practice.[7] Only some discreet methodologic issues that may influence test results in clinical practice are highlighted. For those interested in a detailed methodologic discussion, the authors recommend the recently updated European Respiratory Society (ERS)/ American Thoracic Society (ATS) guidelines.[14]

Do not get lost in translation: whereas the North-American literature refers to "lung diffusing capacity for CO" (D_{LCO} or diffusion factor in mL/min/mm Hg) and "diffusion coefficient" (K_{CO} (D_{LCO}/V_A) in mL/min/mm Hg/L), the European literature prefers "lung transfer capacity for CO" (T_{LCO} or transfer factor in mmol/min/kPa) and "transfer coefficient" (K_{CO} (T_{LCO}/V_A) in mmol/min/kPa/L), respectively. Multiplying T_{LCO} by approximately 3 (2.987) gives D_{LCO}. Owing to its more widespread use in commercial systems, the symbol D_{LCO} is used here.

PHYSIOLOGIC FOUNDATIONS

The ability of the lungs to exchange any inspired gas across the alveolar–capillary boundaries is determined by[14]

a. The gas tension in the inspired air
b. The absolute levels of ventilation and perfusion
c. The uniformity of the distribution of ventilation relative to perfusion, including any effects of (small) airway closure and changes in capillary caliper
d. Mixing and diffusion of gases in the alveolar ducts, air sacs, and alveoli
e. The gas tension in the alveoli relative to respective tension in the capillaries
f. The diffusion characteristics of the membrane, including its thickness and area
g. Diffusion across the interstitial, endothelial, and plasma barriers
h. Diffusion across the red-cell membrane and within the interior of the red blood cell and
i. The concentration and binding properties of hemoglobin (Hb) in the alveolar capillaries

In a merely descriptive sense, steps (f) to (h) (ie, those immediately previous to gas binding to Hb) are grouped under the denomination of the "membrane diffusing capacity" (D_M).[15] D_M is strongly related to the level of lung expansion because greater inflation leads to spherical airspace expansion and unfolding of the surface.[16] On the other hand, the "diffusing capacity of the blood" (step (i)) depends on[15]

- The microvascular ("capillary") blood volume in contact with the inhaled gas (Vc) and
- The rate of its reaction with Hb (represented by the Greek letter theta [θ])

As outlined in **Fig. 1**, the standard method to measure Dʟco using a single O_2 concentration (usually 21%) does not allow the separation of the membrane from the blood component. However, there is convincing evidence that most of the Dʟco signal (∼80%) comes from the blood phase, that is, the number of red cells or the number of open capillary vessels.[17] There is a close interdependence between Dм and Vc, which variably affects their dynamic interaction and, consequently, Dʟco.[2] This important point for Dʟco and Kco interpretation is discussed in the section entitled Kco and the Accessible Vᴀ.

There are at least 2 approaches to estimate the relative contribution of the "membrane" versus the "blood" components to explain a low Dʟco:

a. Making the subject inhale at least 1 hyperoxic mixture in addition to 21% O_2. Considering that under higher alveolar Po₂ more O_2 will compete with CO for the available Hb, the greater the decrease in Dʟco as Po₂ increases, the greater the contribution of the "blood" component to Dʟco.

b. Making the subject inhale, in addition to CO, another gas whose rate of transfer is mainly determined by the "membrane" component (eg, nitric oxide [NO]). Thus, the Dʟno/Dʟco ratio is biased to represent the contribution of the "membrane" component to Dʟco.

Unfortunately, partitioning Dʟco into its "membrane" and "blood" components has failed to date to have an impact on clinical decision making, likely because Dʟco is strongly determined by its "blood" component; moreover, the "blood" component must exist for the "membrane" component to be measured.

METHODOLOGIC BASES

For the measurement of the single-breath Dʟco (**Fig. 2**),[14] a seated subject breathes at tidal volume for a sufficient time to ensure that he/she is comfortable with the mouthpiece and that there are no leaks around the nose clips and mouthpiece. After unforced exhalation to residual volume (RV) (which might take considerable amount of time in patients with airflow limitation), the subject inhales rapidly to total lung capacity (TLC) a gas mixture containing 0.3% CO, 21% O_2, a biologically inert tracer gas (usually helium or methane),

and a balance of nitrogen. The subject is then asked to hold his/her breath for 10 s, avoiding a Valsalva maneuver with subsequent exhalation to RV.[14] The expired concentrations of CO and the tracer gas are measured after allowing washout of the air from the dead space (breathing apparatus plus anatomic) (see **Fig. 2**).[19]

An estimate of the lung gas volume into which CO is distributed (accessible Vᴀ) is obtained by calculating how much the inert gas has been diluted; the lower the expired fraction of this gas, the higher the dilution volume (Vᴀ). Dʟco is then calculated taking into consideration[14]

- The expired fraction of CO relative to its known inspired fraction, thereby allowing the calculation of how much CO has been taken in by the lung capillaries
- The Vᴀ, and
- The breath-hold time

Thus, the lower the expired CO and the higher the Vᴀ for a given breath-hold time, the higher the Dʟco. Key potential errors in the maneuvers required for Dʟco measurements with a greater potential to interfere with measurements are shown in **Table 1**.[14]

CHALLENGES TO INTERPRETATION
Diffusion Coefficient for Carbon Monoxide and the Accessible Alveolar Volume

The concept that Dʟco should increase as the alveoli are distended from functional residual capacity (FRC) to TLC is straightforward: the alveolar surface area for gas exchange increases in tandem with Vᴀ, and secondarily, the alveolar–capillary membrane becomes thinner (ie, ⇑ Dм) (**Fig. 3**A).[20] However, juxtaalveolar capillaries are also progressively compressed by the distended alveoli (ie, ⇓ Vc) although this is more variable due to differential stretching and flattening of alveolar and extraalveolar capillaries (see **Fig. 3**A).[21] Overall, the positive effects of higher Vᴀ on Dм are larger than its negative consequences on Vc. It follows that Dʟco increases and the Dʟco/Vᴀ ratio (Kco) decreases nonlinearly as Vᴀ increases (**Fig. 3**B).[8] In other words, 1 "unit" change in Vᴀ does not lead to 1 "unit" change in Dʟco[22]; thus, it is highly misleading to state that "the Dʟco/Vᴀ ratio represents Dʟco corrected by Vᴀ."

The above-mentioned reasoning also applies to the opposite: as the alveoli shrink with lung deflation (⇓ Vᴀ), the surface area to gas exchange decreases while turning progressively thicker (⇓ Dм) (see **Fig. 3**A).[20] However, the capillaries are also less compressed by the smaller alveoli, and there is a relative predominance of Vc over Dм (see **Fig. 3**A).[21] Overall, the negative effects of lower

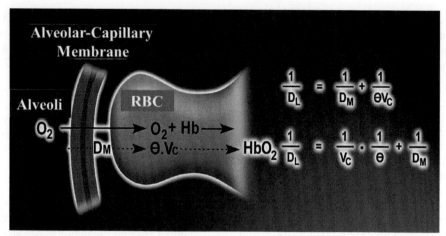

Fig. 1. The resistance to oxygen (O_2) transfer from alveolar gas to hemoglobin (Hb) in the red blood cell (RBC) depends on the diffusion resistance from the epithelial surface to the RBC membrane (D_M) and the RBC resistance to O_2 uptake, the latter being lower the higher the affinity of Hb to O_2 (θ; ie, the rate of O_2 uptake per mL of blood) and the greater the amount of Hb available in lung capillaries (V_C; ie, the pulmonary capillary volume).[15] In practice, carbon monoxide (CO) is used to measure the integrity of this process as CO's affinity to Hb is approximately 230 times greater than that of O_2, and there is little CO dissolved in the blood; thus, CO partial pressure in blood is negligible allowing a quick transfer to Hb. Because approximately 80% of the resistance lies in the RBC component,[18] the lung diffusing capacity BT diffusion factor/coefficient (D_{LCO}) has been described as a "window to pulmonary microcirculation."[2]

V_A on D_M are larger than its positive consequences on V_C. It follows that lower lung volumes negatively affect V_A more than D_{LCO}; consequently, the D_{LCO}/V_A ratio (K_{CO}) increases markedly as V_A decreases (see **Fig. 3B**).[8] The same reasoning applies to patients with different V_A values: as shown in **Fig. 4**, K_{CO} increases markedly as V_A decreases. The effects of low V_A on K_{CO} are clinically more relevant as K_{CO} is more useful in the differential diagnosis of a restrictive ventilatory pattern

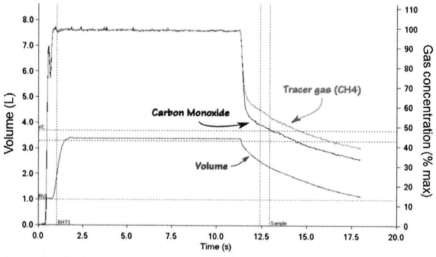

Fig. 2. The key signals for D_{LCO} measurement using a rapid gas analyzer system: volume, [carbon monoxide], [tracer gas] (in this case, methane [CH_4]), and time. After a full exhalation to residual volume (RV) at time "zero," there is a quick inspiration of an air volume greater than 85% vital capacity (V_C). The breath-hold time (BHT) is the time elapsed between the start and the end of gas concentration stability. A virtual "alveolar" sample for analysis of expired concentrations (usually 200 mL) is taken after the total anatomic and equipment dead-space volume has been washed out. Collecting an alveolar gas sample before the point of dead-space washout will underestimate D_{LCO}, whereas delaying sample collection beyond the point of dead-space washout will overestimate D_{LCO}. **Table 1** shows the key potential mistakes on the maneuver that can interfere with the accuracy of results.

Table 1
Key errors in the respiratory maneuvers with greater potential to interfere with DLco measurements

Technical Mistake	Consequences	Recommendation
Failure to reach residual volume before inhalation of the gas mixture Failure to inhale completely from residual volume to total lung capacity	⇓ DLco ⇓⇓ VA ⇑ Kco	The inspired volume should be within 85% of the largest vital capacity and the VA within 200 mL or 5% (whichever is greater) of the highest VA among acceptable maneuvers[14]
Slow inspiration	⇓ DLco Slower lung filling decreases the amount of time the lung is at full inspiration	Inspiration of test gas should be sufficiently rapid such that 85% of the air must be inspired in <4.0 s[14]
Valsalva maneuver during breath hold	⇓ DLco Lower pulmonary blood volume	Avoid the maneuver
Muller maneuver during breath hold	⇑ DLco Higher pulmonary blood volume	Avoid the maneuver

Data from Graham BL, Brusasco V, Burgos F, et al. 2017 ERS/ATS standards for single-breath carbon monoxide uptake in the lung. Eur Respir J 2017;49(1). https://doi.org/10.1183/13993003.00016-2016.

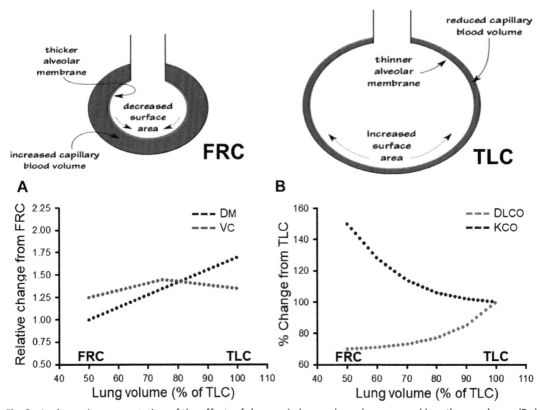

Fig. 3. A schematic representation of the effects of changes in lung volume (*upper panels*) on the membrane (Dм) and capillary (Vc) components of lung diffusing capacity (*A*) and their consequences on the diffusion factor (DLco) and the diffusion coefficient (Kco) (*B*). Note that Dм increases linearly from functional residual capacity (FRC) to total lung capacity (TLC) (*A*) because of the increase in surface area and a thinner membrane as the alveoli are expanded. In contrast, Vc predominates over Dм at FRC because there is less capillary compression in the smaller alveoli (with the opposite being found at TLC) (*upper panels*). The positive effects of a larger Dм lead to an exponential increase in DLco at higher lung volumes although the relatively lower Vc precludes even larger increases in DLco (*B*). The relative predominance of Vc over Dм leads to an exponential increase in Kco as the lung deflates toward FRC (*B*). See the text for further elaboration.

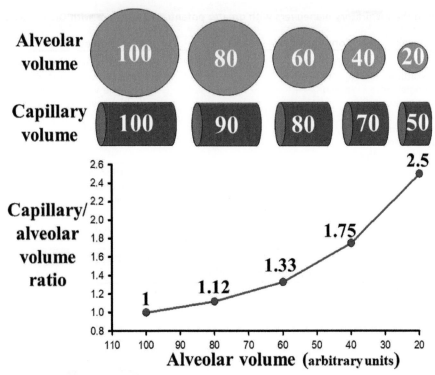

Fig. 4. A simplified representation of the effects of progressively lower alveolar volumes in the capillary volume/alveolar volume ratio in patients with different lung volumes. Typically, the capillary volume decreases less than the alveolar volume as the latter decreases. Moreover, those differences are greater the smaller the alveoli. It follows that there is a curvilinear increase in the capillary/alveolar volume ratio from large to small lung volumes. See the text for further elaboration on the interpretative considerations relative to the diffusion coefficient (Kco) in patients with different values of accessible alveolar volume (VA).

(see the sections on Patterns of Dysfunction and Differential Diagnosis of a Restrictive Ventilatory Defect).

> The DLco/VA ratio does not represent "DLco corrected by VA" because 1 unit change in VA does not lead to 1 unit change in DLco. To avoid confusion and misinterpretation, Kco should always be used instead of DLco/VA.

Another complicating issue is that the fraction of TLC accessed by the inhaled mixture (VA) depends on how well the peripheral units connect with the large airways.[23,24] In most healthy young people, the so-called "poor-communicating fraction" [PCF= (1 − (VA/TLC) × 100)] is a low fraction of plethysmographically determined TLC (~15%–20% or a VA/TLC ratio >0.85[25]–0.80[26]) **(Fig. 5)**. Thus, VA approaches TLC provided that the subject performs a maximal inspiratory maneuver (see **Fig. 2**, **Table 1**). However, in the presence of airway disease and extensive maldistribution of ventilation, VA is a poor representation of the

lungs as a whole (TLC) (see **Fig. 5**).[23] In this context, Kco might turn "normal" (particularly if DLco is only mildly to moderately reduced) despite extensive impairment in gas exchange efficiency because[8]

- Only the better ventilated and perfused alveolar unities had been sampled thereby providing a biased picture toward more preserved areas of the lungs
- The large effect of a low VA value on Kco (1 "unit" decrease in VA leads to more than 1 "unit" increase in DLco; see **Fig. 3**B) (see also sections on Patterns of Dysfunction and Differential Diagnosis of an Obstructive Ventilatory Defect)

> Do not throw the baby out with the bathwater: although interpretation of VA and Kco has pitfalls, they do increase the yield of clinically relevant information provided by isolated DLco measurements. However, a "preserved" Kco should never be interpreted as indication of no major pulmonary abnormalities.

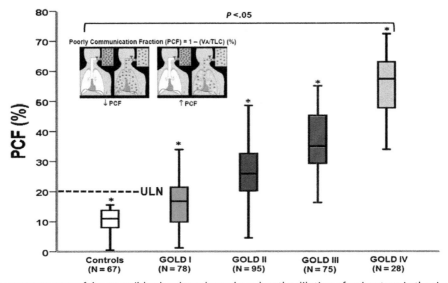

Fig. 5. The measurement of the accessible alveolar volume, based on the dilution of an inert gas in the single-breath DLco maneuver, depends on an adequate transfer of the inhaled gas mixture to the peripheral airways. The "poor-communicating fraction" (PCF) is the inverse of the accessible alveolar volume (VA)/total lung capacity (TLC) ratio expressed as % of TLC $[(1 - (V_A/TLC) \times 100)]$ *(inset)*. Note that the upper limit of normal (ULN as the one-tailed 95% confidence interval) for PCF is 20% (ie, VA/TLC <0.8). PCF increases in tandem with COPD severity because less peripheral units are sampled (lower VA) in patients with worse maldistribution of ventilation, that is, the lesser VA is not a faithful representation of the total intrathoracic gas (TLC). GOLD, Global Initiative for Obstructive Lung Disease. * p<0.05. *(Modified from* Neder JA, O'Donnell CDJ, Cory J, et al. Ventilation distribution heterogeneity at rest as a marker of exercise impairment in mild-to-advanced COPD. COPD 2015;12(3):251; with permission.)

Sources of Variability

Despite its apparent simplicity, the maneuver required for DLco measurement (see section on Methodological Bases) has many potential sources of variability. The potential errors in the performance of the maneuver with greater practical implications are depicted in **Table 1**.[14] In addition

- If the dead space (equipment plus anatomic) is overestimated or underestimated relative to the size of the patient's lungs, DLco will be decreased or increased, respectively. In practice, the equipment dead space (filter, valve, and mouthpiece), frequently forgotten to be considered in the calculations, leads to a high DLco; conversely, the use of a fixed anatomic dead space (eg, 150 mL) instead of the predicted value for the individual's size (~2.2 mL/kg) may lead to a spuriously low DLco.[19]
- DLco is characteristically higher in sites that are not at sea level, likely reflecting the lower PaO$_2$ secondary to lower barometric pressure (and, in high altitude, high [Hb]).[27] Thus, the ERS recommends that recorded values of DLco and Kco should be adjusted to standard pressure (101.3 kPa or 760 mm Hg) before comparison with the predicted values according to the Global Lung Initiative (GLI) equations.[19]

In addition to these technical issues, the biological sources of variability with a greater potential to interfere with DLco include[14]

- Those increasing Vc (eg, exercise, supine position).
- Those decreasing or increasing [Hb] (anemia and polycythemia, respectively). Although DLco should ideally be corrected for the individual's Hb,[28] this is frequently not feasible in practice. If no information is available on current Hb levels, this should be mentioned and taken into consideration in the interpretation of DLco and Kco. The highest value of DLco in women is observed just before the menses and the lowest on the third day of menses.[29] This might explain the significantly higher coefficient of variation of DLco in women than men.[19]
- Those decreasing or increasing Hb affinity for CO; for example, hyperoxia and recent smoking (high CO back-pressure and less bindings sites available for CO)[30] or hypoxia, respectively.

Based on the observed variability of the measurement, the GLI's reference values for DLco established a physiologically relevant difference as 0.3 to 0.8 mmol min kPa (1–2.4 mL/min/mm Hg) or 10% relative change (or even higher in the elderly).[19]

Reference Values

Several comparative studies reported a large variability among D_{LCO} prediction equations (as recently reviewed by Stanojevic and colleagues[19]) The above-mentioned GLI consortium advises the use of large datasets with values and 95% confidence intervals expressed as z scores.[31] The GLI-endorsed reference values for whites aged 5 to 85 years are characteristically lower than those predicted by older studies.[19] This might partially explain why low thresholds (D_{LCO} <60%–70% predicted) were associated with negative clinical outcomes in the past.[32] However, the residuals along the mean D_{LCO} predicted values are symmetrically distributed around the mean regression line in adults from 20 to 85 years.[19] Thus, a given threshold for an abnormal test result as a percentage of predicted (eg, 70%) is more likely to represent a false-positive for abnormality in the elderly than in younger people. To date, there have been no GLI studies involving nonwhites. For those populations, the use of a prediction equation that best fits the observed values in a local sample of normal individuals of both genders with a large variability in body size and age is recommended.[14]

PATTERNS OF DYSFUNCTION
Low Diffusion Coefficient for Carbon Monoxide

A low K_{CO} signals inefficient gas exchange, most commonly at the lung level (**Fig. 6**).[8] The term "inefficient" here is merely descriptive; it indicates that the rate of CO transfer from alveolar air to Hb was less than expected for the volume of the gas exchanging units that received the inhaled gas mixture. The differential diagnosis of a low K_{CO} should take into consideration the following:

- When V_A is preserved, there is a high negative predictive value for restriction (because V_A is always a fraction of TLC; thus, if V_A is normal, so is TLC in the most subjects).[33] If obstruction were present, it would decrease V_A secondary to a low V_A/TLC (see **Fig. 5**).[34] It follows that a preserved V_A, when associated with a low K_{CO} (provided there is no anemia or recent smoking) (scenario 1 in **Fig. 7**), suggests pulmonary vascular disease or intrapulmonary right-to-left shunting (see **Fig. 6**).

There are at least 2 scenarios in which obstruction can coexist with a normal V_A:

- The patient with mild airflow limitation in whom the distributive abnormalities are not severe enough to decrease V_A/TLC less than 0.8 (eg, mild emphysema, smokers with microvascular impairment),[26,35] and, conversely
- The severely hyperinflated patient (high TLC)[36] in whom V_A may still lie in the normal range despite a low V_A/TLC (eg, TLC = 140%, V_A/TLC = 0.62, V_A = 85%) (note the asterisks in **Fig. 7**). In any case, the

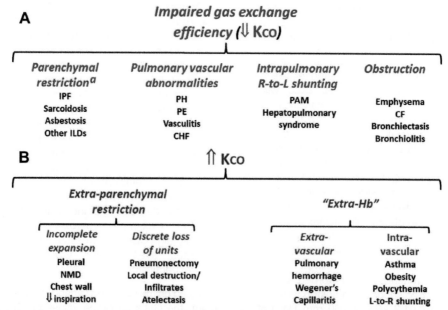

Fig. 6. The most frequent causes of low (A) and high (B) diffusion coefficient for carbon monoxide (K_{CO}) according to specific pathophysiologic mechanisms. [a] The pattern of "parenchymal restriction" may coexist with normal K_{CO}. See the text for further elaboration. CF, cystic fibrosis; CHF, chronic heart failure; ILD, interstitial lung disease; IPF, interstitial pulmonary fibrosis; L, left; NMD, neuromuscular disease; PAM, pulmonary arteriovenous malformation; PE, pulmonary embolism; PH, pulmonary hypertension; R, right.

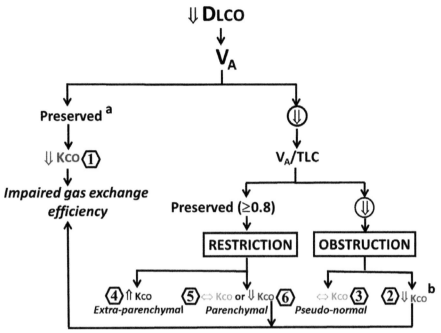

Fig. 7. A simplified algorithm to further interpret the meaning of a low (⇊) DLCO (< lower limit of normal) taking into consideration the caveats outlined in the text. If the accessible alveolar volume (VA) is preserved (⇔), the DLCO/VA ratio (KCO) will be low, that is, there is impaired gas exchange efficiency due to pulmonary vascular disease, right-to-left shunt or mild emphysema, and others (scenario 1). If VA is reduced, the next step is to check whether the VA/TLC ratio is low due to ventilation maldistribution secondary to an obstructive airway disease. A low VA/TLC may "normalize" KCO, precluding any further interpretation of this index (scenario 3); however, if KCO is reduced despite a low VA/TLC, there is impaired gas exchange efficiency (eg, extensive emphysema) (scenario 2). Conversely, if VA is preserved, there is not restriction because VA is always a fraction of TLC, that is, if VA is preserved so is TLC. A high (⇑) KCO here signals extraparenchymal restriction (scenario 4), that is, capillary volume is relatively greater than alveolar volume (eg, neuromuscular, pleural, and chest wall disease). Parenchymal restriction (eg, interstitial lung disease) may be associated either with preserved KCO (scenario 5) or a low KCO (scenario 6). Whereas scenario 5 does not allow further mechanistic elaboration (because of the trend of a low VA to normalize KCO), scenario 6 also indicates impaired pulmonary gas exchange efficiency. [a] A normal VA may coexist with airflow obstruction in a patient with mild airflow limitation in whom the distributive abnormalities are not severe enough to decrease VA/TLC less than 0.8; [b] VA may still lie in the normal range despite a low VA/TLC in a severely hyperinflated patient (high TLC).

interpretation does not change; there is impaired gas exchange efficiency despite a low VA/TLC (usually seen in severe emphysema) (see **Fig. 6**).

- When VA is low, it is crucial to check the VA/TLC ratio; if it is low (<0.8) indicating obstruction with ventilation distribution abnormalities, the KCO might seem preserved (pseudonormal). In this scenario (scenario 3 in **Fig. 7**), no further valid inferences can be made regarding KCO. However, if despite those caveats (which would otherwise conspire to increase VA/TLC) (see **Fig. 4**), KCO is low, there is extensive impairment in pulmonary gas exchange efficiency; for example, severe emphysema (scenario 2 in **Fig. 7**). On the other hand, a low VA in the presence of a normal VA/TLC implies restriction; a low KCO points to intraparenchymal restriction with impaired gas exchange efficiency (scenario 6 in **Fig. 7**).

The first step in the interpretation of KCO in the presence of a low VA is to check whether VA has significantly underestimated TLC; this is indicated by a VA/TLC ratio less than 0.8.

High Diffusion Coefficient for Carbon Monoxide

A high KCO indicates, at closer inspection, a predominance of VC over DM either due to extraparenchymal restriction (scenario 4 in **Fig. 7**) or the presence of extra Hb either inside or outside the lung vessels (see **Fig. 6**). The extraparenchymal pattern may happen due to[8]

- Incomplete alveolar expansion on a background of otherwise normal lung parenchyma; for example, pleural, chest wall and neuromuscular disease; or

- Discrete loss of units with overperfusion of the remaining units; for example, pneumonectomy, local infiltrates, atelectasis.

Some investigators propose the discrimination of "incomplete alveolar expansion" from "discrete loss of units" as a cause of the extraparenchymal pattern based on the fact that the former is associated with higher K_{CO} at a given V_A.[8–10] This stems from the assumption that preservation of V_C, for a given V_A, leads to higher DL_{CO} and K_{CO} in the incomplete alveolar expansion situation than for discrete loss of alveolar units.[8] In practice, however, there is substantial overlap of K_{CO} values in a given patient; thus, it is frequently complex to differentiate those 2 scenarios leading to a high K_{CO}. In any case, it is instructive to be aware that the pattern of extraparenchymal restriction, particularly if milder than expected for the level of impairment in V_A, may be associated with an intrapulmonary process, for example, local alveolar infiltrate or collapse, consolidation, or local destruction.[8]

> Before making any mechanistic inferences on a high K_{CO} due to a low V_A, it is crucial to rule out submaximal inspiration as the cause of a low V_A.

Normal Diffusion Coefficient for Carbon Monoxide

A normal K_{CO}, in the presence of a low DL_{CO}, is invariably associated with an equally low V_A. Again, it is crucial to assess the V_A/TLC ratio before jumping to any interpretative conclusion:[8]

- If V_A is low secondary to restriction (ie, preserved V_A/TLC), this is consistent with intraparenchymal restriction with normal K_{CO} (scenario 5 in **Fig. 6**). This is the most common finding in patients with high-resolution computed tomography (CT) abnormalities showing a pattern consistent with idiopathic interstitial pneumonia.[37] Thus, it is beyond debate that a normal K_{CO} should never be misinterpreted as indicating "no interstitial lung disease [ILD]."[13,38] In this context, a normal K_{CO} may either indicate that the main mechanism underlying the low DL_{CO} is loss of lung volume (eg, fibrotic ILD) or the low V_A led to a normalization of K_{CO} due to the curvilinear increase in K_{CO} as V_A decreases (see **Figs. 3** and **4**). Conversely,

- If V_A is low secondary to obstruction (ie, low V_A/TLC), there is a pseudonormal K_{CO}. As mentioned, no meaningful interpretation can be elaborated regarding the efficiency of pulmonary gas exchange (scenario 3 in **Fig. 7**).[11]

CLINICAL USEFULNESS

Key recommendations for the clinical interpretation of DL_{CO} in different scenarios are shown in **Table 2**.

Dyspnea of Unknown Origin

Chronic dyspnea despite normal spirometry, chest radiograph, and resting echocardiogram is a frequent and challenging scenario in the chest physician's office (further discussion the topic is provided in Unraveling the Causes of Unexplained Dyspnea: The Value of Exercise Testing).[39–41] Preserved DL_{CO} might be reassuring that major respiratory disease is not present,[13] particularly if associated with normal static lung volumes. Occasionally, a low uncorrected DL_{CO} identifies anemia that was missed in previous investigations.[28] A pattern of "extraparenchymal restriction" ($\Downarrow DL_{CO}$, $\Downarrow\Downarrow V_A$, $\Leftrightarrow V_A/TLC$, $\Uparrow K_{CO}$) (see **Fig. 7**) should raise the suspicion of a neuromuscular cause of dyspnea in a patient without pleural or chest wall disease (Case 1). (further discussion the topic is provided in Respiratory Muscle assessment in Clinical Practice)[2] A pattern of "impaired gas exchange efficiency" ($\Downarrow DL_{CO}$, $\Leftrightarrow V_A$, $\Leftrightarrow V_A/TLC$, $\Downarrow K_{CO}$) (see **Fig. 7**) in the absence (or out of proportion to) emphysema on CT chest should prompt further investigations to exclude pulmonary vascular disease or shunt (Case 2).[42] As mentioned, a "preserved DL_{CO}" in patients in whom a high DL_{CO} would be otherwise expected (eg, morbid obesity)[43] may signal a concurrent pathologic process causing an impairment in pulmonary gas exchange (Case 3).

In patients with multiple potential causes of dyspnea, DL_{CO} is less useful because there is a high probability of a low value with an ample differential. DL_{CO} (and, to a lesser extent, K_{CO}) is frequently low in patients with moderate to severe heart failure with reduced ejection fraction (HFrEF) (further discussion the topic is provided in Pulmonary Limitations in Heart Failure).[44] Thus, the severity of an underlying respiratory disease may be overestimated based on DL_{CO} impairment.[45] As in other circumstances, a low V_A/TLC in HFrEF signals ventilation distribution abnormalities, largely due to COPD, which may coexist with a preserved FEV_1 (Case 4).[45]

Case 1: A 59-year-old man with dyspnea Medical Research Council (MRC) score 2 in the preceding 6 months, normal chest radiograph and spirometry showing a moderate and proportional decrease in forced expiratory volume in first second of expiration (FEV_1) and forced vital capacity (FVC) before and after inhaling bronchodilator (nonspecific pattern).

DLco (% Predicted)	VA/TLC	TLC (% Predicted)	VA (% Predicted)	Kco (% Predicted)
61[a]	0.97	50[a]	44[a]	145[a]

[a]Abnormal test result.

Interpretation: Mildly decreased DLco and supranormal Kco, in the context of restriction and preserved VA/TLC, indicates extraparenchymal restriction (more likely incomplete alveolar expansion). A neuromuscular protocol is recommended.

Follow-up: Myasthenia gravis.

Case 2: A 48-year-old woman, long-term smoker, dyspnea MRC score 2, chronic obstructive pulmonary disease (COPD) despite normal spirometry before and after inhaling bronchodilator.

DLco (% Predicted)	VA/ TLC	TLC (% Predicted)	VA (% Predicted)	Kco (% Predicted)
54[a]	0.86	91	82	64[a]

[a]Abnormal test result.

Interpretation: Moderately decreased DLco and low Kco, in the context of preserved VA/TLC, indicates impaired pulmonary gas exchange efficiency.

Follow-up: Idiopathic pulmonary arterial hypertension.

Case 3: A 68-year-old woman, body mass index = 67.2 kg/m^2, dyspnea MRC score 4 in the preceding few months with normal chest radiograph and spirometry showing a mild and proportional decrease in FEV_1 and FVC before and after inhaling bronchodilator.

DLco (% Predicted)	VA/TLC	TLC (% Predicted)	VA (% Predicted)	Kco (% Predicted)
74	0.84	76[a]	64[a]	105

[a]Abnormal test result.

Interpretation: Preserved DLco and Kco with mild restriction likely due to severe obesity. Kco is not increased as it would be anticipated by patient's body mass index. Further investigation recommended to rule out a cause of poor gas exchange efficiency.

Follow-up: Lobar and multi-segmental pulmonary embolism.

Case 4: An 84-year-old man, left ventricular ejection fraction of 31%, long-term smoker, 11% emphysema on CT chest, spirometry showing low FEV_1/FVC and mid-expiratory flows but preserved FEV_1 before and after inhaling bronchodilator.

DLco (% Predicted)	VA/TLC	TLC (% Predicted)	VA (% Predicted)	Kco (% Predicted)
48[a]	0.62[a]	114	67[a]	71

[a]Abnormal test result.

Interpretation: Moderately reduced DLco. Low VA/TLC indicating ventilation distribution abnormalities; thus, Kco cannot be appropriately interpreted. Disproportionally low DLco for patient's emphysema burden likely indicates the combined deleterious effects of heart failure and COPD on pulmonary gas exchange.

Follow-up: Comorbid HFrEF and COPD.

Table 2
Selected scenarios in which DLco measurements are more likely to provide clinically relevant information

Clinical Scenarios	Usefulness
Dyspnea of unknown origin	• Preserved DLco might be reassuring that major respiratory disease is not present • A low uncorrected DLco may uncover missed anemia • A pattern of "extraparenchymal restriction" should raise the suspicion of a neuromuscular cause of dyspnea in a patient without pleural or chest wall disease • A pattern of "intraparenchymal restriction" should prompt more detailed chest imaging, for example, high-resolution CT • A pattern of "impaired gas exchange efficiency" in the absence of (or out-of-proportion) emphysema on CT chest may prompt further investigations to exclude pulmonary vascular disease or shunt
Dyspnea and exercise Intolerance in COPD	• A low DLco is associated with dyspnea and poor tolerance of effort across the whole spectrum of disease severity (including in symptomatic smokers) • A low DLco is an independent predictor of reduced physical activity in daily life in COPD • A severely reduced DLco (<45% predicted) with precapillary pulmonary hypertension, despite only moderate airflow limitation, and a pattern of circulatory limitation to exercise characterizes a "pulmonary vascular phenotype" of COPD • A low DLco predicts negative clinical outcomes in patients with COPD with co-morbid cardiovascular disease
Differential diagnosis of obstruction	• A normal DLco is not consistent with the emphysema phenotype of COPD • A high DLco (and Kco) is commonly seen in asthma • The diagnosis of coexistent COPD (emphysema phenotype) should be considered in a smoker with established asthma who presents with a low DLco
Differential diagnosis of restriction	• Useful in differentiating "extraparenchymal" from "parenchymal" restriction
Management of interstitial lung disease (ILD)	• Early detection (screening) of lung disease in patients who are at increased risk (eg, environmental or drug exposure, systemic diseases, radiation therapy to the chest) or have respiratory symptoms with apparent spirometric restriction • Definition of the severity of ILD (magnitude of impairment and risk of morbidity and mortality) • Follow up the course of the disease or the response to a given therapy
Prediction of perioperative risk	• A predicted postoperative (ppo) DLco <60% should prompt further evaluation in the form of an incremental cardiopulmonary exercise test • A ppoDLco $\geq$60% (and a ppoFEV$_1$) $\geq$60% defines a low-risk patient
High Kco	• Provided there is no underestimation of predicted values or obesity, in the right clinical context, a disease associated with increased pulmonary blood volume (either intraalveolar or extraalveolar) or inflammation (such as asthma) should be suspected

Dyspnea and Exercise Intolerance in Chronic Obstructive Pulmonary Disease

There is increasing evidence that a low DLco is associated with the severity of exertional breathlessness in smokers with largely preserved FEV$_1$ (Case 5),[46] even those without obstruction on spirometry.[47,48] Impairment in DLco might also be detected during exercise in the latter group.[49] Despite similar gas trapping (increased RV/TLC ratio), only smokers with COPD had reduced Kco and emphysema on chest CT scans compared with never smokers with COPD.[50]

The link of DLco with dyspnea might stem from the fact that a low value is related to the fraction of breath wasted in the dead space.[51,52] Higher emphysema burden[47,53] or impaired microvascular pulmonary blood flow[54,55] may lead to areas with high ventilation/perfusion mismatch,[56,57] that is, high physiologic dead space.[58] Thus, patients with low DLco need to ventilate in excess for a given metabolic load (ie, poor ventilatory efficiency) to overcome an enlarged physiologic dead space (further discussion the topic is provided in

---

Case 5: A 71-year-old-man, dyspnea MRC score 3, which progressed from score 1 in the past 5 years with chest radiograph suggesting mild hyperinflation and spirometry showing a mild obstructive ventilatory defect with preserved FEV$_1$.

D$_{LCO}$ (% Predicted)	V$_A$/TLC	TLC (% Predicted)	V$_A$ (% Predicted)	K$_{CO}$ (% Predicted)
59[a]	0.72[a]	91	68[a]	82

[a]Abnormal test result.

Interpretation: Moderately reduced D$_{LCO}$. Low V$_A$/TLC indicating ventilation distribution abnormalities; thus, K$_{CO}$ cannot be appropriately interpreted.

Follow-up: Cardiopulmonary exercise test revealing moderately impaired exercise tolerance with poor ventilatory efficiency and limiting dyspnea (Borg score 7/10). Normal cardiovascular response to exertion. Treated as symptomatic stage 1 COPD.

The Pathophysiology of Dyspnea and Exercise Intolerance in COPD).[59] Patients with low D$_{LCO}$ (<50% predicted) are also at higher risk of developing[60] (or worsening)[61] hypoxemia on exertion (further discussion the topic is provided in Physiologic Effects of O$_2$ Supplementation during Exercise in Chronic Obstructive Pulmonary Disease). The attendant increase in neural drive due to multiple chemical afferent stimuli is then centrally interpreted as dyspnea.[62]

are consistent with the notion that a low D$_{LCO}$ signals the presence of pulmonary vascular destruction or dysfunction in COPD.[69] Thus, a low D$_{LCO}$ (<45% predicted) in a patient with pre-capillary pulmonary hypertension despite only moderate airflow limitation who presents with no or mild hypercapnia and a pattern of circulatory limitation to exercise may characterize a "pulmonary vascular phenotype" of COPD (Case 6).[69]

Case 6: A 78-year-old man, long-term dyspnea MRC score 4, CT chest consistent with COPD plus pulmonary artery trunk diameter of 36 mm, mild airflow limitation before and after inhaling bronchodilator.

D$_{LCO}$ (% Predicted)	V$_A$/TLC	TLC (% Predicted)	V$_A$ (% Predicted)	K$_{CO}$ (% Predicted)
39[a]	0.61[a]	112	59[a]	61[a]

[a]Abnormal test result.

Interpretation: Severely reduced D$_{LCO}$. Despite low V$_A$/TLC indicating ventilation distribution abnormalities, K$_{CO}$ is also reduced. The pattern is consistent with severe impairment in pulmonary gas exchange efficiency in a patient with obstruction.

Follow-up: Resting Pa$_{CO_2}$ = 52 mm Hg. Estimated systolic pulmonary arterial pressure on resting echocardiogram = 58 mm Hg. Cardiopulmonary exercise test revealing severely impaired exercise tolerance. Poor ventilatory efficiency and an abnormal cardiovascular response to exertion, absence of critical submaximal inspiratory volume constraints and preserved peak ventilatory reserve. Conclusion: Out-of-proportion pulmonary vascular disease in a patient with COPD.

These physiologic derangements and their sensory consequences likely explain why a low D$_{LCO}$ is an independent predictor of reduced physical activity in daily life in COPD.[63]

The cross-relationships among low D$_{LCO}$, high dyspnea, and poor exercise capacity has also been found in more advanced COPD.[64–66] Increased pulmonary arterial pressures[67] and enlarged pulmonary arteries on CT[68] have been consistently related to a low D$_{LCO}$; these findings

The ability of a low D$_{LCO}$ to predict negative clinical outcomes persists in patients with COPD with left-sided cardiac diseases. For instance, patients with COPD with coronary artery disease who presented with poorer ventilatory efficiency had lower D$_{LCO}$ than their counterparts who ventilated less on exertion.[70] In patients with comorbid COPD HFrEF, D$_{LCO}$ was particularly reduced in a subset of more dyspneic patients in whom chronic afferent stimuli led to a downward displacement of the Pa_{CO_2} set point and poor ventilatory efficiency.[71]

points to severe impairment in gas exchange efficiency as seen in cystic fibrosis with diffuse parenchymal destruction and emphysema.[55]

Case 7: A 61-year-old woman, dyspnea MRC score 2, chronic productive cough and wheezing, long-term smoker (38 pack-years) with spirometry showing mild airflow limitation before and after inhaling bronchodilator.

D_{LCO} (% Predicted)	V_A/TLC	TLC (% Predicted)	V_A (% Predicted)	K_{CO} (% Predicted)
112	0.86	98	84	123[a]

[a]Abnormal test result.

Interpretation: Despite the presence of an obstructive ventilatory defect on spirometry and extensive smoking history, D_{LCO} is normal–high and K_{CO} is high. These results are not consistent with the emphysema phenotype of COPD.

Follow-up: Airway disease with no emphysema on CT chest. Conclusion: asthma.

Differential Diagnosis of an Obstructive Ventilatory Defect

Differentiation of asthma from COPD is a frequent cause of referral to a PFT laboratory.[7] Unfortunately, there are few scenarios in which spirometry, reversibility tests, bronchoprovocation, and body plethysmography allow unequivocal discrimination.[7] Frequently forgotten, however, is the fact that a normal or high D_{LCO} speaks against the emphysema phenotype of COPD, unless associated obesity led to D_{LCO} normalization (Case 3).[72] On the other hand, a high D_{LCO} is frequently seen in asthma (Case 7), provided that there is not extensive mucous plugging, severe ventilation distribution abnormalities, and comorbid COPD. Low D_M associated with the severity of parenchymal destruction on CT has been consistently observed in cystic fibrosis.[73] As discussed earlier, however, a low V_A/TLC is an important confounder of the K_{CO} interpretation in cystic fibrosis, as in any airway disease.[73] A low K_{CO} despite a low V_A/TLC

Differential Diagnosis of a Restrictive Ventilatory Defect

A judicious use of D_{LCO}, V_A, V_A/TLC ratio, and K_{CO} might be helpful in discriminating an "extraparenchymal" (eg, loss of alveolar expansion) (Case 1) from a "parenchymal" (eg, diffuse loss of gas exchanging units) (Case 8) cause of restriction (see **Fig. 6**). As the restriction worsens, K_{CO} % predicted will suggest less impairment than D_{LCO} % predicted because K_{CO} is inversely related to V_A (see **Fig. 4**). Unless some complex adjustments are made (not feasible in clinical practice),[10] it is therefore advisable to always grade the level of functional impairment based on D_{LCO}, not on K_{CO}. Substantially more complex, however, is the coexistence of "extraparenchymal" and "parenchymal" causes of restriction in a given patient; longitudinal analysis of serial measurements might prove useful to uncover the dominant mechanism of restriction at a given point in time (Case 9).

Case 8: An 84-year-old man, rapidly progressing dyspnea (currently MRC score 3), bilateral reticular infiltrates with ground-glass opacities and spirometry suggesting a moderately severe restrictive ventilatory defect.

D_{LCO} (% Predicted)	V_A/TLC	TLC (% Predicted)	V_A (% Predicted)	K_{CO} (% Predicted)
45[a]	0.85	65[a]	54[a]	68[a]

[a]Abnormal test result.

Interpretation: Moderate to severe decrease in D_{LCO} with low K_{CO} in the context of mildly impaired TLC and preserved V_A/TLC. Overall, consistent with an intraparenchymal restrictive ventilatory defect with impaired gas exchange efficiency.

Follow-up: Nonspecific interstitial pneumonia, drug toxicity.

Case 9: A 62-year-old woman with worsening dyspnea, cough, and chest pain in the preceding 6 months (currently dyspnea MRC score 2–3), bilateral ground-glass opacities, and spirometry suggesting a mild restrictive ventilatory defect.

D~LCO~ (% Predicted)	V~A~/TLC	TLC (% Predicted)	V~A~ (% Predicted)	K~CO~ (% Predicted)
62[a]	0.90	67[a]	64[a]	88

Admitted 15 days later to the intensive care unit with hypoxic respiratory failure leading to prolonged invasive mechanical ventilation. Measurements 1 month after discharge:

D~LCO~ (% Predicted)	V~A~/TLC	TLC (% Predicted)	V~A~ (% Predicted)	K~CO~ (% Predicted)
59[a]	0.88	53[a]	49[a]	141[a]

[a]Abnormal test result.

Interpretation: D~LCO~ is moderately impaired and V~A~/TLC is preserved in both evaluations. However, there was longitudinal worsening of restriction with a normal K~CO~ turning supranormal in the second assessment. Results consistent with intraparenchymal restriction followed by extraparenchymal restriction.

Follow-up: Lupus pneumonitis followed by severe respiratory muscle weakness after long-term intensive care unit stay and high doses of corticosteroids.

D~LCO~, not K~CO~, should be used to gradate the level of functional impairment (exception made to the patient with normal D~LCO~ but low K~CO~; eg, mild emphysema).

Management of Interstitial Lung Disease

A low D~LCO~ is a key finding in patients with ILD (see also Exercise Pathophysiology in Interstitial Lung Disease). Depending on the specific disease, the mechanisms may involve

- Microvascular obliterations and destruction[74]
- Alveolar ventilation–capillary perfusion mismatch,[75] and, secondarily
- Extensive fibrosis with thickening of the alveolar–capillary membrane[76]

D~LCO~ was more sensitive in demonstrating gas exchange abnormalities in fibrotic lung disease than resting Pao$_2$, peak exercise P(A-a) o$_2$, or pulse oximetry during a 6-minute walking test.[37] Established clinical indications for D~LCO~ measurements in the context of ILD include[14]

1. Early detection (screening) of lung disease in patients who are at increased risk (eg, environmental or drug exposure, systemic diseases, radiation therapy to the chest) or have respiratory symptoms with apparent spirometric restriction (low Vc but normal FEV$_1$/Vc); as mentioned, however, a "preserved" K~CO~ should never be used to rule out the presence of ILD

2. Assessment of the severity of ILD (magnitude of impairment and risk of morbidity and mortality), and
3. Follow-up the course of the disease or the response to a given therapy

D~LCO~ (in association with FVC and TLC) is a key prognostic marker in idiopathic pulmonary fibrosis (IPF).[77] Whereas baseline FVC showed contradictory results, baseline D~LCO~ was a more reliable predictor of mortality; a cutoff around 40% predicted has been consistently associated with an increased risk of mortality.[78] A simple model (the Gender, Age and Physiology model [GAP]) to predict mortality risk in 1 to 3 years includes D~LCO~ (and FVC).[79] A decline in D~LCO~ (15%) has also been associated with decreased survival in IPF although less consistently than a decline in FVC (10%).[78,79]

The D~LCO~ has also an important role in ILD associated with occupational exposure. For instance, D~LCO~ is the most sensitive marker of functional and anatomic[80] impairment in nonmalignant asbestos-related disorders, and is useful to detect longitudinal changes[81] even in patients with mild asbestosis.[82] As expected, however, smoking and asbestos exposure do interact in reducing D~LCO~,[83] which indicates that careful emphysema quantification is important before fully ascribing a given impairment to the occupational lung disease. Patients with isolated diffuse pleural thickness typically present with the pattern of extraparenchymal restriction, that is, ⇓ D~LCO~, ⇓⇓ V~A~, ⇔ V~A~/TLC, ⇑K~CO~.[84]

The D_{LCO} has also an important role in the clinical management of sarcoidosis.[85] In most patients with stage 2 or greater sarcoidosis, there is a variable (usually mild–moderate) decrement in D_{LCO} with low normal K_{CO}.[86] A decrease in D_M (mainly due to ventilation–perfusion mismatch)[75,87] seems to dominate over V_C. D_{LCO} is the best resting predictor of exertional gas exchange abnormalities in sarcoidosis, with significant exertional hypoxemia associated with values less than 50% to 55% predicted.[88] D_{LCO} and (secondarily) exertional O_2 desaturation on exercise are the closest correlates with the severity of sarcoidosis scores.[89] The relative importance of a low V_C to explain a low D_{LCO} increases as disease progresses; there is a significant correlation between D_{LCO} less than 50% and mean pulmonary arterial pressure.[90] In a large series, D_{LCO} was severely impaired in sarcoid patients with pulmonary hypertension

of both interstitial fibrosis and emphysema to the decrease in gas exchange.[93] The distribution of emphysema (isolated or mixed with fibrotic tissue) has an important physiologic impact in CPFE; when emphysema and fibrosis coexist, contraction of the interstitial connective tissue framework may pull small airways open,[94] leading to ventilation of emphysematous airspaces with consequent preservation of FVC and V_A. Thus, preservation of V_A by admixed emphysema was associated with a low K_{CO}, whereas the extent of "pure" ILD did not.[93] There is also recent evidence that in patients with CPFE with a larger emphysema burden (10%), D_{LCO}, not FVC, is the strongest predictor of mortality.[95] The confounding effects of emphysema on D_{LCO} as a marker of ILD severity, however, may interfere with the relationship between D_{LCO} and pulmonary vascular disease, which can be attributed to scleroderma.[96]

Case 10: An 80-year-old man, long-term diagnosis of COPD, worsening dyspnea in the preceding 2 years (currently dyspnea MRC score 4) showing reticular opacities with honeycombing on both lung bases. FVC = 81% predicted.

D_{LCO} (% Predicted)	V_A/TLC	TLC (% Predicted)	V_A (% Predicted)	K_{CO} (% Predicted)
35[a]	0.59[a]	82	57[a]	66[a]

[a]Abnormal test result.

Interpretation: Severe impairment in D_{LCO} with low K_{CO} and V_A/TLC in the context of preserved TLC. Suspicious for a mixed disorder (obstruction with associated restriction leading to FVC and TLC preservation) contributing to impaired D_{LCO}.

Follow-up: CPFE.

---

by right heart cathererization.[91] After the diagnosis, most experts recommend a follow-up visit every 3 to 6 months with clinical, radiographic, and functional assessment that should include D_{LCO}.[85] An out-of-proportion decrease in D_{LCO}, taking into account the extension of pulmonary infiltration and anemia (if present), should prompt further assessment for potential pulmonary hypertension (further discussion the topic is provided in Pulmonary Hypertension and Exercise).[91]

Impairment in gas exchange is also a key feature in the growing population of patients with combined pulmonary fibrosis and emphysema (CPFE). These patients characteristically present with preserved lung volume and markedly impaired D_{LCO}, that is, high FVC/D_{LCO} ratio (Case 10).[92] Thus, the D_{LCO} is the cardinal functional index in CPFE because it reflects the contribution

Prediction of Perioperative Risk

Impaired gas exchange, as suggested by a low D_{LCO}, has been widely recommended to predict morbidity and mortality associated with lung resection.[97–100] The enthusiasm for D_{LCO} followed the earlier disappointing results with the isolated use of FEV_1 to predict a negative outcome.[97] This is probably not surprising because D_{LCO} adds important information regarding gas exchange and cardiovascular reserves, which are critical to the trans- and postoperative stresses.[99]

In this context, predicting postoperative D_{LCO} (ppoD_{LCO}) based on the extension of the resection has been specifically emphasized. An isolated ppoD_{LCO} less than 60% is currently the most accepted cutoff to refer a patient for further assessment, usually an incremental cardiopulmonary exercise test (CPET).[98] Conversely, a ppoDLco $\geq$60% (and ppoFEV$_1$ $\geq$60%) defines a low-risk patient who does not need an exercise stress test.[97–100] There is, however, some disagreement about the threshold ppoDLco value to refer a patient for CPET. For instance, the Japanese[100] and the British[101] guidelines for risk assessment of lung resection recommend a stricter criterion for CPET referral (ppoDLco <40%). Part of the lower risk associated with a more preserved ppoDLco might be explained by its inverse relationship with exercise ventilatory inefficiency,[102] another CPET variable (in addition to low peak O_2 uptake)[103] that discriminates patients at greater risk of complications.[104] There is also some recent evidence that Kco % predicted is a relevant predictor of respiratory morbidity.[105]

In the context of lung volume reduction surgery for diffuse emphysema, a Cochrane review found that a preoperative DLco less than 20% predicted defined an unacceptable high risk.[106] However, this cutoff might not necessarily be applicable to selected extremely hyperinflated patients with heterogeneous emphysema.[107] Despite the recognized relevance of DLco in the assessment of operative risk in thoracic surgery with lung resection in patients with and without COPD, a recent European audit indicated only 24% compliance with the guidelines for preoperative DLco evaluation.[108]

The Clinical Meaning of a High Resting Diffusing Capacity for Carbon Monoxide

A high, supraphysiologic DLco is more commonly due to underestimation of predicted values (see the section on Reference Values), obesity or, in the right clinical context, a disease associated with increased pulmonary blood flow or inflammation (such as asthma) (see **Fig. 6**). Supranormal DLco in a patient presenting with new lung infiltrates, particularly patchy ground-glass opacities or a pattern of alveolar consolidation, should raise the suspicion of alveolar hemorrhage.[8] Other conditions associated with a high DLco include polycythemia[109] and left-to-right cardiac shunt (see **Fig. 6**).

SUMMARY

Despite the remarkable advances in molecular biology, classic PFTs, such as single-breath DLco measurements, have survived the test of time.[4] This article provided a physiologic framework to assist the chest physician in maximizing the yield of information derived from a judicious use of DLco, VA, and Kco. As is the case with any laboratory-based investigation, however, test results should always be appreciated in the light of the pretest likelihood of abnormality and relevant clinical information.

REFERENCES

1. Comroe JH. Pulmonary diffusing capacity for carbon monoxide (DLCO). Am Rev Respir Dis 1975; 111(2):225–8.
2. Hughes JMB. The single breath transfer factor (Tl,co) and the transfer coefficient (Kco): a window onto the pulmonary microcirculation. Clin Physiol Funct Imaging 2003;23(2):63–71.
3. Blakemore WS, Forster RE, Morton JW, et al. A standardized breath holding technique for the clinical measurement of the diffusing capacity of the lung for carbon monoxide. J Clin Invest 1957; 36(1 Part 1):1–17.
4. Hughes JMB, Borland CDR. The centenary (2015) of the transfer factor for carbon monoxide (T(LCO)): Marie Krogh's legacy. Thorax 2015;70(4):391–4.
5. Hughes JMB, Bates DV. Historical review: the carbon monoxide diffusing capacity (DLCO) and its membrane (DM) and red cell (Theta.Vc) components. Respir Physiol Neurobiol 2003;138(2–3):115–42.
6. Krogh M. The diffusion of gases through the lungs of man. J Physiol 1915;49(4):271–300.
7. Pellegrino R, Viegi G, Brusasco V, et al. Interpretative strategies for lung function tests. Eur Respir J 2005;26(5):948–68.
8. Hughes JM, Pride NB. In defence of the carbon monoxide transfer coefficient Kco (TL/VA). Eur Respir J 2001;17(2):168–74.
9. Frans A, Nemery B, Veriter C, et al. Effect of alveolar volume on the interpretation of single breath DLCO. Respir Med 1997;91(5):263–73.
10. Stam H, Splinter TA, Versprille A. Evaluation of diffusing capacity in patients with a restrictive lung disease. Chest 2000;117(3):752–7.
11. Cotes JE. Carbon monoxide transfer coefficient KCO (TL/VA): a flawed index. Eur Respir J 2001; 18(5):893–4.
12. Graham BL, Brusasco V, Burgos F, et al. DLCO: adjust for lung volume, standardised reporting and interpretation. Eur Respir J 2017;50(2).
13. Enright Md P. Office-based DLCO tests help pulmonologists to make important clinical decisions. Respir Investig 2016;54(5):305–11.
14. Graham BL, Brusasco V, Burgos F, et al. 2017 ERS/ATS standards for single-breath carbon monoxide uptake in the lung. Eur Respir J 2017;49(1). https://doi.org/10.1183/13993003.00016-2016.
15. Roughton FJ, Forster RE. Relative importance of diffusion and chemical reaction rates in determining rate of exchange of gases in the human lung, with special reference to true diffusing capacity of pulmonary membrane and volume of blood in the lung capillaries. J Appl Physiol 1957;11(2): 290–302.
16. Tamhane RM, Johnson RL, Hsia CC. Pulmonary membrane diffusing capacity and capillary blood

volume measured during exercise from nitric oxide uptake. Chest 2001;120(6):1850–6.

17. Hughes JMB, Dinh-Xuan AT. The DLNO/DLCO ratio: physiological significance and clinical implications. Respir Physiol Neurobiol 2017;241:17–22.

18. Borland CDR, Dunningham H, Bottrill F, et al. Significant blood resistance to nitric oxide transfer in the lung. J Appl Physiol 2010;108(5):1052–60.

19. Stanojevic S, Graham BL, Cooper BG, et al. Official ERS technical standards: global Lung Function Initiative reference values for the carbon monoxide transfer factor for Caucasians. Eur Respir J 2017;50(3). https://doi.org/10.1183/13993003.00010-2017.

20. Weibel ER. Morphometric estimation of pulmonary diffusion capacity. I. Model and method. Respir Physiol 1970;11(1):54–75.

21. Stam H, Versprille A, Bogaard JM. The components of the carbon monoxide diffusing capacity in man dependent on alveolar volume. Bull Eur Physiopathol Respir 1983;19(1):17–22.

22. Johnson DC. Importance of adjusting carbon monoxide diffusing capacity (DLCO) and carbon monoxide transfer coefficient (KCO) for alveolar volume. Respir Med 2000;94(1):28–37.

23. Ross JC, Ley GD, Krumholz RA, et al. A technique for evaluation of gas mixing in the lung: studies in cigarette smokers and nonsmokers. Am Rev Respir Dis 1967;95(3):447–53.

24. Davis C, Sheikh K, Pike D, et al. Ventilation heterogeneity in never-smokers and COPD: comparison of pulmonary functional magnetic resonance imaging with the poorly communicating fraction derived from plethysmography. Acad Radiol 2016;23(4):398–405.

25. Cotes JE. Assessment of distribution of ventilation and of blood flow through the lung, . Lung function. assessment and application in medicine. Oxford (United Kingdom): Blackwell Scientific Publications; 1993. p. 213–62.

26. Neder JA, O'Donnell CDJ, Cory J, et al. Ventilation distribution heterogeneity at rest as a marker of exercise impairment in mild-to-advanced COPD. COPD 2015;12(3):249–56.

27. Gray G, Zamel N, Crapo RO. Effect of a simulated 3,048 meter altitude on the single-breath transfer factor. Bull Eur Physiopathol Respir 1986;22(5):429–31.

28. Marrades RM, Diaz O, Roca J, et al. Adjustment of DLCO for hemoglobin concentration. Am J Respir Crit Care Med 1997;155(1):236–41.

29. Sansores RH, Abboud RT, Kennell C, et al. The effect of menstruation on the pulmonary carbon monoxide diffusing capacity. Am J Respir Crit Care Med 1995;152(1):381–4.

30. Sansores RH, Pare PD, Abboud RT. Acute effect of cigarette smoking on the carbon monoxide diffusing capacity of the lung. Am Rev Respir Dis 1992;146(4):951–8.

31. Quanjer PH, Pretto JJ, Brazzale DJ, et al. Grading the severity of airways obstruction: new wine in new bottles. Eur Respir J 2014;43(2):505–12.

32. Crapo RO, Forster RE. Carbon monoxide diffusing capacity. Clin Chest Med 1989;10(2):187–98.

33. Odo NU, Mandel JH, Perlman DM, et al. Estimates of restrictive ventilatory defect in the mining industry. Considerations for epidemiological investigations: a cross-sectional study. BMJ Open 2013;3(7). https://doi.org/10.1136/bmjopen-2013-002561.

34. Punjabi NM, Shade D, Wise RA. Correction of single-breath helium lung volumes in patients with airflow obstruction. Chest 1998;114(3):907–18.

35. Hueper K, Vogel-Claussen J, Parikh MA, et al. Pulmonary microvascular blood flow in mild chronic obstructive pulmonary disease and emphysema. The MESA COPD study. Am J Respir Crit Care Med 2015;192(5):570–80.

36. Langer D, Ciavaglia CE, Neder JA, et al. Lung hyperinflation in chronic obstructive pulmonary disease: mechanisms, clinical implications and treatment. Expert Rev Respir Med 2014;8(6):731–49.

37. Wallaert B, Wemeau-Stervinou L, Salleron J, et al. Do we need exercise tests to detect gas exchange impairment in fibrotic idiopathic interstitial pneumonias? Pulm Med 2012;2012:657180.

38. van der Lee I, Zanen P, van den Bosch JMM, et al. Pattern of diffusion disturbance related to clinical diagnosis: the K(CO) has no diagnostic value next to the DL(CO). Respir Med 2006;100(1):101–9.

39. Weisman IM, Zeballos RJ. Clinical evaluation of unexplained dyspnea. Cardiologia 1996;41(7):621–34.

40. DePaso WJ, Winterbauer RH, Lusk JA, et al. Chronic dyspnea unexplained by history, physical examination, chest roentgenogram, and spirometry. Analysis of a seven-year experience. Chest 1991;100(5):1293–9.

41. Martinez FJ, Stanopoulos I, Acero R, et al. Graded comprehensive cardiopulmonary exercise testing in the evaluation of dyspnea unexplained by routine evaluation. Chest 1994;105(1):168–74.

42. Delcour KS, Singla A, Jarbou M, et al. Does reduced lung diffusing capacity for carbon monoxide predict the presence of pulmonary hypertension? Am J Med Sci 2010;340(1):54–9.

43. Oppenheimer BW, Berger KI, Ali S, et al. Pulmonary vascular congestion: a mechanism for distal lung unit dysfunction in obesity. PLoS One 2016;11(4):e0152769.

44. Apostolo A, Giusti G, Gargiulo P, et al. Lungs in heart failure. Pulm Med 2012;2012:952741.

45. Neder JA, Rocha A, Alencar MCN, et al. Current challenges in managing comorbid heart failure

and COPD. Expert Rev Cardiovasc Ther 2018; 16(9):653–73.

46. Elbehairy AF, Faisal A, Guenette JA, et al. Resting physiological correlates of reduced exercise capacity in smokers with mild airway obstruction. COPD 2017;14(3):267–75.

47. Kirby M, Owrangi A, Svenningsen S, et al. On the role of abnormal DL(CO) in ex-smokers without airflow limitation: symptoms, exercise capacity and hyperpolarised helium-3 MRI. Thorax 2013; 68(8):752–9.

48. Walter Barbosa G, Neder JA, Utida K, et al. Impaired exercise ventilatory efficiency in smokers with low transfer factor but normal spirometry. Eur Respir J 2017;49(3). https://doi.org/10.1183/13993003.02511-2016.

49. Rizzi M, Tarsia P, La Spina T, et al. A new approach to detect early lung functional impairment in very light smokers. Respir Physiol Neurobiol 2016; 231:1–6.

50. Tan WC, Sin DD, Bourbeau J, et al. Characteristics of COPD in never-smokers and ever-smokers in the general population: results from the CanCOLD study. Thorax 2015;70(9):822–9.

51. Mahut B, Chevalier-Bidaud B, Plantier L, et al. Diffusing capacity for carbon monoxide is linked to ventilatory demand in patients with chronic obstructive pulmonary disease. COPD 2012;9(1): 16–21.

52. O'Donnell DE, Webb KA. Breathlessness in patients with severe chronic airflow limitation. Physiologic correlations. Chest 1992;102(3):824–31.

53. Jones JH, Zelt JT, Hirai DM, et al. Emphysema on thoracic CT and exercise ventilatory inefficiency in mild-to-moderate COPD. COPD 2016. https://doi.org/10.1080/15412555.2016.1253670.

54. Behnia M, Wheatley CM, Avolio A, et al. Alveolar-capillary reserve during exercise in patients with chronic obstructive pulmonary disease. Int J Chron Obstruct Pulmon Dis 2017;12:3115–22.

55. Barr RG. The epidemiology of vascular dysfunction relating to chronic obstructive pulmonary disease and emphysema. Proc Am Thorac Soc 2011;8(6): 522–7.

56. Barbera JA, Ramirez J, Roca J, et al. Lung structure and gas exchange in mild chronic obstructive pulmonary disease. Am Rev Respir Dis 1990;141(4 Pt 1):895–901.

57. Barbera JA, Roca J, Ramirez J, et al. Gas exchange during exercise in mild chronic obstructive pulmonary disease. Correlation with lung structure. Am Rev Respir Dis 1991;144(3 Pt 1):520–5.

58. Robertson HT. Dead space: the physiology of wasted ventilation. Eur Respir J 2015;45(6): 1704–16.

59. Neder JA, Berton DC, Müller PT, et al. Ventilatory inefficiency and exertional dyspnea in early chronic obstructive pulmonary disease. Ann Am Thorac Soc 2017. https://doi.org/10.1513/AnnalsATS.201612-1033FR.

60. Andrianopoulos V, Franssen FME, Peeters JPI, et al. Exercise-induced oxygen desaturation in COPD patients without resting hypoxemia. Respir Physiol Neurobiol 2014;190:40–6.

61. Knower MT, Dunagan DP, Adair NE, et al. Baseline oxygen saturation predicts exercise desaturation below prescription threshold in patients with chronic obstructive pulmonary disease. Arch Intern Med 2001;161(5):732–6.

62. Mahler DA, O'Donnell DE. Recent advances in dyspnea. Chest 2015;147(1):232–41.

63. Garcia-Aymerich J, Serra I, Gómez FP, et al. Physical activity and clinical and functional status in COPD. Chest 2009;136(1):62–70.

64. Farkhooy A, Janson C, Arnardóttir RH, et al. Impaired Carbon Monoxide Diffusing Capacity is the strongest lung function predictor of decline in 12 minute-walking distance in COPD; a 5-year follow-up study. COPD 2015;12(3):240–8.

65. Behnia M, Wheatley C, Avolio A, et al. Influence of resting lung diffusion on exercise capacity in patients with COPD. BMC Pulm Med 2017; 17(1):117.

66. Díaz AA, Pinto-Plata V, Hernández C, et al. Emphysema and DLCO predict a clinically important difference for 6MWD decline in COPD. Respir Med 2015;109(7):882–9.

67. Chaouat A, Bugnet A-S, Kadaoui N, et al. Severe pulmonary hypertension and chronic obstructive pulmonary disease. Am J Respir Crit Care Med 2005;172(2):189–94.

68. Lindenmaier TJ, Kirby M, Paulin G, et al. Pulmonary artery abnormalities in ex-smokers with and without airflow obstruction. COPD 2016;13(2):224–34.

69. Kovacs G, Agusti A, Barberà JA, et al. Pulmonary vascular involvement in chronic obstructive pulmonary disease. Is there a pulmonary vascular phenotype? Am J Respir Crit Care Med 2018;198(8): 1000–11.

70. Thirapatarapong W, Armstrong HF, Bartels MN. Comparison of cardiopulmonary exercise testing variables in COPD patients with and without coronary artery disease. Heart Lung 2014;43(2):146–51.

71. Rocha A, Arbex FF, Sperandio PA, et al. Excess ventilation in COPD-heart failure overlap: implications for dyspnea and exercise intolerance. Am J Respir Crit Care Med 2017. https://doi.org/10.1164/rccm.201704-0675OC.

72. O'Donnell DE, Ciavaglia CE, Neder JA. When obesity and chronic obstructive pulmonary disease collide. Physiological and clinical consequences. Ann Am Thorac Soc 2014;11(4):635–44.

73. Young IH, Bye PTP. Gas exchange in disease: asthma, chronic obstructive pulmonary disease,

cystic fibrosis, and interstitial lung disease. Compr Physiol 2011;1(2):663–97.

74. Agustí AG, Roca J, Gea J, et al. Mechanisms of gas-exchange impairment in idiopathic pulmonary fibrosis. Am Rev Respir Dis 1991;143(2):219–25.

75. Eklund A, Broman L, Broman M, et al. V/Q and alveolar gas exchange in pulmonary sarcoidosis. Eur Respir J 1989;2(2):135–44.

76. Jernudd-Wilhelmsson Y, Hörnblad Y, Hedenstierna G. Ventilation-perfusion relationships in interstitial lung disease. Eur J Respir Dis 1986;68(1):39–49.

77. Ley B, Collard HR, King TE. Clinical course and prediction of survival in idiopathic pulmonary fibrosis. Am J Respir Crit Care Med 2011;183(4): 431–40.

78. Raghu G, Collard HR, Egan JJ, et al. An official ATS/ERS/JRS/ALAT statement: idiopathic pulmonary fibrosis: evidence-based guidelines for diagnosis and management. Am J Respir Crit Care Med 2011;183(6):788–824.

79. Ley B, Ryerson CJ, Vittinghoff E, et al. A multidimensional index and staging system for idiopathic pulmonary fibrosis. Ann Intern Med 2012;156(10):684–91.

80. Sette A, Neder JA, Nery LE, et al. Thin-section CT abnormalities and pulmonary gas exchange impairment in workers exposed to asbestos. Radiology 2004;232(1):66–74.

81. Wang X, Wang M, Qiu H, et al. Longitudinal changes in pulmonary function of asbestos workers. J Occup Health 2010;52(5):272–7.

82. Nogueira CR, Nápolis LM, Bagatin E, et al. Lung diffusing capacity relates better to short-term progression on HRCT abnormalities than spirometry in mild asbestosis. Am J Ind Med 2011;54(3): 185–93.

83. Abejie BA, Wang X, Kales SN, et al. Patterns of pulmonary dysfunction in asbestos workers: a cross-sectional study. J Occup Med Toxicol 2010;5:12.

84. Kee ST, Gamsu G, Blanc P. Causes of pulmonary impairment in asbestos-exposed individuals with diffuse pleural thickening. Am J Respir Crit Care Med 1996;154(3 Pt 1):789–93.

85. Valeyre D, Bernaudin J-F, Jeny F, et al. Pulmonary sarcoidosis. Clin Chest Med 2015;36(4):631–41.

86. Gibson GJ, Prescott RJ, Muers MF, et al. British Thoracic Society Sarcoidosis study: effects of long term corticosteroid treatment. Thorax 1996; 51(3):238–47.

87. Zwijnenburg A, Alberts C, Jansen HM, et al. Distribution of ventilation-perfusion ratios in pulmonary sarcoidosis. Sarcoidosis 1987;4(2):122–8.

88. Karetzky M, McDonough M. Exercise and resting pulmonary function in sarcoidosis. Sarcoidosis Vasc Diffuse Lung Dis 1996;13(1):43–9.

89. Carrington CB. Structure and function in sarcoidosis. Ann N Y Acad Sci 1976;278:265–83.

90. Mirsaeidi M, Omar HR, Baughman R, et al. The association between BNP, 6MWD test, DLCO% and pulmonary hypertension in sarcoidosis. Sarcoidosis Vasc Diffuse Lung Dis 2016;33(4): 317–20.

91. Baughman RP, Shlobin OA, Wells AU, et al. Clinical features of sarcoidosis associated pulmonary hypertension: results of a multi-national registry. Respir Med 2018;139:72–8.

92. Cottin V. The impact of emphysema in pulmonary fibrosis. Eur Respir Rev 2013;22(128):153–7.

93. Jacob J, Bartholmai BJ, Rajagopalan S, et al. Functional and prognostic effects when emphysema complicates idiopathic pulmonary fibrosis. Eur Respir J 2017;50(1). https://doi.org/10.1183/13993003.00379-2017.

94. Strickland NH, Hughes JM, Hart DA, et al. Cause of regional ventilation-perfusion mismatching in patients with idiopathic pulmonary fibrosis: a combined CT and scintigraphic study. AJR Am J Roentgenol 1993;161(4):719–25.

95. Yoon H-Y, Kim TH, Seo JB, et al. Effects of emphysema on physiological and prognostic characteristics of lung function in idiopathic pulmonary fibrosis. Respirology 2018. https://doi.org/10.1111/resp.13387.

96. Antoniou KM, Margaritopoulos GA, Goh NS, et al. Combined pulmonary fibrosis and emphysema in scleroderma-related lung disease has a major confounding effect on lung physiology and screening for pulmonary hypertension. Arthritis Rheumatol 2016;68(4):1004–12.

97. Colice GL, Shafazand S, Griffin JP, et al. Physiologic evaluation of the patient with lung cancer being considered for resectional surgery: ACCP evidenced-based clinical practice guidelines (2nd edition). Chest 2007;132(3 Suppl): 161S–77S.

98. Brunelli A, Kim AW, Berger KI, et al. Physiologic evaluation of the patient with lung cancer being considered for resectional surgery: diagnosis and management of lung cancer, 3rd ed: American College of Chest Physicians evidence-based clinical practice guidelines. Chest 2013;143(5 Suppl): e166S–90S.

99. Salati M, Brunelli A. Risk stratification in lung resection. Curr Surg Rep 2016;4(11):37.

100. Sawabata N, Nagayasu T, Kadota Y, et al. Risk assessment of lung resection for lung cancer according to pulmonary function: republication of systematic review and proposals by guideline committee of the Japanese association for chest surgery 2014. Gen Thorac Cardiovasc Surg 2015; 63(1):14–21.

101. Lim E, Baldwin D, Beckles M, et al. Guidelines on the radical management of patients with lung cancer. Thorax 2010;65(Suppl 3):iii1–27.

102. Neder JA, Arbex FF, Alencar MCN, et al. Exercise ventilatory inefficiency in mild to end-stage COPD. Eur Respir J 2015;45(2): 377–87.

103. Shafiek H, Valera JL, Togores B, et al. Risk of post-operative complications in chronic obstructive lung diseases patients considered fit for lung cancer surgery: beyond oxygen consumption. Eur J Cardiothorac Surg 2016. https://doi.org/10.1093/ejcts/ezw104.

104. Brunelli A, Belardinelli R, Pompili C, et al. Minute ventilation-to-carbon dioxide output (VE/VCO2) slope is the strongest predictor of respiratory complications and death after pulmonary resection. Ann Thorac Surg 2012;93(6): 1802–6.

105. Cerfolio RJ, Bryant AS. Different diffusing capacity of the lung for carbon monoxide as predictors of respiratory morbidity. Ann Thorac Surg 2009; 88(2):405–10 [discussion: 410–11].

106. van Agteren JE, Carson KV, Tiong LU, et al. Lung volume reduction surgery for diffuse emphysema. Cochrane Database Syst Rev 2016;(10): CD001001.

107. Caviezel C, Schneiter D, Opitz I, et al. Lung volume reduction surgery beyond the NETT selection criteria. J Thorac Dis 2018;10(Suppl 23):S2748–53.

108. Salati M, Brunelli A, Decaluwe H, et al. Report from the European Society of Thoracic Surgeons Database 2017: patterns of care and perioperative outcomes of surgery for malignant lung neoplasm. Eur J Cardiothorac Surg 2017;52(6): 1041–8.

109. Greening AP, Patel K, Goolden AW, et al. Carbon monoxide diffusing capacity in polycythaemia rubra vera. Thorax 1982;37(7):528–31.

Respiratory Muscle Assessment in Clinical Practice

Michael I. Polkey, MB ChB, PhD, FRCP

KEYWORDS

- Diaphragm • Sniff nasal inspiratory pressure • Magnetic phrenic nerve stimulation
- Expiratory muscle strength

KEY POINTS

- Inspiratory muscle weakness should always be considered in unexplained breathlessness, respiratory failure, or an inability to wean from mechanical ventilation.
- Inspiratory muscle weakness can often be excluded by simple tests.
- Inspiratory muscle strength is a continuous variable. Even where proven neuromuscular disease exists, values may be normal.
- Expiratory muscle weakness is prevalent in neurologic disease and increases susceptibility to chest infections.

INTRODUCTION

Respiratory muscle weakness is relatively rare in clinical practice and, therefore, it is seldom a clinician's first thought. However, it should always be considered where a patient has unexplained breathlessness see, for instance, cases # 5 and #6 Unraveling the Causes of Unexplained Dyspnea: The Value of Exercise Testing, respiratory failure, or experiences difficulty weaning from mechanical ventilation (see also in The Control of Breathing during Mechanical Ventilation). Particular vigilance must be exercised when managing patients with known neuromuscular disease. The aim of this article was to explain normal physiology and suggest a hierarchical approach whereby respiratory muscle weakness may be excluded or included in the differential diagnosis.

Normal Physiology

Unlike cardiac muscle, which has an inherent rhythmicity, respiratory muscle is histologically and functionally composed of skeletal muscle, identical at a molecular level to, for example, the quadriceps. The inspiratory muscles contract only in response to signals received via motor nerves, of which the most important are the 2 phrenic nerves, which innervate each hemidiaphragm. Automatic control of the respiratory muscles occurs at the brainstem, which is sensitive in particular to increasing levels of carbon dioxide, but can be overridden by the cortex to permit speech and other functions. Importantly, all volitional tests of respiratory muscle function require intact cortical function and subnormal values are obtained where cortical disease is present or where the patient is unable (or indeed unwilling) to make a fully maximal effort.

> All volitional tests of respiratory muscle function require intact cortical function and subnormal values are obtained where cortical disease is present or where the patient is unable (or indeed unwilling) to make a maximal effort.

Disclosure Statement: Dr M.I. Polkey discloses personal and or institutional financial support for advice or research, lecture fees from the following companies: Novartis, Biomarin, Amicus, Orion, GSK, and Genzyme-Sanofi.
Department of Respiratory Medicine, Royal Brompton & Harefield NHS Foundation Trust, Fulham Road, London SW3 6NP, UK
E-mail address: m.polkey@rbht.nhs.uk

Clin Chest Med 40 (2019) 307–315
https://doi.org/10.1016/j.ccm.2019.02.015
0272-5231/19/© 2019 Elsevier Inc. All rights reserved.

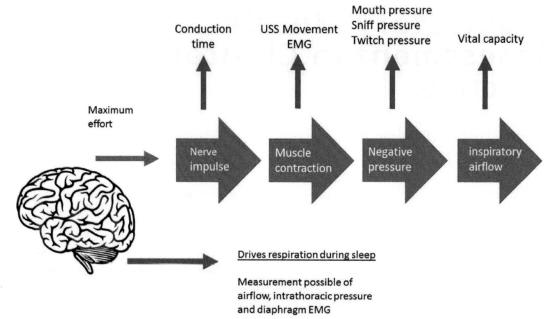

Fig. 1. Overview of normal physiology (*blue*); measurement opportunities indicated by *red arrows*. EMG, electromyogram; USS, ultrasound scan.

Anatomically, the inspiratory muscles are composed of the 2 hemidiaphragms and the extra-diaphragmatic muscles (scalenes, sternomastoid, and intercostals). Traditionally, the diaphragm is thought to account for 60% to 70% of lung volume change,[1] but there is sufficient capacity in the non-diaphragmatic muscles that patients with bilateral diaphragm paralysis can manage without ventilatory support.[2] During inspiratory muscle contraction, the dome of the diaphragm is pulled caudally, which increases lung volume both through its own craniocaudal movement, but also through outward movement of the rib cage mediated by transmission of the rising intrabdominal pressure through the zone of apposition.[3] The increased volume within the thorax leads to a subatmospheric pressure, which in turn results in inward airflow. Expiration is passive at rest in normal humans, but may be increased, in the absence of flow limitation,[4] by expiratory muscle contraction. Expiratory muscles are also necessary to generate the supraatmospheric intrathoracic pressures associated with an effective cough.[5] Understanding physiology in turn leads to identification of the ways in which respiratory muscle strength may be measured (**Fig. 1**).

Because the respiratory muscles are striated skeletal muscle, they are influenced by factors known to influence other skeletal muscles. Of these factors, the most important is length; in isolated skeletal muscle, there is an optimal length at which tension is generated and lower tensions are elicited at lengths shorter, and to some extent, longer than this[6]; in practice, in human respiratory muscle the greatest pressures are elicited close to the residual volume and the lowest at total lung capacity,[7] so reduced tension generation owing to lengthening is not an issue. Shortening of the diaphragm is a consequence of hyperinflation that accompanies chronic obstructive pulmonary disease. Hyperinflation also decreases the effective transmission of tension to reduce intrathoracic pressure and reduces the size of the zone of apposition.

Clinical Causes of Respiratory Muscle Weakness

The causes of respiratory muscle weakness are summarized in **Table 1**. Broadly speaking from a clinician's perspective, respiratory muscle weakness may either be a known and anticipated feature of an existing diagnosis (eg, as in muscular dystrophy) or may be a cause of a new presentation with breathlessness or respiratory failure.

Clinical features suggesting respiratory muscle weakness include breathlessness characteristically worse when bending forward (eg, when tying shoelaces or getting out of a car) or lying flat,

During inspiratory muscle contraction, the dome of the diaphragm is pulled caudally, which increases lung volume (60%–70% of total change at rest) through (a) its own craniocaudal movement and (b) outward movement of the rib cage mediated by transmission of the rising intrabdominal pressure through the zone of apposition.

Table 1
Causes of respiratory muscle weakness

Pathology	Nerve	Neuromuscular Junction	Muscle
	Amyotrophic lateral sclerosis	Myasthenic syndromes	Muscular dystrophies
	Guillain Barre	Botulism	ICUAW
	ICUAW	Lambert Eaton syndrome	Pompes (Acid Maltase def.)
	Enevnomation	Poisoning (nerve agents)	Hypokalemia/other biochemical
	Polio		

by speed of onset	Rapid Onset (h/d)		Slow Onset (mo/y)
	Evenomation		Past polio syndrome
	Guillin Barrre		Muscular dystrophies
	Myasthenic decompensation		Amyotrophic lateral sclerosis
	Hypokalemia/other biochemical		Pompes
	Acute polio		
	Poisoning (nerve agents)		
	Organophosphates		
	ICUAW		

Abbreviation: ICUAW, intensive care unit–acquired weakness.

although the latter can be feature of other cardio-respiratory conditions. Classically, patients with diaphragm weakness are more breathless in water,[8] although many patients referred for assessment do not swim for other reasons. An examination may yield signs consistent with more generalized neurologic disease, but the cardinal feature of isolated diaphragm weakness—paradoxic abdominal motion—is only present where intact extradiaphragmatic muscles remain.

> Clinical features suggesting respiratory muscle weakness include breathlessness characteristically worse when bending forward (eg, when tying shoelaces or getting out of a car) or lying flat although the latter can be feature of other cardiorespiratory conditions.

Standard Clinical Investigations

Respiratory muscle weakness is associated with a reduced vital capacity, which occurs because inspiratory muscle weakness decreases total lung capacity and expiratory muscle weakness increases residual volume. Clinician should be aware that substantial inspiratory muscle weakness may be present with a near normal vital capacity.[9] The normal change in vital capacity on adopting the supine position (<20%) may be increased in respiratory muscle weakness and an unequivocally normal supine vital capacity excludes important respiratory muscle weakness. The lung transfer factor for carbon monoxide is typically reduced but its coefficient adjusted for lung volume is classically supernormal (see also

J. Alberto Neder and colleagues' article, "Incorporating Lung Diffusing Capacity for Carbon Monoxide in Clinical Decision Making in Chest Medicine," in this issue).[10]

Chest radiography may show elevation of one or both hemidiaphragms, although the latter is difficult to distinguish from a submaximal inspiration. Chest radiography is only moderately predictive of hemidiaphragm function when judged against the gold standard of phrenic nerve stimulation.[11]

Bedside Tests

Bedside measurement of respiratory muscle strength can be obtained by measuring pressure. Classically, pressure is measured during a maximal inspiratory effort against a closed shutter (maximum inspiratory pressure) undertaken near the residual volume and during an expiratory effort (maximum expiratory pressure) undertaken at total lung capacity. The American Thoracic Society guidelines stipulate that the highest 1-second average be recorded, as opposed to the highest individual pressure[12] (**Fig. 2**). An alternative test of inspiratory muscle function is the sniff nasal inspiratory pressure, which intuitively one might imagine is easier for patients to do; unlike the static maneuver, the highest single value observed is recorded. Limits of agreement between the sniff nasal inspiratory pressure and maximum inspiratory pressure are wide[13,14] and thus both tests can be used together on the basis that it is impossible to get a falsely high result. Several reference equations are available to define normality but Rodrigues and colleagues[15] showed recently that 3 of the equations available provided the best

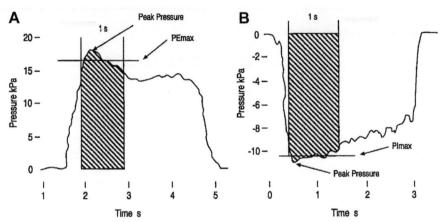

Fig. 2. Measurement of maximum inspiratory (*A*) and expiratory (*B*) mouth pressures. (*From* American Thoracic Society/European Respiratory Society. ATS/ERS Statement on respiratory muscle testing. Am J Respir Crit Care Med 2002;166(4):518–624.)

correspondence to patients with a phenotype of inspiratory muscle weakness.

Advanced Tests

Pressures

Greater insight into the performance of the respiratory muscles can be obtained by measurement of intrathoracic pressure by measurement of pressure in the esophagus (P_{oes}). This is often combined with measurement of pressure in the stomach (P_{gas}) and the arithmetical difference P_{gas}–P_{oes} is the transdiaphragmatic pressure (P_{di}). Although P_{oes} and P_{di} can be measured during both static and sniff maneuvers, for the assessment of strength they seldom offer an advantage over noninvasive measurements (indeed this is the basis for validating noninvasive measures). Occasionally, however, nasal obstruction (owing to polyps) or glottic dysfunction (common in some neurologic diseases) can result in significant underestimation of intrathoracic pressure by nasal or mouth pressure measurements.

Continuous monitoring of pressures during a stress (eg, exercise) can provide insights into respiratory mechanics. The work done by the respiratory muscles, if expressed as a product of pressure and time (pressure–time product) can then be used to measure the impact of therapeutic interventions, such as noninvasive ventilation (**Fig. 3**).

> Greater insight into the performance of the respiratory muscles can be obtained by measurement of intrathoracic pressure: P_{oes}, in the stomach (P_{gas}) and the arithmetical difference (P_{gas}–P_{oes}) representing P_{di}.

Phrenic nerve stimulation (PNS) can test the function of the nerve–diaphragm unit. PNS was originally undertaken with electrical stimulation, but reproducible values are hard to achieve even in experienced hands[16] and, except where the patient has implanted ferrous metal, has been superseded by magnetic nerve stimulation. A detailed discussion of this technique is beyond the scope of this review (fuller details may be found in Man and colleagues[17]), but briefly a strong magnetic field is created over the phrenic nerve that induces a nerve impulse that travels to the diaphragm. The operator may then measure either the pressure change termed twitch P_{di} (Tw P_{di}) or the action potential elicited by diaphragm contraction (discussed elsewhere in this article). Stimulation may be given to one or the other phrenic nerve in isolation or to both nerves together. The indications for PNS are shown in **Box 1**. The unpotentiated the Tw P_{di} in healthy adults, depending to some extent on the technique used should be greater than 18 to 20 cm H_2O and for unilateral stimulation values greater than 7 cm H_2O may be considered normal; the effect of age is modest,[18] but normal values in the very elderly remain unknown. Where the technique is used to follow sequential change (with disease or treatment) or to detect fatigue it is important to rigorously control for the other factors that affect Tw P_{di}, principally prior contractile activity[19] (a phenomenon termed potentiation) and lung volume.[20] **Fig. 4** shows an example of pressures elicited by bilateral PNS in a patient with chronic obstructive pulmonary disease.

As is the case with the sniff the esophageal pressure elicited by PNS may be measured in the upper airways as twitch mouth pressure,[21] or in intubated patients as endotracheal or tracheotomy pressure.[22] One problem with this approach

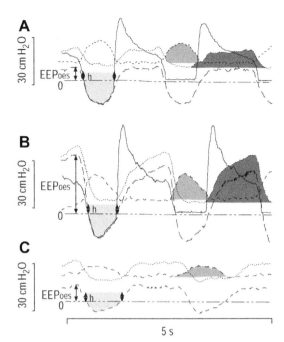

Fig. 3. The areas subtended by P_{oes} (*broad dashed line*). P_{gas} (*dots*), and P_{di} (*short dashed line*) can be measured to calculate the pressure–time product. Flow is shown with the *solid line* and is necessary to separate inspiratory and expiratory phases. (*A*) A patients with chronic obstructive pulmonary disease at rest. (*B*) The same patient at the end of exercise. (*C*) The same patient at the end of a similar exercise task where breathing was supported by noninvasive ventilation, with a demonstrable decrease in respiratory muscle work. (*Reproduced with permission of the © ERS 2019. From Kyroussis D, Polkey MI, Hamnegard CH, et al. Respiratory muscle activity in patients with COPD walking to exhaustion with and without pressure support. Eur Respir J. 2000 Apr;15(4):649–55.*)

is that, as noted, the esophageal component of Tw P_{di} is disproportionately influenced by lung volume change so this variable must be carefully controlled.

Box 1
Indications for phrenic nerve stimulation studies

- Measurement of phrenic nerve conduction time (in demyelinating neuropathies)
- Evaluation of hemidiaphragm function
- Evaluation of bilateral diaphragm function where
  - Submaximal patient effort is suspected
  - Patient cooperation is impossible (eg, intensive care unit, cognitive difficulties)

Magnetic phrenic nerve stimulation can be used to follow sequential change (with disease or treatment) or to detect fatigue. However, it is important to rigorously control for factors such as prior contractile activity (potentiation) and lung volume, which can interfere with the pressure change induced by muscle activation (twitch P_{di})

Electromyogram

Like pressure, the electrical activity of the diaphragm may be measured continuously or in response to stimulation. Electrodes may be placed on the skin surface,[23] in the diaphragm as a needle, or recorded from the crural diaphragm using an esophageal electrode. Needle electrodes are favored by some neurophysiologists, but are not widely used in patients with respiratory disease because of the fear of pneumothorax; surface electrodes can be contaminated by extradiaphragmatic muscles even where great care is exercised. Consequently, recent studies have favored esophageal electromyography, which has been reviewed in detail elsewhere.[24] Normal phrenic nerve conduction times depend on the stimulation modality used,[25] so it is important to observe local normal ranges.

When used for continuous monitoring, diaphragm electromyogram has been used to demonstrate the relationship between respiratory muscle activity and breathlessness in lung disease and obesity and to show, in the case of dynamic hyperinflation, that neural drive, rather than minute ventilation, best tracks dyspnea,[26] leading to the concept of neuromechanical dissociation (**Fig. 5**) (further discussion on the topic is provided in also discussed in The Pathophysiology of Dyspnea and Exercise Intolerance in COPD). The technique has also been used to evaluate upper airway resistance[27] and to adjudicate whether apneas or central or obstructive in nature during sleep.[28]

When used for continuous monitoring, diaphragm electromyogram has been used to demonstrate that, in the case of dynamic hyperinflation, inspiratory neural drive, rather than minute ventilation best tracks intensity of dyspnea.

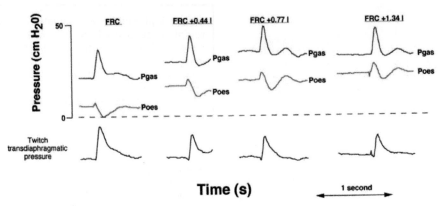

Fig. 4. Twitch pressures from a patient with severe chronic obstructive pulmonary disease. Note even at functional residual capacity (FRC), the end-expiratory P_{oes} is positive owing to air trapping. Twitches recorded at increasing lung volumes shows no impact on Tw P_{gas} but a decrease in Tw P_{oes} and consequently Tw P_{di}. (Image from the author's own thesis.)

Imaging

As noted, an elevated hemidiaphragm has only a modest relationship with hemidiaphragm function assessed using phrenic nerve stimulation.[11] Ultrasound examination (and previously fluoroscopy) can be used to track diaphragm movement, but this approach is not quantitative and a 6% false-positive rate for the detection of abnormal movement has been reported.[29]

The first identification of the diaphragm using ultrasound was reported in 1979[30] and was soon followed by the observation that its movement following phrenic nerve stimulation could be detected by ultrasound examination.[31] Diaphragm thickness, when measured by experienced operators, has a good relationship with measured

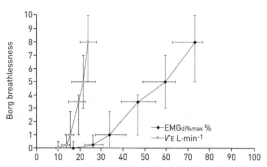

Fig. 5. Data relate breathlessness to the electromyogram (EMG) signal (*solid line*) and minute ventilation in a group of patients with chronic obstructive pulmonary disease during an exercise protocol. Because minute ventilation cannot increase (owing to ventilatory constraints), the relationship with dyspnea is poor, but well-captured by an EMG. (*Data from* Jolley CJ, Luo YM, Steier J, et al. Neural respiratory drive and breathlessness in COPD. E Respir J 2015;45(2):355–64.)

thickness[32] and the shortening during inspiration can be quantified.[33] Ultrasound examination has several features that make it an attractive method for assessing respiratory muscle strength; specifically, it is radiation free and suitable for use at the bedside. It has been particularly studied for the purpose of predicting weaning success; in 2014 DiNino and associates[34] reported the outcomes of 63 patients undergoing mechanical ventilation. They measured diaphragm thickening during a trial of either spontaneous breathing or pressure support ventilation and showed that those able to mount a greater increase (>30%) in diaphragm thickening with inspiration were more likely to successfully wean. Both diaphragm thinning and decreased excursion occur soon after the initiation of mechanical ventilation[35] and are associated with a poor prognosis and a prolonged stay in the intensive care unit.[36] One study has compared diaphragm ultrasound data with the endotracheal tube pressure elicited by phrenic nerve stimulation in critically ill patients; Dubé and colleagues[37] found that the best correlates of Tw P_{tr} were thickening and excursion rather than thickness. Of note, and as might be expected, data recorded during assist control ventilation did not convey prognostic information. Their cutoff value for diaphragm thickening which indicated a good prognosis was very similar to that of DiNino and coworkers.

> Ultrasound examination (and previously fluoroscopy) can be used to track diaphragm movement. The method can also be used to assess diaphragm thickness and to quantify shortening during inspiration.

Assessment of Respiratory Muscle Function in Children

Experienced operators can pass esophageal and gastric balloons in older children to measure respiratory muscle function and mechanics,[38] but few centers globally possess this ability. Therefore, except for intubated and sedated children in whom phrenic nerve stimulation is possible,[39] minimally invasive tests are preferred. Children over the age of approximately 6 years are usually able to undertake the sniff maneuver and normal values for this age range are available.[40,41]

Expiratory Muscle Function

Although the expiratory muscles are not used for quiet respiration in healthy adults, they are activated during exercise[42] and are necessary for coughing, which serves as a useful protection against foreign body intrusion into the airway and for expectoration of secretions. The most widespread method of measuring expiratory muscle function is as maximum expiratory pressure (discussed elsewhere in this article), but many units prefer to measure the peak cough expiratory flow; reduced values (<270 L/min is used by many units) are considered to be associated with an increased risk of chest infection and, consequently, in patients with neuromuscular disease, an indication for the use of mechanical insufflation–exsufflation (MI-E), although the threshold for MI-E is typically <160 L/min.[43] However, physiologically speaking, the peak cough expiratory flow is a slightly unsatisfactory measure because it is determined also by lung volume and, thus, inspiratory muscle strength. Alternatives are cough gastric pressure[44] or the whistle mouth pressure[45]; although the latter may be attractive especially for children, users should be aware that diaphragm tonicity sometimes results in the imperfect transmission of gastric pressure to the thorax.[5,44] The thoracic nerve roots that innervate the abdominal muscles can also be stimulated by magnetic nerve stimulation,[5,46] but it would be unfair to describe this test as routine in clinical practice. An effective cough is thought to be associated with transient supramaximal flow, which creates shear forces propelling mucus cranially. Data from patients with amyotrophic lateral sclerosis suggest a critical level of strength necessary to achieve this is a cough P_{gas} of greater than 50 cm H_2O.[47]

Assessment for Diaphragm Pacing

Although few centers offer diaphragm pacing, it is of reported value where the connection between

the brain and spinal motor neurons is irreversibly interrupted, but the path of the phrenic nerve itself is intact; a classical example is a high spinal lesion as a result of trauma. A demonstration of the integrity of the peripheral nerve is straightforward using the techniques as described, but assessing the integrity of the corticospinal pathway was more problematic. Historically, although electrical stimulation of the cortex was possible,[48] the small size of the diaphragm motor area made the technique unsuitable for clinical use. However, it has been reported that magnetic stimulation of the cortex can reliably detect a corticospinal pathway that, in some patients, will eventually recover, rendering a diaphragm pacemaker unnecessary.[49]

SUMMARY

In general clinical practice, diaphragm weakness can often be ruled out by careful application of history, examination, and noninvasive bedside tests. However, more quantitative tests also exist that can be of value in the research environment and for patients requiring sequential assessment. In conditions where the predominant problem is respiratory muscle weakness these tests convey useful prognostic information,[36,37,50] which can be used both for the management of an individual patient but also to enrich study populations allowing reduced sample size in clinical trials.

REFERENCES

1. Mead J, Loring SH. Analysis of volume displacement and length changes of the diaphragm during breathing. J Appl Physiol Respir Environ Exerc Physiol 1982;53:750–5.
2. Laroche CM, Carroll N, Moxham J, et al. Clinical significance of severe isolated diaphragm weakness. Am Rev Respir Dis 1988;138(4):862–6.
3. Urmey WF, De Troyer A, Kelly KB, et al. Pleural pressure increases during inspiration in the zone of apposition of diaphragm to rib cage. J Appl Physiol (1985) 1988;65:2207–12.
4. Hyatt RE, Schilder DP, Fry DL. Relationship between maximum expiratory flow and degree of lung inflation. J Appl Physiol 1958;13:331–6.
5. Polkey MI, Luo Y, Guleria R, et al. Functional magnetic stimulation of the abdominal muscles in humans. Am J Respir Crit Care Med 1999;160(2):513–22.
6. Abbott BC, Aubert XM. The force exerted by active striated muscle during and after change of length. J Physiol 1952;117(1):77–86.
7. Polkey MI, Hamnegard C-H, Hughes PD, et al. Influence of acute lung volume change on contractile properties of the human diaphragm. J Appl Physiol (1985) 1998;85:1322–8.

8. Schoenhofer B, Koehler D, Polkey MI. Influence of immersion in water on muscle function and breathing pattern in patients with severe diaphragm weakness. Chest 2004;125(6):2069–74.

9. Gordon PH, Corcia P, Lacomblez L, et al. Defining survival as an outcome measure in amyotrophic lateral sclerosis. Arch Neurol 2009;66(6):758–61.

10. Hart N, Cramer D, Ward SP, et al. Effect of pattern and severity of respiratory muscle weakness on carbon monoxide gas transfer and lung volumes. Eur Respir J 2002;20(4):996–1002.

11. Chetta A, Rehman AK, Moxham J, et al. Chest radiography cannot predict diaphragm function. Respir Med 2005;99(1):39–44.

12. American Thoracic Society/European Respiratory Society. ATS/ERS Statement on respiratory muscle testing. Am J Respir Crit Care Med 2002;166(4): 518–624.

13. Hart N, Polkey MI, Sharshar T, et al. Limitations of sniff nasal pressure in patients with severe neuromuscular weakness. J Neurol Neurosurg Psychiatry 2003;74(12):1685–7.

14. Steier J, Kaul S, Seymour J, et al. The value of multiple tests of respiratory muscle strength. Thorax 2007;62(11):975–80.

15. Rodrigues A, Da Silva ML, Berton DC, et al. Maximal inspiratory pressure: does the choice of reference values actually matter? Chest 2017;152(1):32–9.

16. Control of breathing: assessment in intact man. Proc R Soc Med 1975;68:237–46.

17. Man WD, Moxham J, Polkey MI. Magnetic stimulation for the measurement of respiratory and skeletal muscle function. Eur Respir J 2004;24(5): 846–60.

18. Polkey MI, Harris ML, Hughes PD, et al. The contractile properties of the elderly human diaphragm. Am J Respir Crit Care Med 1997;155(5):1560–4.

19. Wragg S, Hamnegard C, Road J, et al. Potentiation of diaphragmatic twitch after voluntary contraction in normal subjects. Thorax 1994;49(12):1234–7.

20. Similowski T, Yan S, Gauthier AP, et al. Contractile properties of the human diaphragm during chronic hyperinflation. N Engl J Med 1991;325:917–23.

21. Similowski T, Gauthier AP, Yan S, et al. Assessment of diaphragm function using mouth pressure twitches in chronic obstructive pulmonary disease patients. Am Rev Respir Dis 1993;147:850–6.

22. Watson AC, Hughes PD, Louise Harris M, et al. Measurement of twitch transdiaphragmatic, esophageal, and endotracheal tube pressure with bilateral anterolateral magnetic phrenic nerve stimulation in patients in the intensive care unit. Crit Care Med 2001;29(7):1325–31.

23. Verin E, Straus C, Demoule A, et al. Validation of improved recording site to measure phrenic conduction from surface electrodes in humans. J Appl Physiol (1985) 2002;92:967–74.

24. Luo YM, Moxham J, Polkey MI. Diaphragm electromyography using an oesophageal catheter: current concepts. Clin Sci 2008;115(8):233–44.

25. Similowski T, Mehiri S, Duguet A, et al. Comparison of magnetic and electrical phrenic nerve stimulation in assessment of phrenic nerve conduction time. J Appl Physiol (1985) 1997;82: 1190–9.

26. Jolley CJ, Luo YM, Steier J, et al. Neural respiratory drive and breathlessness in COPD. Eur Respir J 2015;45(2):355–64.

27. Luo YM, He BT, Wu YX, et al. Neural respiratory drive and ventilation in patients with chronic obstructive pulmonary disease during sleep. Am J Respir Crit Care Med 2014;190(2):227–9.

28. Luo YM, Tang J, Jolley C, et al. Distinguishing obstructive from central sleep apnea events: diaphragm electromyogram and esophageal pressure compared. Chest 2009;135(5):1133–41.

29. Alexander C. Diaphragm movements and the diagnosis of diaphragmatic paralysis. Clin Radiol 1966; 17:79–83.

30. Callen PW, Filly RA, Sarti DA, et al. Ultrasonography of the diaphragmatic crura. Radiology 1979;130(3): 721–4.

31. McCauley RG, Labib KB. Diaphragmatic paralysis evaluated by phrenic nerve stimulation during fluoroscopy or real-time ultrasound. Radiology 1984; 153(1):33–6.

32. Cohn D, Benditt JO, Eveloff S, et al. Diaphragm thickening during inspiration. J Appl Physiol (1985) 1997;83(1):291–6.

33. Boussuges A, Gole Y, Blanc P. Diaphragmatic motion studied by m-mode ultrasonography: methods, reproducibility, and normal values. Chest. 2009; 135(2):391–400.

34. DiNino E, Gartman EJ, Sethi JM, et al. Diaphragm ultrasound as a predictor of successful extubation from mechanical ventilation. Thorax 2014;69(5): 423–7.

35. Goligher EC, Fan E, Herridge MS, et al. Evolution of diaphragm thickness during mechanical ventilation. Impact of Inspiratory Effort. Am J Respir Crit Care Med 2015;192(9):1080–8.

36. Goligher EC, Dres M, Fan E, et al. Mechanical ventilation-induced diaphragm atrophy strongly impacts clinical outcomes. Am J Respir Crit Care Med 2018;197(2):204–13.

37. Dubé BP, Dres M, Mayaux J, et al. Ultrasound evaluation of diaphragm function in mechanically ventilated patients: comparison to phrenic stimulation and prognostic implications. Thorax 2017;72(9): 811–8.

38. Nicot F, Hart N, Forin V, et al. Respiratory muscle testing: a valuable tool for children with neuromuscular disorders. Am J Respir Crit Care Med 2006; 174(1):67–74.

39. Rafferty GF, Greenough A, Manczur T, et al. Magnetic phrenic nerve stimulation to assess diaphragm function in children following liver transplantation. Pediatr Crit Care Med 2001;2:122–6.

40. Rafferty GF, Leech S, Knight L, et al. Sniff nasal inspiratory pressure in children. Pediatr Pulmonol 2000;29(6):468–75.

41. Stefanutti D, Fitting J-W. Sniff nasal inspiratory pressure. Reference values in children. Am J Respir Crit Care Med 1999;159:107–11.

42. Campbell EJM, Green JH. The behaviour of the abdominal muscles and the intraabdominal pressure during quiet breathing and increased pulmonary ventilation. a study in man. J Physiol 1955; 127:423–6.

43. Bach JR. Mechanical Insufflation-Exsufflation. Comparison of peak expiratory flows with manually assisted and unassisted coughing techniques. Chest 1993;104:1553–62.

44. Man WD, Kyroussis D, Fleming TA, et al. Cough gastric pressure and maximum expiratory mouth pressure in humans. Am J Respir Crit Care Med 2003;168(6):714–7.

45. Chetta A, Harris ML, Lyall RA, et al. Whistle mouth pressure as test of expiratory muscle strength. Eur Respir J 2001;17(4):688–95.

46. Kyroussis D, Mills GH, Polkey MI, et al. Abdominal muscle fatigue after maximal ventilation in humans. J Appl Physiol (1985) 1996;81:1477–83.

47. Polkey MI, Lyall RA, Green M, et al. Expiratory muscle function in amyotrophic lateral sclerosis. Am J Respir Crit Care Med 1998;158:734–41.

48. Gandevia SC, McKenzie DK, Plassman BL. Activation of human respiratory muscles during different voluntary manoeuvres. J Physiol Lond 1990;428: 387–403.

49. Similowski T, Straus C, Attali V, et al. Assessment of the motor pathway to the diaphragm using cortical and cervical magnetic stimulation in the decision making process of phrenic pacing. Chest 1996; 110:1551–7.

50. Polkey MI, Lyall RA, Yang K, et al. Respiratory muscle strength as a predictive biomarker for survival in amyotrophic lateral sclerosis. Am J Respir Crit Care Med 2017;195(1):86–95.

Pathogenesis of Obstructive Sleep Apnea

Magdy Younes, MD, FRCPC, PhD*

KEYWORDS

- Phenotyping • Targeted therapy • Effective recruitment threshold • Arousal

KEY POINTS

- Arousal is not required to open the airway in most patients.
- For a given degree of upper airway collapsibility, obstructive sleep apnea severity is largely determined by how the respiratory control system responds to the obstructive event.
- Factors that promote instability include arousal threshold; response of respiratory drive to asphyxia; and, probably most importantly, the increase in chemical drive required to open the airway without arousal.
- Factors that promote stability include prominent afterdischarge in upper airway dilator muscles' activity, ability to increase the fraction of time occupied by inspiration (T_I/T_{TOT}), and fast sleep recovery following arousals.
- Phenotyping the traits that affect severity may open the way to pharmacologic therapy in selected patients.

INTRODUCTION

Relative to other medical disorders, obstructive sleep apnea (OSA) is a newly described disorder beginning with anecdotal reports in the 1960s[1] that showed occurrence of airway obstruction in patients with the pickwickian syndrome, what is now called the obesity-hypoventilation syndrome (gross obesity, somnolence, and respiratory failure). Dramatic improvements in somnolence, respiration, and (if present) congestive heart failure following tracheostomy confirmed the upper airway location of obstruction.

Over the past 50 years:

- There has been increased recognition of the tendency of the upper airway to obstruct during sleep in some people who are neither obese nor hypercapnic.

- It has been shown that OSA can impair quality of life[2] and is a risk factor for accidents[3]; cardiovascular,[4,5] metabolic,[6] and cognitive[7] disorders; and even malignancy.[8]
- Testing for OSA has become common. It is now clear that OSA is a major public health problem, with moderate to severe OSA (apnea-hypopnea index [AHI] >15/h) affecting 10% to 17% of adult men and 3% to 9% of adult women.[9]

Because of the substantial change in clinical presentation of OSA since its first description, the pathogenesis and, by extension, the approach to therapy has also changed considerably over time. Although early concepts emphasized the need for mechanical support of the upper airway (UA), current emphasis is on identifying which of several possible mechanisms is

Disclosure: The author receives consultation fees and royalties from Cerebra Health (https://cerebrahealth.com/), a Manitoba company that provides sleep diagnostic services. The royalties are for a license the company received from me for scoring technology I developed.
Department of Medicine, University of Manitoba, Winnipeg, Manitoba, Canada
* 1001 Wellington Crescent, Winnipeg, Manitoba R3M 0A7, Canada.
E-mail address: mkyounes@shaw.ca

Clin Chest Med 40 (2019) 317–330
https://doi.org/10.1016/j.ccm.2019.02.008

(are) responsible in individual patients (phenotyping) with the therapeutic aim of targeting the specific offending mechanisms by nonmechanical means (individualized medicine). This newer approach to therapy is particularly driven by the poor tolerance to mechanical approaches.

> An easily collapsible, narrower UA (largely caused by low pharyngeal muscle dilator activity) predisposes to obstructive events seen when the wakefulness drive is reduced (ie, during sleep) in patients with OSA.

WHY DOES THE UPPER AIRWAY OBSTRUCT DURING SLEEP?

While awake, patients with OSA have no problem breathing, even at very high levels of ventilation. The reason the UA collapses during sleep is that activity in pharyngeal dilators is reduced at sleep onset.[10] As a percentage of wake activity, this sleep-induced reduction in dilator activity is larger in patients with OSA.[10] However, patients with OSA have much higher activity during wakefulness,[11] such that, even with the greater percentage reduction, residual activity is still higher than in subjects without OSA. Thus, it is clear that the airway in patients with OSA requires more dilator activity to remain sufficiently open during sleep. The corollary of this observation is that the passive airway in patients with OSA is more collapsible that in normal subjects.

Several methods have been developed to study the mechanical characteristics of the passive pharynx. These methods made it possible to determine the luminal pressure at which the passive UA closes (P_{CLOSE}) and the luminal area (or maximum flow) at different distending pressures.[12–14] Studies using these methods confirmed that, on average, the passive UA in patients with OSA closes completely at a higher pressure than in control subjects, and the luminal area or maximum flow is less than in controls at the same distending pressure.[12–14] In many patients with OSA, closing pressure is considerably more than atmospheric pressure, indicating that, without a substantial dilating force (dilator muscle activity or continuous positive airway pressure [CPAP]), the airway would completely close. Furthermore, these studies showed that, even if closing pressure is less than atmospheric pressure, the maximum flow at atmospheric pressure in the passive pharynx is not sufficient to allow normal ventilation.[15] Thus, the essential problem in OSA is that the pharynx is narrower and requires a dilating force to remain sufficiently open to permit adequate ventilation. During wakefulness the pharyngeal dilators compensate adequately but this compensation is lost at sleep onset, resulting in airway collapse.

WHY IS THE AIRWAY NARROWED IN PATIENTS WITH OBSTRUCTIVE SLEEP APNEA?

Hundreds of studies using a variety of imaging techniques have been performed to determine the reason for airway narrowing in patients with OSA.[16,17] Briefly, the size of the pharynx is the difference between the dimensions of the cavity enclosed by craniofacial bony structures and the volume occupied by the soft tissues (tongue and other muscles, palate, lymphoid tissue, blood, and fat). Thus, a narrow pharynx results whenever the bony structure is relatively small or the soft tissues are relatively large. Both factors have been found to contribute to the narrowing but the contribution of bony structure and soft tissue volume differ among individuals and particularly among different ethnic groups.[18,19] No single abnormality in either category has been found to substantially explain the narrowing. Craniofacial abnormalities most commonly found in patients with OSA are: (1) a shorter maxilla with a narrow tapered arch, (2) small retroposed mandible, and (3) inferiorly displaced hyoid.[16] The total volume of soft tissues surrounding the airway is, on average, larger in patients with OSA, and all soft tissue components were found to be larger, on average, in patients with OSA.[16] The amount of fat within the oral cavity increases significantly with obesity[20] and this accounts, in part, for the increased risk of OSA in obese people.[21]

CLINICAL EVALUATION OF ANATOMIC FACTORS IN PATIENTS WITH OBSTRUCTIVE SLEEP APNEA

Quantitative computed tomography and MRI scans have been extensively used in research studies but simpler methods are available to assess the collapsibility of the UA in clinical practice. The most direct, practical, and reliable method of evaluating collapsibility of the passive pharynx is determination of the P_{CLOSE}.[14] The basis for this test is that UA dilator muscle activity is minimal or absent while patients are on therapeutic CPAP,[22,23] and their activity does not increase for 2 to 3 breaths on inducing an obstructive episode by transiently reducing CPAP pressure.[14,23]

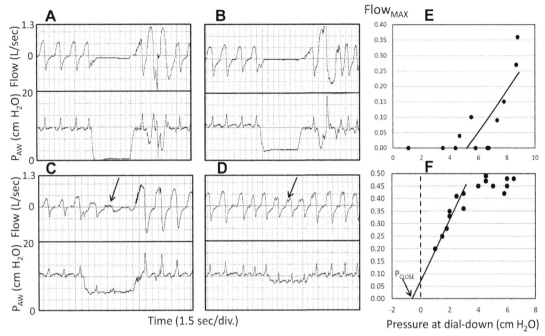

Fig. 1. Method for determining pressure at which the airway closes in the absence of dilator muscle activity (P_{CLOSE}) in the clinical laboratory. A CPAP device capable of reducing pressure to 1 cm H_2O is used. During stable sleep, the pressure is dropped to different levels for 2 to 4 breaths (*A–D*). Pressure and peak flow in flow-limited breaths are measured in the second or third breath and the data are plotted as in (*E*) and (*F*). A regression line is drawn for the data with flow limitation. The intercept is P_{CLOSE}. (*A*) Data from the patient of (*A*) to (*D*). P_{CLOSE} is greater than 0. (*F*) Data from a patient with a negative P_{CLOSE}. div, division.

Fig. 1 illustrates the procedure, which can be performed during a CPAP titration or a split study. If neither study is planned, CPAP may be titrated in the last hour of the study simply for this purpose. The patient should ideally be in the position associated with more severe OSA. The procedure requires the use of CPAP devices that allow reduction of pressure to less than or equal to 1 cm H_2O. A limitation of this approach is that, to avoid rebreathing, most commercial CPAP devices do not allow such low pressures. However, CPAP manufacturers can provide such devices for investigational purposes (minimum pressure of 1 cm H_2O was standard before the US Food and Drug Administration increased the minimum set pressure).

After determining the pressure required to eliminate respiratory events and flow limitation, and while the patient is in stable sleep, CPAP pressure is decreased to 1 cm H_2O for 3 breaths and then increased again to the therapeutic level (**Fig. 1**A). Once stable breathing resumes, CPAP is briefly dialed down again to a slightly higher pressure (eg, **Fig. 1**B). This process is repeated at progressively higher dial-down pressure until there is no change in inspiratory flow during the dial-down.

The whole sequence is repeated 2 or 3 times. Sleep technologists can easily be trained to perform this procedure. Following the study, the relation between dial-down pressure and maximum flow, preferably measured in the second dial-down breath, is determined from a scatter plot of these values, as shown in **Fig. 1**E (for a patient with positive P_{CLOSE}) and **Fig. 1**F (for a patient with negative P_{CLOSE}).

Another approach is to determine the Mallampati score. Based on the observation that patients with OSA are more difficult to intubate, it was suggested that the Mallampati score, an index long used by anesthetists to predict intubation difficulty,[24] should be used as a screening test for OSA. The procedure and scoring method are illustrated in **Fig. 2**.[25] The score correlates weakly with the severity of OSA as measured by the AHI ($r = 0.20$–0.35).[25,26] However, the correlation between P_{CLOSE} and the AHI is also weak (discussed later). The writer is not aware of studies that have directly correlated the Mallampati score with P_{CLOSE}. Such a study would help determine whether this simple score is a reliable index of the severity of the anatomic abnormality.

> The contribution of a small bony structure versus a large mass of soft tissues to narrowing of the pharynx varies markedly in patients with OSA of similar severity.

EARLY CONCEPTS OF OBSTRUCTIVE SLEEP APNEA PATHOGENESIS

The hallmark of OSA is that obstructive events are repetitive. Remmers and colleagues[27] were the first to undertake a systematic physiologic study to determine why patients with OSA develop repetitive obstructions. In their landmark 1978 study, they recorded pharyngeal pressure ($P_{PHARYNX}$) and electrical activity of the tongue (genioglossus [GG] activity) during obstructive episodes. They noted that at the beginning of the event GG activity was low and $P_{PHARYNX}$ was slightly negative, indicating weak inspiratory efforts. As the obstruction continued, GG activity increased but $P_{PHARYNX}$ also became more negative, thereby exerting more suction on the tongue. This situation continued until there was a disproportionate increase in GG activity associated with cortical arousal. At this point the airway opened, there was excessive ventilation in response to increased chemical drive, GG activity decreased, the airway

obstructed again, and the cycle repeated. The investigators concluded that the airway does not open despite the increase in GG activity because the increase in protrusion force resulting from this activity is countered by the simultaneous increase in suction pressure produced by increasing inspiratory efforts against a closed airway. Only when an arousal-induced disproportionate increase in GG activity occurs does the balance of forces favor airway opening.[27]

The balance of forces theory and the essentiality of arousal to open the airway remained unchallenged for a quarter century. The implication of this theory is that, unless UA dilators increase their activity more than that of the diaphragm in response to asphyxia, treatment must rely on mechanical means (CPAP, mandibular advancement devices, surgery) that counter the tendency of the passive UA to collapse during sleep. This implication was further supported by several studies showing that response of UA dilator muscles in patients with OSA is normal.[10,11]

NEW CONCEPTS REGARDING OBSTRUCTIVE SLEEP APNEA PATHOGENESIS

Along with the increased testing for OSA, there has been a major change in the clinical presentation of patients with OSA; the original presentation

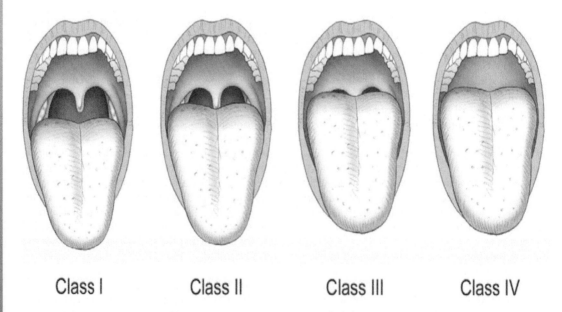

Class I   Class II   Class III   Class IV

Fig. 2. Mallampati airway classification (I–IV scale). During assessment, patients are instructed to open their mouths as wide as possible, while protruding the tongue as far as possible. Patients are instructed to not emit sounds during the assessment. Class I, soft palate and entire uvula visible; class II, soft palate and portion of uvula visible; class III, soft palate visible (may include base of uvula); class IV, soft palate not visible. (*From* Nuckton TJ, Glidden DV, Browner WS, et al. Physical examination: Mallampati score as an independent predictor of obstructive sleep apnea. Sleep 2006;29:903–8.)

(obesity-hypoventilation syndrome) now accounts for less than 10% of all diagnosed patients and many patients have no somnolence or, paradoxically, complain of insomnia.[4] In the early 2000s, Younes[28,29] noted several features in patients with OSA that were inconsistent with the balance of forces theory and essentiality of arousals:

- Most patients currently diagnosed with OSA have periods of stable breathing, with no arousals, in the same body position and sleep stage in which recurrent OSA is seen.[15,28] The periods of stable breathing could not be explained by less UA collapsibility (eg, caused by changes in head position). Jordan and colleagues[30] later confirmed that GG activity during these stable periods is increased relative to the periods of repetitive events. These observations indicated that most patients currently diagnosed with OSA can overcome the obstruction without arousal.
- Many patients with positive P_{CLOSE} (ie, severe collapsibility) had extensive amounts of stable

breathing and sleep, whereas many patients with mild collapsibility had periods of recurrent events (**Fig. 3**). UA collapsibility accounted for only a third of the variability in amount of stable breathing without arousals. This observation indicated that the response to a given degree of obstruction varies from patient to patient and from time to time in the same patient, and that, although a collapsible UA is a prerequisite for development of OSA, the response to obstructive events is a major, if not the most important, determinant of OSA severity when the UA is collapsible.

- Some obstructive events in the same patient are relieved without arousal, whereas, in others, arousals occur before or seconds after the event was terminated (**Fig. 4**).[29]
- The ventilatory overshoot at UA opening is directly related to arousal intensity (**Fig. 5**), and the more intense the arousal, the more severe the next hypopnea is.[29] These observations suggested that, in most currently

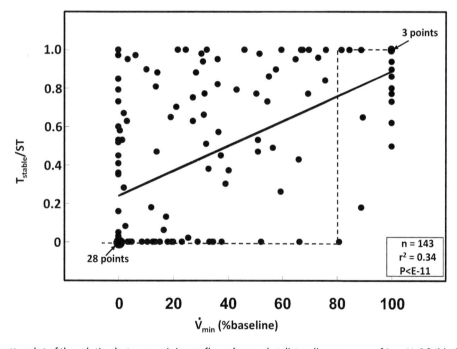

Fig. 3. Scatter plot of the relation between minimum flow observed at distending pressure of 1 cm H_2O [V(dot)min] and the fraction of sleep time in stable breathing (Tstable/ST) in the same patient and same body position. V(dot)min of 0 indicates that P_{CLOSE} was greater than 1.0 cm H_2O. Some patients had observations in both the supine and lateral positions accounting for n being 143 when the number of patients was 82. The dashed line represents the expected Tstable/ST according to the balance of forces theory, whereby upper airway does not open in the absence of arousal. This prediction assumes that when V(dot)min is greater than 80% baseline stable breathing can develop without arousal. Note that most of the points to the left of the 80% vertical line show periods of stable time, indicating that these patients were able to mount effective compensation without arousal for at least part of the time. (*Reprinted* with permission of the American Thoracic Society. Copyright © 2019 American Thoracic Society. Younes M. Contributions of upper airway mechanics and control mechanisms to severity of obstructive apnea. Am J Respir Crit Care Med 2003;168:652. The American Journal of Respiratory and Critical Care Medicine is an official journal of the American Thoracic Society.)

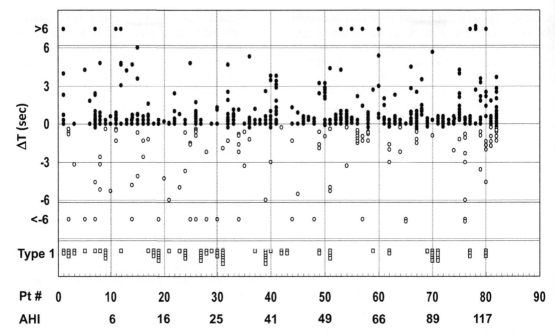

Fig. 4. Time difference between UA opening and onset of arousal (ΔT) in individual dial-downs in each of 82 patients. Patients are arranged in order of increasing AHI (AHI) during polysomnography. The AHI at selected patient numbers is shown in the lower legend. Solid circles, arousal occurs at or before the time of upper airway opening; open circles, arousal occurs after upper airway opening; open squares, no arousal before or after airway opening. ΔT values greater than 6 and less than or equal to 6 are assigned a single value to help expand the vertical axis. Note that most patients showed more than 1 type and that ΔT was highly inconsistent between and within patients. There is no tendency for the mix of types to change as AHI increases. Pt, patient. (*Reprinted* with permission of the American Thoracic Society. Copyright © 2019 American Thoracic Society. Younes M. Role of arousals in the pathogenesis of obstructive sleep apnea. Am J Respir Crit Care Med 2004;169:623–33. The American Journal of Respiratory and Critical Care Medicine is an official journal of the American Thoracic Society.)

diagnosed patients, rather than being essential for opening the airway, arousals help perpetuate the obstructive events though promoting greater postevent ventilation and greater reduction in respiratory drive.

Meanwhile several studies had established that respiratory drive, as reflected in the negative pharyngeal pressure during obstruction, is a common stimulus both for activation of UA dilator muscles and for arousal.[16] These findings, along with his own findings,[28,29] led Younes[29] to propose a new schema for the pathogenesis of OSA (**Fig. 6**). This schema allows for UA opening to occur without arousal (if the threshold for sufficient activation of UA dilators is reached first) or with arousal (if arousal threshold is reached first) but with additional inputs that help synchronize arousal with UA opening, leading to the belief that arousals are responsible for UA opening. Also, given that arousal threshold varies during the night as sleep depth changes,[31] it allows for some events to terminate with or without arousal in the same individual. This model was subsequently experimentally validated.[32]

The response to obstruction is of major relevance in determining the severity of OSA when the UA is collapsible. UA opening and arousal may or may not occur simultaneously, depending on the activation of these independent events. It follows that arousal is not a sine qua non phenomenon in the pathogenesis of OSA.

IMPLICATIONS OF THE CHANGE IN PATHOGENESIS

Before the findings discussed earlier, cortical arousal was considered a necessary evil. The necessity is that the increase in UA dilators' activity cannot overcome the simultaneously increasing suction pressure unless dilator activity increases disproportionately, and this was thought to require arousal.[27] The evil is sleep fragmentation. The new findings indicated that, in most currently diagnosed patients and under the right circumstances (discussed later), the increase in UA dilator activity in response to OSA-associated asphyxia can overcome the suction pressure without arousal

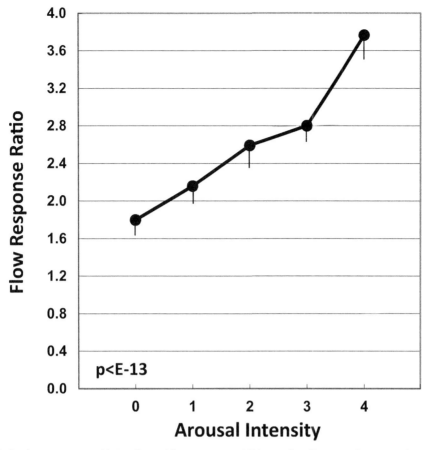

Fig. 5. Relation between arousal intensity and flow response at UA opening. Response is expressed as a ratio of peak flow during the open phase to the initial decline in flow. A response ratio of 1 is ideal. Bars are standard error of the mean. (*Reprinted* with permission of the American Thoracic Society. Copyright © 2019 American Thoracic Society. Younes M. Role of arousals in the pathogenesis of obstructive sleep apnea. Am J Respir Crit Care Med 2004;169:627. The American Journal of Respiratory and Critical Care Medicine is an official journal of the American Thoracic Society.)

and that premature arousal preempts the orderly increase in this activity that would, otherwise, open the airway without disrupting sleep and with a lesser likelihood of recurrence. This realization stimulated further research into the relation between arousal threshold and UA opening threshold (see **Fig. 6**) in individual patients as well as into other factors that may augment postevent ventilatory overshoot, the main culprit in promoting recurrence of events. The ultimate goal of these investigations was to be able to identify, and correct, the main mechanisms responsible for increased postevent ventilatory overshoot in individual patients.

FURTHER INVESTIGATIONS INTO DETERMINANTS OF POSTEVENT VENTILATORY OVERSHOOT

Postevent overshoot is primarily determined by the intrathoracic negative pressure at the time of opening and the extent of UA opening (UA resistance) at that time. Because UA cannot open until

the dilators are sufficiently activated by reflex or arousal-related inputs (see **Fig. 6**), respiratory drive and, by extension, intrathoracic inspiratory negative pressure at opening are largely determined by UA opening threshold.

- In the absence of arousal, UA opening threshold is determined by the increase in chemical drive required to provide threshold activation to the dilators through mechanoreceptors and chemoreceptors (see **Fig. 6**).
- In the presence of arousal, chemical drive at opening may be lower because the event is terminated sooner. However, arousal increases respiratory drive independent of chemical drive,[33] so the net effect of arousal on intrathoracic pressure at opening may be bidirectional.
- However, arousal is associated with a disproportionate increase in UA dilator activity[27] that may be expected to cause a greater opening (lower UA resistance), and hence greater overshoot, than would otherwise occur.

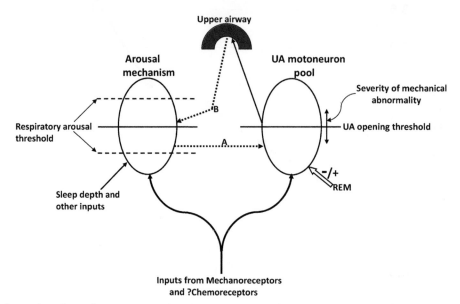

Fig. 6. Schema for relation between arousal and UA opening. Both the arousal mechanism and UA motoneuron pool receive excitatory input from mechanoreceptors and likely also from chemoreceptors. The excitation required to cause arousal is, on average, the same as the excitation required to activate the UA motoneuron pool enough to independently open UA. However, because the two systems are subject to different influences, one can occur before the other. There are 2 additional inputs that help enhance the association (synchronizing inputs). When arousal occurs first, an additional excitatory input (input A) is conveyed to UA motoneuron pool, which helps bring it to threshold. When UA opening occurs first, UA opening provides additional arousal promoting inputs (sound, vibration, and so forth; input B) that increase the probability of arousal occurring. REM, rapid eye movement. (*Reprinted* with permission of the American Thoracic Society. Copyright © 2019 American Thoracic Society. Younes M. Role of arousals in the pathogenesis of obstructive sleep apnea. Am J Respir Crit Care Med 2004;169:630. The American Journal of Respiratory and Critical Care Medicine is an official journal of the American Thoracic Society.)

- Furthermore, as a result of the lung to carotid circulation delay, the chemoreceptors are always responding to gas tensions that existed in the lungs several seconds before (see also Update on Chemoreception: Influence on Cardiorespiratory Regulation and Patho-Physiology). Accordingly, at opening, blood gas tensions in the lungs are worse relative to the levels required to effect opening at the chemoreceptor level. Thus, blood gas tensions at the chemoreceptor continue to deteriorate for several seconds beyond opening, further increasing the overshoot. As informed by studies on Cheyne-Stokes breathing[34] the extent to which the overshoot increases as a result of circulation delay depends on the magnitude of the lung-carotid delay, how much gas tensions deteriorate during this delay (plant gain), and the ventilatory response to these gas tension (controller gain) (further discussion on the topic is provided in Pulmonary Limitations in Heart Failure and Exertional periodic breathing in heart failure: mechanisms and clinical implications).

The factors that determine the extent of overshoot are, accordingly, complicated and may vary among individual patients with OSA. Because some of these variables are amenable to modification by nonmechanical means, the opportunity exists for identifying the responsible factors in individual patients (phenotyping) and for targeted therapy.

In 2007, Younes and colleagues[35] determined the range of the following variables in individual patients with OSA:

1. Increase in chemical drive required to cause arousal in the absence of obstruction (arousal threshold [T_A], expressed as multiples of baseline ventilation on CPAP)
2. Circulation delay
3. Ventilatory response to transient fixed-duration asphyxia in the absence of obstruction or arousal (a combined measure of plant and controller gains, Δ ventilation [V_E] expressed in multiples of baseline V_E on CPAP
4. Increase in chemical drive required to prevent obstruction at atmospheric pressure in the absence of arousal (called effective recruitment

pressure [T_{ER}], which is essentially UA opening threshold in the absence of arousal inputs, also expressed in multiples of baseline V_E).

With the exception of circulation time, which was normal, all variables ranged widely among individuals: arousal threshold ranged from 62% to greater than 268% of baseline V_E, T_{ER} ranged from 0 (ie, the UA remained open at 1 cm H_2O without any increase in chemical drive) to greater than 170% of baseline V_E (ie, UA remained closed at 1 cm H_2O despite near-trebling of chemical drive) and the increase in V_E on CPAP during 30 seconds of breathing air at alveolar gas tensions (to simulate asphyxia) ranged from 56% to 477% of baseline V_E. More importantly, there was little correlation between the different variables, indicating that the dominant mechanism for instability varies considerably among patients. These findings set the stage for phenotyping studies and targeted therapy.

In further studies, Loewen and colleagues[36] observed that in most patients the GG response to increasing chemical drive is highly nonlinear, with an initial phase in which the response is nearly flat, followed by a phase with brisk responses. The threshold increase in chemical drive at which GG began responding briskly varied considerably among patients, and in some patients it was in excess of triple baseline (**Fig. 7**).[36] Differences in the increase in chemical drive required to open the airway (T_{ER}) were largely related to the differences in this activation threshold.

> There is large interpatient variability in the mechanisms of the postevent ventilatory overshoot seen in patients with OSA: the arousal threshold, the plant and controller gains in the absence of obstruction or arousal, and the sensitivity of the chemoreceptors to hypoxia and hypercapnia in the absence of arousal.

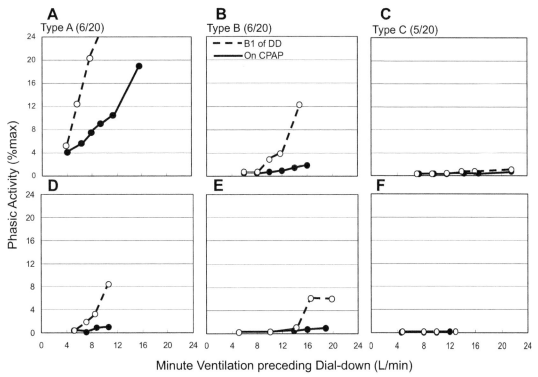

Fig. 7. Response of phasic GG activity to increasing chemical drive on CPAP (*solid lines*) and during the first obstructed breath in 6 patients. (A and D) GG activity increases as soon as chemical drive (ventilation on CPAP) increases both before and after lowering CPAP pressure to induce an obstruction. Difference between the dashed and solid lines reflects mechanoreceptor feedback related to the difference in pharyngeal pressure between the two states. (B and E) Minimal GG response to increasing drive on CPAP but GG activity during occlusion increases briskly when chemical drive exceeds a threshold (low in B, high in E). (C and F) Two patients with no response up to the maximum value of stimulation that could be achieved without arousal. Note that there was virtually no recruitment even when chemical drive was increased to 3 times baseline. (*From* Loewen A, Ostrowski M, Laprairie J, et al. Response of genioglossus muscle activity to increasing chemical drive. Sleep 2011;34:1061–73; with permission.)

PHARMACOLOGIC THERAPY, PHENOTYPING, AND TARGETED THERAPY

Based on the revised role of arousals in the pathogenesis of OSA, increasing the arousal threshold with hypnotics/sedatives became a primary target for pharmacologic therapy. In patients with low arousal threshold, eszopiclone[37] and trazodone[38] marginally but significantly increased arousal threshold ($\approx$30%). AHI decreased $\approx$30% with eszopiclone but not with trazodone. In both cases the arousal threshold, although higher, remained low and there was considerable individual variability, with some patients experiencing an increase in AHI. In another study using trazodone, the opposite was reported: AHI decreased without an increase in arousal threshold.[39] Tiagabine, an anticonvulsant that increases slow wave activity (with anticipated increase in arousal threshold), had no effect on arousal threshold or AHI.[40] These findings indicate that although common sedatives tend to work in the right direction, their effects, in therapeutic doses, on arousal threshold and AHI are, on average, small.

The other target of pharmacologic therapy was reduction of ventilatory response to asphyxia in an effort to attenuate postevent overshoot. Oxygen breathing reduced AHI by 53% $\pm$ 33% in 6 patients with high loop gain (more unstable chemical control) but AHI on oxygen remained high (34 ± 30 h^{-1}) and some of the AHI reduction was caused by prolongation of events.[41] Diamox reduced the ventilatory overshoot and the AHI, but AHI on acetazolamide remained unacceptable (>15 h^{-1} in 10 of 12 patients tested).[42]

The combination of eszopiclone and oxygen was tested in 20 patients with severe OSA.[43] AHI decreased in 19 patients (95%) and average AHI decreased from 49 ± 6 to 26 ± 5 h^{-1}. In 9 patients, AHI on treatment was less than 15 h^{-1} but it was less than 5 h^{-1} in only 2 (10%). Responders had lower baseline AHI and therapeutic CPAP level was lower, indicating milder anatomic abnormalities.[43]

Although the findings discussed earlier confirm that arousability and ventilatory responses to asphyxia play a role in determining OSA severity, they also show that only a small minority of patients can be treated effectively by currently available measures that target these traits. It is possible that measures to reduce T_{ER} will be more effective because it is T_{ER} (chemical drive just before arousal-free opening) that primarily determines the magnitude of the overshoot at the time of opening. There are currently no effective pharmacologic means to reduce T_{ER}, although hypoglossal nerve stimulation may be effective in patients with very high T_{ER}.

Success of targeted therapy will ultimately depend on finding more effective means to alter the responsible traits and simple, reliable methods for phenotyping that can be implemented in the clinical laboratory. Available phenotyping methods that reliably estimate all these traits in the same patient (which is needed for proper evaluation because most patients have more than 1 abnormal trait) are either too complex to be implemented during routine polysomnography (PSG)[35] or require invasive internal catheters. At present, only 2 of the 4 relevant traits can be measured during routine PSG. P_{CLOSE} can be measured using the procedure described in **Fig. 1** and arousal threshold can be measured using the odds-ratio product (ORP), a continuous index of depth derived from the electroencephalogram that shows excellent correlation with arousability.[44]

Recently, a noninvasive approach was proposed to evaluate all the currently known traits using routine PSG signals.[45] This approach is based on a mathematical model previously described by the investigators[46] that estimates breath-by-breath respiratory drive (the equivalent of diaphragmatic pressure) across the changing ventilation during and after obstructive events. A detailed critique of this study is given here in anticipation of the high impact it is expected to have on future research in this area.

This approach relies on untenable simplifications, namely:

1. UA resistance in the open phase is normal. However, many patients snore and have flow limitation in the open phase. Residual UA narrowing during the open phase leads to underestimation of ventilatory drive. Furthermore, airway resistance increases breath by breath during that open phase,[47] which clearly affects the time course of ventilation during the open phase and, by extension, confounds the estimated time constant of the change in respiratory drive, a most important variable in estimating the traits.

2. Arousals are assumed to provide a constant input to ventilatory drive regardless of their intensity and are treated as simply present or absent.[46] However, heart rate[48] and ventilatory[29] responses vary with arousal intensity and arousal intensity is not the same in different people or in different events within the same person,[48] and even visually varies within the same arousal.

To compound matters, as described,[45] the methods are very brief and validation results miss important information (eg, the direct relation between estimated and electromyogram [EMG]-derived respiratory drive) and model results are validated against the results of methods that themselves rely on untenable assumptions. For example, how can $V_{PASSIVE}$ (collapsibility of the passive pharynx) be determined from the gold-standard EMG method without knowledge of UA dilator activity, or how can no compensation simply be inferred because flow did not increase during the event when it is clearly established that flow does not increase, or decreases, in the course of obstructive events despite increases in dilator activity.[27,32]

> Pharmacologic attempts to increase the arousal threshold or decrease the ventilatory response to asphyxia have shown only limited benefit in patients with OSA. There is currently no effective pharmacologic means of decreasing the chemical drive just before arousal-free UA opening.

OTHER RECENTLY DISCOVERED TRAITS THAT INFLUENCE STABILITY

1. Rate of sleep recovery following cortical arousal. The idea that a given patient has a unique arousal threshold is no longer tenable. The arousal threshold changes continuously during sleep.[31] The rate at which sleep depth progresses following arousals is highly variable. It is given by average sleep depth during the 9 seconds immediately following arousal (ORP-9).[49] Because obstructive events occur soon after arousals, in patients with slow rate of sleep recovery, obstructive events occur when sleep is still light (ie, before it had time to progress to deep sleep) and are, therefore, more likely to arouse soon after the event starts. There is a significant correlation between ORP-9 and AHI as well as between ORP-9 and arousal index in patients with OSA.[49] Measures to speed up sleep recovery may help reduce OSA severity.

2. Short-term potentiation and the afterdischarge.[50,51] Afterdischarge is a phenomenon whereby muscles continue to be active for a while after the stimulus has ended.[52] This phenomenon was recently demonstrated in the GG of sleeping patients with OSA but its magnitude varied considerably among patients.[52] The GG is strongly activated at the end of respiratory events, whether by arousal or increased respiratory drive.[16] Continued activity beyond the hyperventilatory phase would protect against recurrent obstruction during the low-drive phase that follows. Measures to promote the afterdischarge may also help reduce OSA severity. The afterdischarge was recently found to be enhanced in stage N3 (delta sleep).[53] Along with the increase in arousal threshold, this finding helps explain the tendency of OSA to stop during that stage.

3. Respiratory duty cycle (T_I/T_{TOT}). Prolongation of inspiration with an increase in T_I/T_{TOT} is a well-known response to increased inspiratory resistance in conscious people.[54] It also occurs in snorers, but the magnitude of increase in duty cycle is variable[55] and likely genetically determined.[56] An important increase in the fraction of time spent in inspiration makes it possible to reach tolerable (ie, without arousal) levels of tidal volume and, by extension, ventilation at lower flow rates.[28] The importance of this response in promoting stable breathing has recently been recognized.[28]

HOW PHYSIOLOGIC TRAITS DETERMINE CLINICAL PRESENTATION

Not all individuals with a collapsible UA develop the usual OSA. The spectrum of clinical presentations ranges from no abnormalities to intermittent snoring, to steady snoring with normal sleep, to steady snoring with increased sleep fragmentation (UA resistance syndrome), to recurrent OSA with varying degrees of severity but with normocapnia, to obesity-hypoventilation syndrome with or without recurrent OSA. An attempt at identifying the responsible physiologic mechanisms in each of these categories has been made (**Fig. 8**).[28]

Apart from PSG manifestations, patients with the same OSA severity, as measured by AHI, have different complaints (no complaints, somnolence, or insomnia) and differ in their susceptibility to cardiovascular disease.[4,57] Large studies are currently underway to identify physiologic and/or biochemical traits that predispose to specific OSA complications. The ultimate intent of these studies is to identify subsets of patients with OSA who are not symptomatic and have little risk for complications. In those patients, treatment may not be necessary.

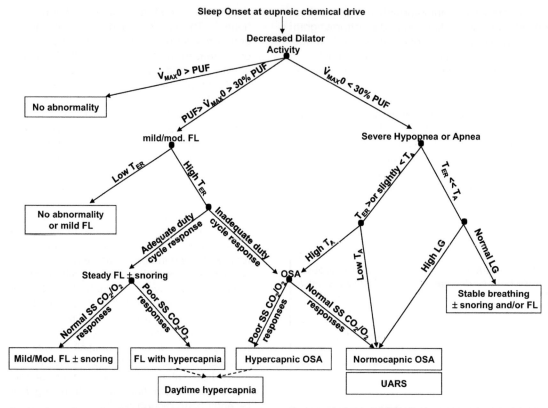

Fig. 8. Flow chart showing how different polysomnographic presentations (*boxed terms*) can arise following sleep-induced obstructive events. FL, flow limitation; LG, loop gain; OSA, obstructive sleep apnea; PUF, peak unobstructed flow rate; SS, steady state; UAR, upper airway resistance syndrome; V(dot)_MAX0, maximum flow at atmospheric pressure in the absence of pharyngeal dilator activity. (*From* Younes M. Role of control mechanisms in the pathogenesis of obstructive sleep disorders. J Appl Physiol (1985) 2008;105:1389–405; with permission.)

SUMMARY

The pathogenesis of OSA has undergone major revisions since it was first described in 1978.[27] Recent studies have identified several traits that promote stable or unstable responses to the obstructive events. Some of these traits are potentially amenable to pharmacologic therapy. Further studies are underway to determine underlying factors responsible for differences in symptoms and complications of this common disorder.

REFERENCES

1. Gastaut H, Tassinari CA, Duron B. Polygraphic study of the episodic diurnal and nocturnal manifestations of the Pickwick syndrome. Brain Res 1966;1:167–86.
2. Bjornsdottir E, Keenan BT, Eysteinsdottir B, et al. Quality of life among untreated sleep apnea patients compared with the general population and changes after treatment with positive airway pressure. J Sleep Res 2015;24:328–38.
3. Sassani A, Findley LJ, Kryger M, et al. Reducing motor-vehicle collisions, costs, and fatalities by treating obstructive sleep apnea syndrome. Sleep 2004;27:453–8.
4. Lim DC, Pack AI. Obstructive sleep apnea: update and future. Annu Rev Med 2017;68:99–112.
5. Pack AI, Gislason T. Obstructive sleep apnea and cardiovascular disease: a perspective and future directions. Prog Cardiovasc Dis 2009;51:434–51.
6. Davies SK, Ang JE, Revell VL, et al. Effect of sleep deprivation on the human metabolome. Proc Natl Acad Sci U S A 2014;111:10761–6.
7. Yaffe K, Laffan AM, Harrison SL, et al. Sleep-disordered breathing, hypoxia, and risk of mild cognitive impairment and dementia in older women. JAMA 2011;306:613–9.
8. Nieto FJ, Peppard PE, Young T, et al. Sleep-disordered breathing and cancer mortality: results from the Wisconsin Sleep Cohort Study. Am J Respir Crit Care Med 2012;186:190–4.
9. Peppard PE, Young T, Barnet JH, et al. Increased prevalence of sleep-disordered breathing in adults. Am J Epidemiol 2013;177:1006–14.

10. Mezzanotte WS, Tangel DJ, White DP. Influence of sleep onset on upper-airway muscle activity in apnea patients versus normal controls. Am J Respir Crit Care Med 1996;153:1880–7.

11. Mezzanotte WS, Tangel DJ, White DP. Waking genioglossal electromyogram in sleep apnea patients versus normal controls (a neuromuscular compensatory mechanism). J Clin Invest 1992; 89:1571–9.

12. Isono S, Morrison DL, Launois SH, et al. Static mechanics of the velopharynx of patients with obstructive sleep apnea. J Appl Physiol (1985) 1993;75: 148–54.

13. Isono S, Remmers JE, Tanaka A, et al. Anatomy of pharynx in patients with obstructive sleep apnea and in normal subjects. J Appl Physiol (1985) 1997;82:1319–26.

14. Schwartz AR, O'Donnell CP, Baron J, et al. The hypotonic upper airway in obstructive sleep apnea: role of structures and neuromuscular activity. Am J Respir Crit Care Med 1998;157:1051–7.

15. Younes M. Contributions of upper airway mechanics and control mechanisms to severity of obstructive apnea. Am J Respir Crit Care Med 2003;168:645–8.

16. White DP, Younes MK. Obstructive sleep apnea. Compr Physiol 2012;2:2541–94.

17. Strohl KP, Butler JP, Malhotra A. Mechanical properties of the upper airway. Compr Physiol 2012;2: 1853–72.

18. Sutherland K, Lee RW, Cistulli PA. Obesity and craniofacial structure as risk factors for obstructive sleep apnoea: impact of ethnicity. Respirology 2012;17:213–22.

19. Watanabe T, Isono S, Tanaka A, et al. Contribution of body habitus and craniofacial characteristics to segmental closing pressures of the passive pharynx in patients with sleep-disordered breathing. Am J Respir Crit Care Med 2002;165:260–5.

20. Kim AM, Keenan BT, Jackson N, et al. Tongue fat and its relationship to obstructive sleep apnea. Sleep 2014;37:1639–48.

21. Isono S. Obesity and obstructive sleep apnoea: mechanisms for increased collapsibility of the passive pharyngeal airway. Respirology 2012;17:32–42.

22. Strohl KP, Redline S. Nasal CPAP therapy, upper airway muscle activation, and obstructive sleep apnea. Am Rev Respir Dis 1986;134:555–8.

23. Launois SH, Feroah TR, Campbell WN, et al. Site of pharyngeal narrowing predicts outcome of surgery for obstructive sleep apnea. Am Rev Respir Dis 1993;147:182–9.

24. Mallampati SR, Gatt SP, Gugino LD, et al. A clinical sign to predict difficult tracheal intubation: a prospective study. Can Anaesth Soc J 1985;32:429–34.

25. Nuckton TJ, Glidden DV, Browner WS, et al. Physical examination: Mallampati score as an independent predictor of obstructive sleep apnea. Sleep 2006; 29:903–8.

26. Friedman M, Hamilton C, Samuelson CG, et al. Diagnostic value of the Friedman tongue position and Mallampati classification for obstructive sleep apnea: a meta-analysis. Otolaryngol Head Neck Surg 2013;148:540–7.

27. Remmers JE, deGroot WJ, Sauerland EK, et al. Pathogenesis of upper airway occlusion during sleep. J Appl Physiol Respir Environ Exerc Physiol 1978; 44:931–8.

28. Younes M. Role of control mechanisms in the pathogenesis of obstructive sleep disorders. J Appl Physiol (1985) 2008;105:1389–405.

29. Younes M. Role of arousals in the pathogenesis of obstructive sleep apnea. Am J Respir Crit Care Med 2004;169:623–33.

30. Jordan AS, White DP, Lo YL, et al. Airway dilator muscle activity and lung volume during stable breathing in obstructive sleep apnea. Sleep 2009;32:361–8.

31. Berry RB, Asyali MA, McNellis MI, et al. Within-night variation in respiratory effort preceding apnea termination and EEG delta power in sleep apnea. J Appl Physiol (1985) 1998;85:1434–41.

32. Younes M, Loewen AH, Ostrowski M, et al. Genioglossus activity available via non-arousal mechanisms vs. that required for opening the airway in obstructive apnea patients. J Appl Physiol (1985) 2012;112:249–58.

33. Horner RL. Autonomic consequences of arousal from sleep: mechanisms and implications. Sleep 1996;19(10 Suppl):S193–5.

34. Khoo MC, Kronauer RE, Strohl KP, et al. Factors inducing periodic breathing in humans: a general model. J Appl Physiol (1985) 1982;53:644–59.

35. Younes M, Ostrowski M, Atkar R, et al. Mechanisms of ventilatory instability in individual patients with obstructive sleep apnea. J Appl Physiol (1985) 2007;103:1929–41.

36. Loewen A, Ostrowski M, Laprairie J, et al. Response of genioglossus muscle activity to increasing chemical drive. Sleep 2011;34:1061–73.

37. Eckert DJ, Owens RL, Kehlmann GB, et al. Eszopiclone increases the respiratory arousal threshold and lowers the apnoea/hypopnoea index in obstructive sleep apnoea patients with a low arousal threshold. Clin Sci 2011;120:505–14.

38. Eckert DJ, Malhotra A, Wellman A, et al. Trazodone increases the respiratory arousal threshold in patients with obstructive sleep apnea and a low arousal threshold. Sleep 2014;37:811–9.

39. Smales ET, Edwards BA, Deyoung PN, et al. Trazodone effects on obstructive sleep apnea and Non-REM arousal threshold. Ann Am Thorac Soc 2015; 12:758–64.

40. Taranto-Montemurro L, Sands SA, Edwards BA, et al. Effects of tiagabine on slow wave sleep and

arousal threshold in patients with obstructive sleep apnea. Sleep 2017;40(2):1–7.

41. Wellman A, Malhotra A, Jordan AS, et al. Effect of oxygen in obstructive sleep apnea: role of loop gain. Respir Physiol Neurobiol 2008;162:144–51.

42. Edwards BA, Sands SA, Eckert DJ, et al. Acetazolamide improves loop gain but not the other physiological traits causing obstructive sleep apnoea. J Physiol 2012;590:1199–211.

43. Edwards BA, Sands SA, Owens RL, et al. The combination of supplemental oxygen and a hypnotic markedly improves obstructive sleep apnea in patients with a mild to moderate upper airway collapsibility. Sleep 2016;39:1973–83.

44. Younes M, Ostrowski M, Soiferman M, et al. Odds ratio product of sleep EEG as a continuous measure of sleep state. Sleep 2015;28:641–54.

45. Sands SA, Edwards BA, Terrill PI, et al. Phenotyping pharyngeal pathophysiology using polysomnography in patients with obstructive sleep apnea. Am J Respir Crit Care Med 2018;197:1187–97.

46. Terrill PI, Edwards BA, Nemati S, et al. Quantifying the ventilatory control contribution to sleep apnoea using polysomnography. Eur Respir J 2015;45:408–18.

47. Martin RJ, Pennock BE, Orr WC, et al. Respiratory mechanics and timing during sleep in occlusive sleep apnea. J Appl Physiol (1985) 1980;48:432–7.

48. Azarbarzin A, Ostrowski M, Hanly P, et al. Relationship between arousal intensity and heart rate response to arousal. Sleep 2014;37:645–53.

49. Younes M, Hanly PJ. Immediate post-arousal sleep dynamics: an important determinant of sleep stability in obstructive sleep apnea. J Appl Physiol 2016;120:801–8.

50. Younes M, Loewen A, Ostrowski M, et al. Short-term potentiation in the control of pharyngeal muscles in obstructive apnea patients. Sleep 2014;37:1833–49.

51. Younes M. What short-term potentiation is and why it may be relevant to obstructive sleep apnoea. J Physiol 2018;596:5075–6.

52. Eldridge FL, Gill-Kumar P. Lack of effect of vagal afferent input on central neural respiratory afterdischarge. J Appl Physiol (1985) 1978;45:339–44.

53. Taranto-Montemurro L, Sands SA, Grace KP, et al. Neural memory of the genioglossus muscle during sleep is stage-dependent in healthy subjects and obstructive sleep apnoea patients. J Physiol 2018; 596.5163–73.

54. Iber C, Berssenbrugge A, Skatrud JB, et al. Ventilatory adaptations to resistive loading during wakefulness and non-REM sleep. J Appl Physiol (1985) 1982;52:607–14.

55. Stoohs R, Guilleminault C. Snoring during NREM sleep: respiratory timing, esophageal pressure and EEG arousal. Respir Physiol 1991;85:151–67.

56. Schneider H, Patil SP, Canisius S, et al. Hypercapnic duty cycle is an intermediate physiological phenotype linked to mouse chromosome 5. J Appl Physiol (1985) 2003;95:11–9.

57. Zinchuk AV, Jeon S, Koo BB, et al. Polysomnographic phenotypes and their cardiovascular implications in obstructive sleep apnoea. Thorax 2018;73:472–80.

Respiratory Determinants of Exercise Limitation
Focus on Phrenic Afferents and the Lung Vasculature

Jerome A. Dempsey, PhD

KEYWORDS

- Pulmonary vasculature • Muscle afferents • Muscle fatigue • Congestive heart failure
- Chronic obstructive pulmonary disease

KEY POINTS

- In untrained, healthy subjects, the respiratory system is highly precise and efficient in its response to exercise.
- Intense endurance exercise activates metaboreceptor afferents from both the respiratory and locomotor muscles, which mediate increased sympathetic vasoconstriction.
- The increased sympathetic vasoconstriction limits blood flow to both respiratory and locomotor muscles thereby contributing to their fatigue.
- In the endurance-trained subject capable of working at high Vo_2 and cardiac outputs, pulmonary vascular pressures are markedly elevated, leading to exercise limitation and to maladaptive remodeling of the right heart over time.

INTRODUCTION

The maximal dimensions of the healthy respiratory system including airways, alveolar capillary diffusion surface, respiratory muscles, and the pulmonary vasculature, are generally viewed as adequate or even "overbuilt" to meet the requirements for ventilation and gas exchange demanded by maximum or sustained endurance exercise—at least in the untrained human. However, in the highly trained who undergo substantial adaptations in key determinants of maximal oxygen (O_2) transport such as red cell mass, total circulating blood volume and stroke volume, as well as locomotor muscle mitochondrial volume, and capillary density, there is little evidence that the lung architecture adapts to training-induced increases in demands for O_2 and carbon dioxide (CO_2) transport. Accordingly, as determined previously in significant numbers of highly trained young and older athletes of both sexes, different components of the respiratory system present significant limitations to systemic O_2 transport and exercise performance.[1] These limitations include inadequate oxygen exchange, expiratory flow limitation, high intra-thoracic pressure effects on left ventricular stroke volume, and extra-thoracic airway narrowing. In this brief essay we focus on recent work highlighting respiratory muscle afferents and the pulmonary circulation as additional potential respiratory system limitations to exercise performance, with emphasis on the effects of endurance exercise and training.

PULMONARY VASCULATURE ADAPTATION/MALADAPTATIONS TO EXERCISE
Characteristics/Responses of the Pulmonary Vasculature

The pulmonary vasculature has unique structural and functional characteristics distinct from the

Disclosure Statement: No disclosures.
Department Population Health Sciences, University of Wisconsin-Madison, 707 WARF Building, 610 N. Walnut Street, WI 53726, USA
E-mail address: JDempsey@wisc.edu

Clin Chest Med 40 (2019) 331–342
https://doi.org/10.1016/j.ccm.2019.02.002

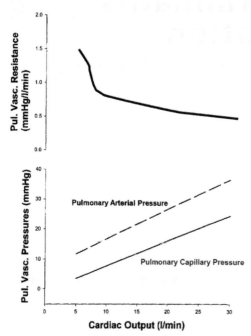

Fig. 1. Pulmonary artery and capillary pressures and pulmonary vascular resistance during steady-state exercise in untrained (up to 15–20 L/min cardiac output) and trained (>20 L/min CO) young adults. (*Data from* Reeves J, Grover RF, Dempsey JA. Pulmonary circulation during exercise. In: Weis E, Reeves J, editors. Pulmonary vascular physiology and pathology. New York: Dekker; 1989. p. 107–33.)

systemic circulation, which seems to make it ideal for an efficient response to exercise, that is, to accept the entirety of the increase in cardiac output (CO) without excessive increases in vascular pressures, which would overburden the right heart and interfere with adequate pulmonary gas exchange. Accordingly, the pulmonary vasculature is thin walled and highly compliant, thus, as pulmonary blood flow increases during exercise vessel caliber is largely "passively" controlled and subject to the pressures imposed by the systemic circulation on the left heart.[2–4] **Fig. 1A, B** shows the increases in pulmonary artery and capillary wedge pressures with increasing CO in healthy young adults. Note that at rest the pulmonary arterial pressures are about 1/20th of those of the systemic circulation, as is pulmonary vascular resistance. With mild intensity exercise pulmonary vascular resistance drops abruptly, likely because of recruitment of previously unperfused vessels in the lung apex. Thereafter, pulmonary capillary blood volume increases exclusively by vessel distention. In turn, vessel distention primarily occurs secondary to increases in left atrial pressure that are transmitted downstream across the pulmonary vascular tree.

Estimates of pulmonary vascular distensibility in vivo during exercise are identical to those obtained in vitro in isolated vessels,[2,5] demonstrating the almost purely passive, "mechanical" control of pulmonary vessel caliber during exercise. This highly compliant and recruitable vascular system bestows 2 major advantages on the exercise response. First, pulmonary capillary and arterial pressures increase at an average rate of about 1 mm Hg per liter increase in CO; thus, at 15 to 20 L max CO in an untrained subject pulmonary capillary pressures increase to about 15 to 20 mm Hg. Given these relatively small increases in capillary pressure combined with a huge capacity of the thoracic lymphatic drainage system, alveolar edema is avoided during exercise, despite an increase of fluid flux from pulmonary capillaries into the lung's interstitial fluid space. Secondly, this low-resistance system also insures adequate alveolar to arterial O_2 exchange with 2 types of adaptations to exercise.[3,6] First, as shown in **Fig. 2**, the pulmonary capillary blood volume expands up to about 2- to 2.5-fold resting levels at 20 L/min CO, thereby limiting the reduction in red cell transit time with an increasing CO and insuring equilibrium of end-pulmonary capillary blood with alveolar P_{O_2}. Secondly, the passively induced distensibility of the pulmonary vasculature with increasing CO seems to be independent of vessel diameter, thus distensibility would be similar across lung regions, ensuring a fairly homogeneous distribution of blood flow (Q) to match alveolar ventilation (V). These adaptations minimize the exercise-induced increased heterogeneity in V/Q distribution and constrains the associated 2- to 2.5-fold increase (>rest) in the alveolar to arterial P_{O_2} difference. Finally, overall V_A increases out of proportion to Q during exercise, ensuring relatively high alveolar and end-capillary P_{O_2} values throughout the lung.

The max dimensions, high compliance, and passively controlled distensibility of the healthy pulmonary vasculature ensure that exercise-induced increases in pulmonary artery and capillary pressures and decreases in red cell transit time throughout the lung are minimized, even up to about a 4-fold increase in cardiac output at max exercise in the untrained healthy adult.

An Underbuilt/Overloaded Pulmonary Vasculature in the Highly Trained?

The endurance-trained athlete with high peak work capacities and correspondingly high CO values, which can reach 35 to 40 L/min at $\dot{V}_{O_2}$ max and be sustained at 80% to 90% of these maximum

↑ VO2max, Cardiac Output in Highly Trained: Effects on Pulmonary Transit Time

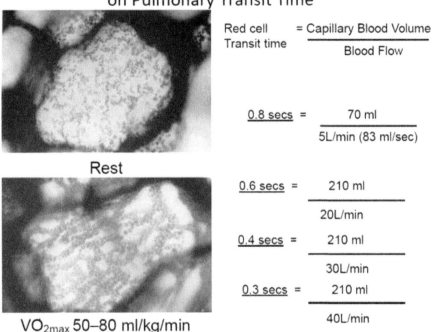

$$\text{Red cell Transit time} = \frac{\text{Capillary Blood Volume}}{\text{Blood Flow}}$$

Rest

$$\underline{0.8 \text{ secs}} = \frac{70 \text{ ml}}{5 \text{L/min (83 ml/sec)}}$$

VO_{2max} 50–80 ml/kg/min

$$\underline{0.6 \text{ secs}} = \frac{210 \text{ ml}}{20 \text{L/min}}$$

$$\underline{0.4 \text{ secs}} = \frac{210 \text{ ml}}{30 \text{L/min}}$$

$$\underline{0.3 \text{ secs}} = \frac{210 \text{ ml}}{40 \text{L/min}}$$

Fig. 2. Exercise-induced changes in pulmonary capillary blood volume, cardiac output, and mean red cell transit time in the lung in healthy young men—untrained (15–20 L/min max CO) and trained (>20 L/min max CO). The max pulmonary capillary blood volumes at max exercise were assumed to be 3× resting values and similar in trained and untrained. The micrographs show the expanded pulmonary capillary blood volume from rest to max exercise. (*Adapted from* Dempsey JA, Miller JD, Romer LM. The respiratory system. In: Tipton C, editor. ACSM Advanced exercise physiology. Philadelphia: Lippincott; 2006. p. 246–99.)

values for prolonged periods, presents specific challenges to the pulmonary circulation. A key difference in the pulmonary versus systemic circulation during exercise is that the latter has a huge reserve for vasodilation within the contracting limb muscles, which receive the major share of the increasing CO in exercise. On the other hand, the pulmonary circulation's reserve for vasodilation is markedly restricted. Accordingly, in heavy-exercise pulmonary vascular resistance is reduced only a small amount below that achieved in moderate intensity exercise (see **Fig. 1A**) and as CO exceeds 30 to 40 L/min pulmonary arterial pressures exceed 40 mm Hg reflecting the effect of the linear increase in blood flow on left atrial pressure, which in turn is transmitted across the pulmonary vasculature. Individual values reported in the study of endurance trained athletes revealed pulmonary arterial pressures in the 35–45 mmHg range coincident with cardiac outputs of 30 l/min.[7]

These elevated pressures present a highly disproportionate load and wall stress on the right ventricle, eliciting marked increases in myocardial O_2 extraction and $\dot{V}O_2$. So this load on the right ventricle at max exercise approximates that

imposed on the left ventricle; however, the load is a "disproportionate one" imposed on the relatively thin-walled right heart. La Gerche and colleagues[8–10] make the point that the human has a pulmonary vasculature that seems to be "adapted" for resting and mild to moderate intensity exercises, as indicated by the low (relative to systemic) pulmonary vascular resistance and capillary pressures under these conditions, but has not been adapted to handle the very high CO values demanded by the high work rates of the endurance-trained athlete. Given the similar slope of increases in pulmonary artery and wedge pressures per liter increase in CO in the trained and untrained, it seems that the athlete's pulmonary vascular distensibility during exercise has also undergone only limited, if any, positive adaptation to chronic physical training (also see later discussion).

Three types of potential short- and long-term maladaptations may result from the effects of high and sustained pulmonary blood flow on the right heart as a result of endurance training. First, whereas it is widely recognized that limitations of left heart stroke volume present a primary limitation to O_2 transport and $\dot{V}O_2$ max, it is worth recalling that right and left heart stoke volumes must be equalized during exercise and that "...the maximum obtainable stoke volume could only be as high as its weakest ventricle."[10] Given the disproportionately high load and wall stress placed on the right ventricle it has been reasoned –but not yet verified—that a major source of stroke volume and therefore CO limitation may well reside in the high work rates and fatigability of the right heart.

Secondly, pulmonary gas exchange and arterial hypoxemia during exercise occur in a significant number of male and female endurance-trained athletes,[1,6] owing primarily to an excessively widened alveolar to arterial O_2 difference. Given the limited expansion of the pulmonary capillary blood volume during exercise, it is conceivable—but not proven—that pulmonary blood flows in excess of 30 to 35 L/min would result in red cell transit times through at least some portions of the lung that are too short to ensure complete alveolar–end-capillary O_2 equilibrium (see **Fig. 2**).[11] Higher capillary pressures and blood flows will also increase lung interstitial fluid turnover and pressure, thereby contributing to V/Q inhomogeneity, and in some rare cases promote red cell movement into the alveolar space.[12]

Thirdly, the long-term effect of repeated bouts of intense endurance exercise results in slightly greater enlargement of the right-sided heart chamber verses the left side.[10,13] A minority of athletes with extremely high endurance training loads develop arrhythmias, and the origin of this arrhythmia is frequently associated with more pronounced remodeling and dysfunction of the right ventricle.[8] An interaction between excessive genetic abnormalities and cardiac structure has been proposed to be manifested in arrhythmogenic cardiomyopathy.

These effects of high pulmonary blood flows on vascular pressures are especially evident during exercise in elderly subjects and in sojourners to high altitude. With aging, starting as early as the third decade, pulmonary vascular compliance begins to decrease, combined with a similar age-dependent decrease in lung elastic recoil, that is, a stiffer pulmonary vasculature resides within a floppier lung. Accordingly Reeves analysis of in vivo distensibility shows significantly lower values in 70-year-olds versus young adult subjects during exercise.[2,4] Similarly, decreased distensibility was also reported for young adults exercising after a few weeks sojourn to high altitude, presumably because of reduced compliance secondary to hypoxic-induced pulmonary vasoconstriction. Thus, in highly trained athletes at advanced age or during high altitude sojourn it might be expected that even greater pulmonary vascular pressures and right ventricular wall stress will occur at even lower absolute workloads and CO values, as previously reported in younger athletes exercising at sea level (see above). In turn, it might also be expected—but not yet tested—that excessive right ventricular remodeling will occur over time with high-intensity training in both the elderly endurance athlete or those who habitually train at high altitudes. During triathlon-type swimming competitions, especially in cold water, elevated pulmonary artery pressures and even hemodynamic-induced pulmonary edema have been reported with increasing prevalence- even in otherwise healthy subjects. These excessive pulmonary vascular pressures have been attributed to central redistribution from the extremities and skin vasculature, which engorges the central veins, heart and lung.[14,15]

An increased slope of the pulmonary artery pressure:Q relationship during exercise will also occur with upstream transmission of high left atrial pressure and in the presence of increased intrathoracic pressure. Accordingly patients with left heart conditions and increased left atrial pressure or chronic obstructive pulmonary disease (COPD) patients who develop expiratory flow limitation, dynamic hyperinflation, and excessive intra-thoracic pressures during exercise will experience steeper slopes of pulmonary arterial presure vs CO.[16,7] In turn, in these patients the right heart will be subjected to excessive, disproportionate loads even during submaximal intensity exercise (see also Clinical and Physiological Implications of Negative Cardiopulmonary Interactions in Coexisting COPD-Heart Failure).

The endurance-trained athlete is capable of achieving and maintaining cardiac outputs in heavy-intensity exercise in excess of 30+ L/min, but pulmonary vasculature recruitment and reductions in vascular resistance are limited. Accordingly, excessive increases occur in pulmonary artery and capillary pressures, thereby placing a disproportionate load on the right heart and—over time—maladaptive ventricular hypertrophy commonly develops. Similar acute and long-term maladaptations may be present during submaximal intensity exercise in older subjects and those sojourning at high altitudes, as well as in patients with COPD and left heart failure conditions.

Finally, the thoroughbred horse epitomizes the ultimate "underbuilt" pulmonary vasculature, because this cursorial animal's lung must accommodate a 400 L/min plus CO during max exercise requiring 160 mL/kg/min plus Vo_2 (**Fig. 3**).[17] Thus, pulmonary arterial pressure exceeds 100 mm Hg

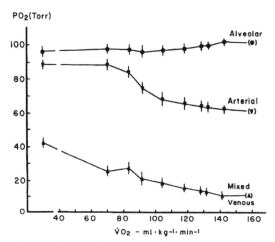
PO$_2$(Torr)

Fig. 3. Effects of incremental exercise (treadmill running) in the thoroughbred horse on alveolar, arterial, and mixed venous PO$_2$. Note the minimal increase in alveolar PO$_2$, the substantial, progressive widening of the alveolar to arterial PO$_2$ difference, and arterial hypoxemia throughout exercise, and the near maximal extraction of O$_2$ by the locomotor muscles. Other max exercise values include Paco$_2$ 50 to 55 mm Hg, arterial pH 7.15, Ppa 120 mm Hg, mixed venous Pco$_2$ 135 mm Hg. (*From* Bayly WM, Hodgson DR, Schulz DA, et al. Exercise-induced hypercapnia in the horse. J Appl Physiol (1985) 1989;67(5):1958–66.)

during heavy-intensity exercise, and excessive pulmonary capillary pressures cause alveolar capillary rupture and pulmonary hemorrhage. Over time, the thickness of the right ventricle approaches that of the left ventricle in the thoroughbred.[10] When these responses in the pulmonary vasculature are combined with evidence of severe arterial hypoxemia and CO$_2$ retention, beginning with even moderate intensity exercise (see **Fig. 3**), it is apparent that the lung and pulmonary vasculature are truly the primary limiting factors to O$_2$ transport and exercise performance in the thoroughbred horse. Furthermore, whereas exercise-induced arterial hypoxemia occurs in a minority of highly trained human athletes (at sea level),[6] it seems to be universal among thoroughbred horses. Indeed, preventing the exercise-induced hypoxemia in the thoroughbred (via supplemental O$_2$) increases Vo$_2$ max ~30% above normoxic room air breathing values.[6]

RESPIRATORY VERSUS LOCOMOTOR MUSCLE AFFERENTS, BLOOD FLOW DISTRIBUTION, AND FATIGUE: A 2-WAY STREET
Exercise-Induced Blood Flow Distribution and Muscle Fatigue

During exercise, an increasing CO is redistributed primarily to contracting skeletal muscle with the amount of blood flow determined by the net effect of 2 opposing mechanisms, namely vasodilation, primarily via release of local metabolites versus sympathetically mediated vasoconstriction. The vasodilation serves O$_2$ transport needs, while the opposing vasoconstriction serves to preserve perfusion pressures in the face of the skeletal muscles' prodigious capabilities for vasodilation if left unopposed.[18] In the following, we present evidence to support the concept that activation of metaboreceptor afferents from both limb locomotor and respiratory muscles are important sources of this exercise-induced sympathetic vasoconstrictor activity, and that they have reciprocal modulatory influences on blood flow distribution to each set of muscles, thereby contributing to each other's exercise-induced fatigue.[19]

Exercise-induced muscle fatigue is quantified objectively by determining the influence of exercise on force output of the muscle in response to supramaximal 1 to 20 Hz stimulation of the motor nerves—phrenic nerves for the diaphragm and femoral nerves for the quadriceps (further discussion in the topic is provided in Respiratory Muscle assessment in Clinical Practice and The Relevance of Limb Muscle Dysfunction In COPD: A Review for Clinicians). For both muscle sets, max force output is reduced significantly immediately following exhaustive endurance exercise at intensities in excess of 80% of max Vo$_2$ in trained and untrained subjects.[20,21] Diaphragm fatigue is first noted about halfway through the high-intensity exercise, is further exacerbated over time and usually, it takes an hour or more for complete recovery. Blood flow and O$_2$ transport are well known to be important determinants of both diaphragm and locomotor muscle fatigue.[21,22]

Muscle metabolite accumulation and fatigue limits performance in 2 ways: (1) by reducing the capability for maximum force output by the muscle, thereby forcing the athlete to work at higher relative intensities of exercise; and (2) by increasing sensory input from the fatiguing muscle supraspinally, which, in turn, will inhibit central locomotor output and "effort," ie, so-called central fatigue.[21] This dual effect of peripheral muscle fatigue of both central and peripheral components of exercise limitation are based on the demonstrated effects of partial blockade of locomotor muscle feedback using intrathecal administration of an opiate agonist. This blockade of muscle afferents promoted a greater central motor drive and force output during a cycling time trial by preventing the normal feedback inhibition of central motor drive. Thus, excessive levels of limb fatigue were achieved at end exercise with blockade than in the presence of muscle feedback and performance time was improved.[21]

Measurements of quadriceps blood flow in humans using thermal dilution techniques showed vascular conductance and flow increasing linearly with CO and plateauing between 90% and 100% of Vo_2 max.[18,23] In ponies exercising at maximum, microsphere measurements of blood flow to all the respiratory muscles averaged 15% to 20% of CO,[24] with similar values estimated in fit humans for respiratory muscle blood flow and the oxygen cost of breathing.[23,25]

Influence of Respiratory Muscle Work and Respiratory Muscle Afferents

Does the high work of breathing incurred during exercise influence blood flow to, and fatigue of, limb locomotor muscles? This question was addressed by a series of studies, all using a unique proportional assist mechanical ventilator in healthy fit young adults to unload the inspiratory muscles during exercise at 80% to 90% of Vo_2 max, which prevented 50% to 70% of the normal exercise-induced increase in respiratory muscle work. The effects of preventing this normally occurring increase in the work of breathing are summarized below and in **Fig. 4**.

- Diaphragm fatigue was prevented, demonstrating the critical importance of the work of the diaphragm during exercise to its own fatigue.[26] Based on these findings we assume that reducing the inspiratory muscle work and preventing their fatigue means that exercise-induced metaboreceptor activation in

inspiratory muscles was also significantly reduced (see later discussion).
- Blood flow and vascular conductance were increased in the working quadriceps muscle[23,27] and decreased in the accessory respiratory muscle, the sternocleidomastoid (**Fig. 5**).[27] These changes in blood flow and vascular conductance with respiratory muscle unloading (and loading) were accompanied by reciprocal changes in norepinephrine spillover across the quadriceps muscle during exercise—indicating changes in sympathetic efferent activity in the quadriceps vasculature.[23]
- Quadriceps muscle fatigue at end exercise—compared with control conditions at equal times and work rates—was reduced, exercise time to exhaustion was prolonged and exercise-induced perception of dyspnea and limb discomfort reduced.

We proposed that the reductions in limb fatigue with respiratory muscle unloading were because of the coincident 5% to 10% increase in limb blood flow and O_2 transport. In turn, we propose that peripheral muscle fatigue and accumulation of locomotor muscle metabolites affect endurance exercise performance by exacerbating both peripheral and central fatigue.[21]

These effects of reducing inspiratory muscle work during exercise and preventing respiratory muscle fatigue on reducing sympathetic vasoconstrictor outflow and increasing locomotor muscle vascular conductance and blood flow are likely

Unloading the Inspiratory Muscles at 85% $\dot{V}O_{2max}$

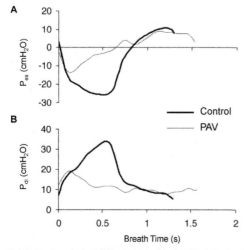

Reducing Diaphragmatic Work via Proportional Assist Mechanical Ventilation (PAV):

- Prevents exercise-induced diaphragm fatigue
- ↓ sympathetic tone, ↑ limb vascular conductance, and ↑ blood flow to limb locomotor muscles
- ↑ blood flow to accessory inspiratory muscles
- ↓ locomotor muscle fatigue
- ↓ perceived sensations of dyspnea and limb discomfort
- ↑ exercise duration to exhaustion

Fig. 4. Summary of effects of reducing the work of breathing during high-intensity exercise in healthy fit subjects (see text for details). The figure shows a typical effect of the proportional assist ventilator on reducing esophageal and transdiaphragmatic pressures during high-intensity exercise (see text for details). (*Adapted from* Sheel AW, Boushel RC, Dempsey JA. Competition for blood flow distribution between respiratory and locomotor muscles: implications for muscle fatigue. J Appl Physiol (1985) 2018;125(3):820–31.)

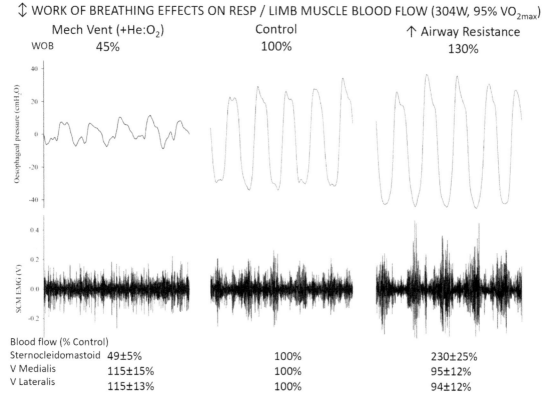

WORK OF BREATHING EFFECTS ON RESP / LIMB MUSCLE BLOOD FLOW (304W, 95% VO$_{2max}$)

	Mech Vent (+He:O$_2$)	Control	↑ Airway Resistance
WOB	45%	100%	130%

Blood flow (% Control)

	Mech Vent	Control	Airway Resistance
Sternocleidomastoid	49±5%	100%	230±25%
V Medialis	115±15%	100%	95±12%
V Lateralis	115±13%	100%	94±12%

Fig. 5. Summary of the effects of respiratory muscle loading and unloading on esophageal pressures, work of breathing (WOB, % of control), raw EMG of the sternoclidomastoid muscle (SCM). Relative changes in muscle blood flows were measured using the combination of iodocyanate dye infusion with near-infrared spectroscopy. (*Adapted from* Dominelli PB, Archiza B, Ramsook AH, et al. Effects of respiratory muscle work on respiratory and locomotor blood flow during exercise. Exp Physiol 2017;102(11):1535–47.)

mediated by the reduced activity of inspiratory muscle type III-IV metaboreceptors. The evidence supporting this postulate includes the following:

- Most fibers in the phrenic nerve are sensory in function and with supraspinal projections to medullary neurons involved in cardiorespiratory control.[28]
- Group IV metaboreceptors in the diaphragm are activated by fatiguing the diaphragm in the rodent.[28]
- Infusion of lactic acid into the phrenic nerve in the exercising dog causes vasoconstriction in the exercising limb and increased mean arterial pressure—effects that were prevented via sympathetic blockade.[29]

We propose that sympathetically mediated vasoconstriction invoked via the respiratory muscle metaboreflex during the course of fatiguing exercise is sufficiently robust to overcome a significant portion of the powerful local vasodilatory influence operative in near maximally contracting locomotor muscle, thereby contributing to limb fatigue and limiting exercise performance.

Influence of Locomotor Muscle Work and Locomotor Muscle Afferents

On the other hand, we need to emphasize that the work of the locomotor muscles also contributes significantly to sympathetically mediated vasoconstriction, blood flow limitation, and fatigue in the respiratory muscles during whole-body exercise. This "2-way street" of sympathetically mediated vasomotor influences between respiratory and limb locomotor muscle is illustrated in **Fig. 6**. The sympathetically mediated vasoconstrictor activity activated via locomotor muscle contraction occurs via group III-IV afferents, which enter the spinal cord through the dorsal roots and make their synapse in the dorsal horn of the gray matter. Babcock and colleagues[30] demonstrated the effect of locomotor muscle exercise on diaphragm fatigue by comparing the effects of high-intensity treadmill running versus a voluntarily produced work of breathing while at rest, which mimicked that during exercise in magnitude and duration (**Fig. 7**). In the resting subject, diaphragm fatigue was less consistent across subjects, substantially less in magnitude, and recovered much more

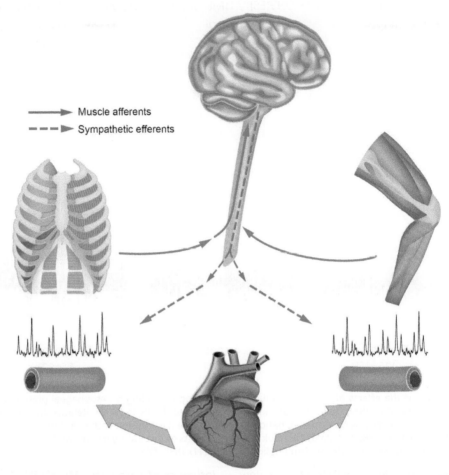

Fig. 6. Schematic illustrating the "2-way street" of muscle afferent reflexes between respiratory and locomotor muscles, which during exercise elicit sympathetically mediated vasoconstriction of the vasculature supplying both sets of muscles, thereby constraining their blood flow and hastening fatigue. (*From* Sheel AW, Boushel RC, Dempsey JA. Competition for blood flow distribution between respiratory and locomotor muscles: implications for muscle fatigue. J Appl Physiol (1985) 2018;125(3):820–31.)

quickly than that experienced as a result of whole-body exercise, that is, when both the limbs and the respiratory muscles were simultaneously active. These data likely reflect the critical influence of limited blood flow distribution to the diaphragm during coincidental limb locomotor muscle exercise, secondary to high levels of sympathetic vasoconstrictor activity emanating from locomotor muscle afferents, thereby contributing to diaphragmatic fatigue.

Just as sympathetically mediated vasoconstriction in the exercising limbs is in part modulated via afferents from the working respiratory muscles, so is vasoconstriction in the diaphragm, in part mediated via metaboreceptor afferent influences from the working limbs.

Prioritization of Blood Flow Distribution during Exercise/Clinical Implications

Is sympatholysis in the face of sympathetically driven vasoconstriction during exercise greater in the diaphragm (and other respiratory muscles) than in limb locomotor muscles … thereby providing a preferential distribution of the available CO to the diaphragm and respiratory muscles versus locomotor muscles? This complex question does not yet have a definitive answer, but there are some hints supporting the hypothesis, including some limited data from clinical investigations.

- A substantially blunted norepinephrine-induced vasoconstrictor response was reported in isolated vessels from the diaphragm versus those from the limb muscle vasculature.[31] This difference was not

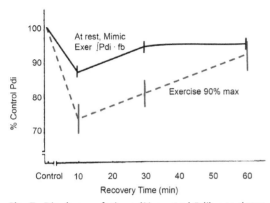

Fig. 7. Diaphragm fatigue (% control Pdi) was determined by supramaximal bilateral electrical stimulation of the phrenic nerves before and in recovery from exhaustive exercise versus before and in recovery from voluntary mimic of the exercise ∫Pdi · fb while at rest. The difference in diaphragm fatigue following whole-body exercise versus mimic of the exercise-induced ∫Pdi · fb while at rest reflects the effects of coincidental locomotor muscle exercise, per se. (*Data from* Babcock MA, Pegelow DF, McClaran SR, et al. Contribution of diaphragmatic power output to exercise-induced diaphragm fatigue. J Appl Physiol (1985) 1995;78(5):1710–19.)

explained by differences in either oxidative capacity or muscle fiber type. Presumably then if this observation held for in vivo conditions a heightened sympathetic nerve activity during exercise would be expected to preferentially affect vasoconstriction more in the limbs than in the diaphragm vasculature[a].

- Congestive heart failure (CHF) is accompanied by high levels of sympathetic nerve activity and also an elevated work of breathing during exercise, achieved via excessive hyperventilation and a reduced lung compliance (further discussion in the topic is provided in Pulmonary Limitations in Heart Failure and Clinical and Physiological Implications of Negative Cardiopulmonary Interactions in Coexisting COPD-Heart Failure). In rodent models of CHF blood flow throughout exercise was shown to be preferentially distributed to the diaphragm versus limb locomotor muscles.[32] In humans

with CHF, unloading the respiratory muscles even during very low intensity submaximal exercise elicited substantial increases in limb vascular conductance and blood flow[33]—similar to the effects previously seen in healthy subjects near maximum exercise.[23,34] Similarly, reducing the work of breathing with mechanical ventilation in COPD patients during mild intensity exercise at 50% of max prevented 25% to 30% of their exercise-induced limb fatigue.[35] That these patients still showed substantial limb fatigue at this mild exercise intensity despite a complete normalization of their work of breathing revealed the markedly compromised aerobic capacity of their locomotor musculature.[35,36]

- Specific training of the respiratory muscles in health and in CHF patients increased vasculature conductance and blood flow and reduced fatigue in exercising limbs.[37,38]
- In the maximum exercising equine, microsphere measures of blood flow distribution showed that maximum vasodilation was achieved in the diaphragm but not in the limb muscle vasculature.[24]

The clinical implications of this 2-way street of muscle metaboreflex effects in such chronic diseases as CHF and COPD pertain to exercise limitation and strategies for rehabilitation. Excessive metaboreflex activity affecting sympathetically mediated vasoconstriction from both the diaphragm and limb afferents during exercise may be expected in these patients because of the excessive work of breathing during exercise and because of the greatly limited aerobic capacity of locomotor muscles. Secondly, these excessive fatigue-producing influences from respiratory and limb muscle may be substantially modified by specific training of the respiratory musculature through resistive breathing treatment procedures, as well as through the use of a single leg extension exercise, which will enhance the aerobic capacity and reduce the fatigability of locomotor muscles—without requiring the dyspneic producing ventilatory response of 2-legged exercise.

---

[a]Although sympatholysis may be greater in the diaphragm versus locomotor muscle vasculature, endurance exercise at high intensity does induce diaphragm fatigue, suggesting that blood flow and O_2 transport to the diaphragm does not precisely match metabolic demand. To this point, although the sympathetically mediated vasoconstrictor response may be less in the diaphragm vasculature it still must occur to a significant extent.

Patients with COPD and CHF are especially suscep-tible to the influence of elevated levels of respiratory muscle work and the accompa-nying metaboreceptor-induced sympathetic acti-vation. Thus, even during low intensity exercise in these patients blood flow is redistributed prefer-entially to the respiratory muscles at the expense of locomotor muscle blood flow and fatigue.

SUMMARY: THE OVERBUILT AND UNDERBUILT RESPIRATORY SYSTEM DURING EXERCISE

The capacity of the lung diffusion surface area, airways, pulmonary vasculature, and respiratory muscle and the precision achieved by the neurochemical ventilatory control system are generally considered to be near-ideal to meet the ventilatory and gas exchange demands of exercise at sea level. Well-documented evidence in support of this generalization is to be found primarily in healthy untrained subjects, as follows:

- The precise control of alveolar ventilation with respect to CO_2 output (Vco_2) and the excess capacity to meet ventilation requirements within the maximum flow: volume envelope.
- The protection from diaphragm fatigue during short-term incremental exercise achieved through the high perfusion and high aerobic capacity of the diaphragm.
- The high compliance and low vascular resis-tance of the pulmonary vasculature minimize increases in pulmonary artery and capillary pressures during exercise.
- The increase in alveolar ventilation in excess of CO insures a high alveolar Po_2 throughout the lung, and an expanded pulmonary capillary blood volume minimizes reductions in red cell transit time as CO increases. These adap-tations ensure that arterial Po_2 is maintained in the face of an exercise-induced increase in V/Q inhomogeneity and a progressively widened alveolar to arterial Po_2 difference.

In our current essay we have focused on 2 sce-narios in which the respiratory system is not opti-mally built to meet the demands of exercise. First, we considered the scenario of respiratory system limitations in endurance-trained athletes whose extraordinary work capacity and accompanying high CO values are not matched by proportional ad-aptations in their pulmonary vasculature. Accord-ingly, during heavy-intensity exercise at high CO values, reductions in pulmonary vascular resistance are limited, excessive increases in pulmonary artery

and capillary pressures are common, as are marked reductions in red cell transit time—both potentially contributing to reduced stroke volume and impaired O_2 exchange. With high-intensity endurance training over time the occurrence of right ventricular remodeling is maladaptive.

Secondly, we considered the dual positive and negative influences of locomotor and respira-tory muscle metaboreflexes on blood flow distribu-tion and muscle fatigue. Activation of locomotor muscle metaboreflexes during moderate and heavy-intensity exercise contributes significantly to increased systemic O_2 transport via increased ventilation and CO and also to sympathetic vaso-constriction to maintain perfusion pressure. On the other hand, these metaboreflex effects also appear to constrain blood flow to the respiratory muscles and hasten diaphragm fatigue. Similarly, excessive sympathetic activation of metabore-flexes from the respiratory muscles during heavy-intensity exercise in normal trained and untrained subjects and even during mild exercise in CHF and COPD patients, or in healthy subjects exer-cising in hypoxia, seems to deprive locomotor mus-cles of optimal blood flow and promotes limb fatigue. Enhanced sympatholysis of respiratory muscle over locomotor muscle vasculature may prevail during exercise, allowing prioritization of blood flow distribution to respiratory muscles. This scenario of a 2-way street metaboreflex effect between locomotor and respiratory muscles occurs during heavy-intensity endurance exercise in trained and untrained healthy subjects and during submaximal exercise in patients with chronic heart and lung disease and in healthy subjects in hypoxia.

ACKNOWLEDGMENTS

The author thanks Anthony Jacques and Ben J. Dempsey for their excellent preparation of the article. The author also acknowledges the signifi-cant scientific contributions of many trainees and faculty colleagues in the Rankin Laboratory, which formed the basis for applying the concept of the respiratory muscle metaboreflex to exercising humans. Original work from the author's labora-tory supported by NHLBI and the American Heart Association.

REFERENCES

1. Dempsey JA, McKenzie DC, Haverkamp HC, et al. Update in the understanding of respiratory limita-tions to exercise performance in fit, active adults. Chest 2008;134(3):613–22.
2. Reeves JT, Linehan JH, Stenmark KR. Distensibility of the normal human lung circulation during

exercise. Am J Physiol Lung Cell Mol Physiol 2005; 288(3):L419–25.

3. Naeije R, Chesler N. Pulmonary circulation at exercise. Compr Physiol 2012;2(1):711–41.

4. Reeves J, Grover RF, Dempsey JA. Pulmonary circulation during exercise. In: Weis E, Reeves J, editors. Pulmonary vascular physiology and pathology. New York: Dekker; 1989. p. 107–33.

5. Lalande S, Yerly P, Faoro V, et al. Pulmonary vascular distensibility predicts aerobic capacity in healthy individuals. J Physiol 2012;590(17):4279–88.

6. Dempsey JA, Wagner PD. Exercise-induced arterial hypoxemia. J Appl Physiol (1985) 1999;87(6): 1997–2006.

7. Naeije R, Vanderpool R, Dhakal BP, et al. Exercise-induced pulmonary hypertension: physiological basis and methodological concerns. Am J Respir Crit Care Med 2013;187(6):576–83.

8. La Gerche A, Robberecht C, Kuiperi C, et al. Lower than expected desmosomal gene mutation prevalence in endurance athletes with complex ventricular arrhythmias of right ventricular origin. Heart 2010; 96(16):1268–74.

9. La Gerche A, Burns AT, Mooney DJ, et al. Exercise-induced right ventricular dysfunction and structural remodelling in endurance athletes. Eur Heart J 2012;33(8):998–1006.

10. La Gerche A, Rakhit DJ, Claessen G. Exercise and the right ventricle: a potential Achilles' heel. Cardiovasc Res 2017;113(12):1499–508.

11. Dempsey JA, Miller JD, Romer LM. The respiratory system. In: Tipton C, editor. ACSM "advanced exercise physiology". Philadelphia: Lippincott; 2006. p. 246–99.

12. Hopkins SR, Schoene RB, Henderson WR, et al. Intense exercise impairs the integrity of the pulmonary blood-gas barrier in elite athletes. Am J Respir Crit Care Med 1997;155(3):1090–4.

13. Aaron CP, Tandri H, Barr RG, et al. Physical activity and right ventricular structure and function. The MESA-Right Ventricle Study. Am J Respir Crit Care Med 2011;183(3):396–404.

14. Moon RE, Martina SD, Peacher DF, et al. Swimming-induced pulmonary edema: pathophysiology and risk reduction with sildenafil. Circulation 2016;133: 988–96.

15. Adir Y, Shupak A, Gil A, et al. Swimming-induced pulmonary edema: clinical presentation and serial lung function. Chest 2004;126:394–9.

16. Naeije R, Boerrigter BG. Pulmonary hypertension at exercise in COPD: does it matter? Eur Respir J 2013; 41(5):1002–4.

17. Bayly WM, Hodgson DR, Schulz DA, et al. Exercise-induced hypercapnia in the horse. J Appl Physiol (1985) 1989;67(5):1958–66.

18. Andersen P, Saltin B. Maximal perfusion of skeletal muscle in man. J Physiol 1985;366:233–49.

19. Sheel AW, Boushel RC, Dempsey JA. Competition for blood flow distribution between respiratory and locomotor muscles: implications for muscle fatigue. J Appl Physiol (1985) 2018;125(3):820–31.

20. Johnson BD, Babcock MA, Suman OE, et al. Exercise-induced diaphragmatic fatigue in healthy humans. J Physiol 1993;460:385–405.

21. Amann M, Dempsey JA. Locomotor muscle fatigue modifies central motor drive in healthy humans and imposes a limitation to exercise performance. J Physiol 2008;586(1):161–73.

22. Supinski G, DiMarco A, Ketai L, et al. Reversibility of diaphragm fatigue by mechanical hyperperfusion. Am Rev Respir Dis 1988;138(3):604–9.

23. Harms CA, Wetter TJ, McClaran SR, et al. Effects of respiratory muscle work on cardiac output and its distribution during maximal exercise. J Appl Physiol (1985) 1998;85(2):609–18.

24. Manohar M. Inspiratory and expiratory muscle perfusion in maximally exercised ponies. J Appl Physiol (1985) 1990;68(2):544–8.

25. Aaron EA, Seow KC, Johnson BD, et al. Oxygen cost of exercise hyperpnea: implications for performance. J Appl Physiol (1985) 1992;72(5): 1818–25.

26. Babcock MA, Pegelow DF, Harms CA, et al. Effects of respiratory muscle unloading on exercise-induced diaphragm fatigue. J Appl Physiol (1985) 2002;93(1):201–6.

27. Dominelli PB, Archiza B, Ramsook AH, et al. Effects of respiratory muscle work on respiratory and locomotor blood flow during exercise. Exp Physiol 2017;102(11):1535–47.

28. Nair J, Streeter KA, Turner SMF, et al. Anatomy and physiology of phrenic afferent neurons. J Neurophysiol 2017; 118(6):2975–90.

29. Rodman JR, Henderson KS, Smith CA, et al. Cardiovascular effects of the respiratory muscle metaboreflexes in dogs: rest and exercise. J Appl Physiol (1985) 2003;95(3):1159–69.

30. Babcock MA, Pegelow DF, McClaran SR, et al. Contribution of diaphragmatic power output to exercise-induced diaphragm fatigue. J Appl Physiol (1985) 1995;78(5):1710–9.

31. Aaker A, Laughlin MH. Diaphragm arterioles are less responsive to alpha1- adrenergic constriction than gastrocnemius arterioles. J Appl Physiol (1985) 2002;92(5):1808–16.

32. Smith JR, Hageman KS, Harms CA, et al. Effect of chronic heart failure in older rats on respiratory muscle and hindlimb blood flow during submaximal exercise. Respir Physiol Neurobiol 2017;243: 20–6.

33. Olson TP, Joyner MJ, Dietz NM, et al. Effects of respiratory muscle work on blood flow distribution during exercise in heart failure. J Physiol 2010;588(Pt 13):2487–501.

34. Dempsey JA, Romer L, Rodman J, et al. Consequences of exercise-induced respiratory muscle work. Respir Physiol Neurobiol 2006;151(2–3): 242–50.

35. Amann M, Regan MS, Kobitary M, et al. Impact of pulmonary system limitations on locomotor muscle fatigue in patients with COPD. Am J Physiol Regul Integr Comp Physiol 2010;299(1):R314–24.

36. Maltais F, LeBlanc P, Whittom F, et al. Oxidative enzyme activities of the vastus lateralis muscle and the functional status in patients with COPD. Thorax 2000;55(10):848–53.

37. McConnell AK, Lomax M. The influence of inspiratory muscle work history and specific inspiratory muscle training upon human limb muscle fatigue. J Physiol 2006;577(Pt 1):445–57.

38. Chiappa GR, Roseguini BT, Vieira PJ, et al. Inspiratory muscle training improves blood flow to resting and exercising limbs in patients with chronic heart failure. J Am Coll Cardiol 2008;51(17):1663–71.

The Pathophysiology of Dyspnea and Exercise Intolerance in Chronic Obstructive Pulmonary Disease

Denis E. O'Donnell, MD, FRCPI, FRCPC, FERS[a],*,
Matthew D. James, BSc[a], Kathryn M. Milne, MD, FRCPC[a,b],
J. Alberto Neder, MD, PhD, FRCPC, FERS[a]

KEYWORDS

• COPD • Dyspnea • Exercise physiology • Inspiratory neural drive • Respiratory mechanics

KEY POINTS

- Multiple studies endorse the proposal that dyspnea rises as inspiratory neural drive (IND) progressively increases in the face of an ever-decreasing capacity of the respiratory system to respond appropriately.
- Increased IND during exercise is primarily linked to mechanical, pulmonary gas exchange, and acid-base abnormalities that worsen as the disease advances.
- Therapeutic interventions such as supplementary oxygen, opiates, and exercise training have the potential to reduce IND but usually positively influence several other pathways relevant to dyspnea and exercise tolerance.
- Acute-on-chronic lung hyperinflation contributes to a rapid and shallow breathing pattern, increased velocity of shortening of the already disadvantaged inspiratory muscles compounding functional muscle weakness, decreased dynamic lung compliance, worsened pulmonary gas exchange (higher physiologic dead space), and possibly negative cardiopulmonary interactions.
- Therapies that reduce lung hyperinflation or counterbalance its negative effects on the inspiratory muscles are associated with reduced dyspnea and improved exercise tolerance.

In the last American Thoracic Society (ATS) statement, dyspnea was defined as "a subjective experience of breathing discomfort that consists of qualitatively distinct sensations that vary in intensity."[1] Dyspnea is the most common symptom in chronic obstructive pulmonary disease (COPD) and often becomes disabling in advanced stages of the disease.[2] Chronic dyspnea erodes perceived health status and diminishes engagement in physical activity, often leading to skeletal muscle deconditioning, anxiety, depression, and social isolation.[3,4] Effective management of dyspnea and exercise intolerance remains an elusive goal. However, a broader understanding of the pathophysiologic underpinnings of this distressing symptom has allowed us to formulate a sound rationale for individualized management. This review examines recent relevant research

Disclosures: Dr D.E. O'Donnell has received research funding via Queen's University from AstraZeneca, Boehringer Ingelheim, Canadian Institutes of Health Research (CIHR), and Canadian Respiratory Research Network (CRRN); and has served on speakers' bureaus, consultation panels, and advisory boards for AstraZeneca, Boehringer Ingelheim, GlaxoSmithKline, and Novartis. There are no conflicts of interest to declare in the publication of this article.
[a] Department of Medicine, Queen's University, Kingston Health Sciences Centre, 102 Stuart Street, Kingston, Ontario K7L 2V6, Canada; [b] Department of Medicine, Clinician Investigator Program, University of British Columbia, Vancouver, British Columbia, Canada
* Corresponding author. 102 Stuart Street, Kingston, Ontario K7L 2V6, Canada.
E-mail address: odonnell@queensu.ca

Clin Chest Med 40 (2019) 343–366
https://doi.org/10.1016/j.ccm.2019.02.007
0272-5231/19/© 2019 Elsevier Inc. All rights reserved.

and provides historical context. The overarching objectives are to consider current constructs of the physiologic mechanisms of activity-related dyspnea and identify specific targets that are amenable to therapeutic manipulation in patients with COPD.

MILESTONES IN DYSPNEA RESEARCH
Early Studies of Afferent and Efferent Signals in Dyspnea

Seminal physiologic studies from the late nineteenth and early twentieth centuries uncovered the anatomic substrate and neurosensory origins of respiratory sensation and pointed to the potential importance of central medullary centers and increased vagal afferent activation.[5,6] Hering and Breuer[5,6] described an inhibitory reflex in animals whereby inspiratory neural drive (IND) is suppressed and the next expiration is promoted by lung inflation: the deeper and faster the inspired breath, the greater the inhibition. The corollary was that interruption of full inspiration was associated with increased medullary respiratory center activity, which may provoke dyspnea. In this context, Wright and Branscomb[7] later suggested that dyspnea was associated with prolonged inspiratory center activation caused by inadequate vagal inhibition. However, in conscious adult humans the specific role of the Hering-Breuer reflex, and indeed of altered pulmonary vagal afferent activity in general, in the genesis of breathing discomfort during rest and exercise remains unknown.[8–10]

Increased reflex chemoreceptor stimulation has long been accorded a central role in the genesis of dyspnea. Haldane and Smith[11] originally demonstrated that a drop in arterial partial pressure of oxygen (Pao_2) by 6 to 8 mm Hg (or 12%), or an increase in partial pressure of carbon dioxide ($Paco_2$) by 1 to 2 mm Hg provoked unpleasant respiratory sensations in healthy humans. In elegant experiments, Fowler[12] in 1954 demonstrated that in healthy volunteers, respiratory distress that escalated at the breakpoint of breath-holding (as $Paco_2$ increased and Pao_2 decreased dramatically) was quickly relieved with resumption of deep inspiration. This relief occurred without correction of the arterial blood gas abnormalities and the attendant continuing and progressive central chemostimulation. Fowler provided the following explanation: "when obstructed breathing movements resume, the afferent pattern changes … the resulting motor activities are more appropriate to the prevailing level of stimulation at the respiratory center, and breathing is less distressing".[12] Subsequently, Flume and colleagues[13] confirmed the original findings of Fowler and postulated that dyspnea relief

coincided with activation of vagal pulmonary stretch receptors during inspiration, which inhibit activation of respiratory midbrain and cortical control centers. The potential role of other sensory mechanoreceptors in the respiratory muscles and chest wall that were also activated by inspiration was not determined. More recently, Gandevia and colleagues[14] showed that an increase in end-tidal CO_2 to 46 mm Hg following addition of CO_2 to the breathing circuit of mechanically ventilated and curarized healthy volunteers was sensed as severe breathing difficulty, even in the absence of activation of the respiratory muscles.

Despite the aforementioned intriguing discoveries, the precise contributions of altered chemical sensory inputs from peripheral and central chemoreceptors to exertional dyspnea, independent of vagal afferent input and respiratory muscle mechanoreceptor activation, have been difficult, if not impossible, to quantify with any precision. What is clear is that activated medullary centers can by themselves cause unpleasant respiratory sensations but that the intensity and quality of the overall sensory experience is profoundly influenced by simultaneous afferent inputs from a multitude of sensory receptors throughout the respiratory system. The study of dyspnea becomes even more challenging in patients with lung diseases during the stress of physical activity when dynamic respiratory mechanical and chemical perturbations are abruptly amplified and breathing discomfort can quickly escalate to intolerable levels. Despite these challenges, modern psychophysical studies, which consider the multidimensional components of dyspnea, have yielded important new mechanistic insights into causation.

> The relative contributions of altered chemical sensory inputs from peripheral and central chemoreceptors to exertional dyspnea, independent of vagal afferent input and respiratory muscle mechanoreceptor activation, have been difficult, if not impossible, to quantify with any precision.

Quantitative Dyspnea Measurement

One of the most important advances in dyspnea research has been the application of psychophysical principles to its measurement.[15–19] Many studies have now confirmed that respiratory sensation can be measured as accurately as other sensory phenomena (eg, light intensity, loudness, pain) using techniques such as sensory detection thresholds and open magnitude scaling during added standardized chemical and mechanical loading. Moreover, Stevens[15,16] showed that intensity of unpleasant respiratory sensation increases as a power function of the provocative stimulus. Influenced by his mentor, Tenney,[19] Borg[20–22] developed and validated a semiquantitative, category scale with ratio properties to measure dyspnea intensity during standardized stimuli such as external loading and exercise. Killian and coworkers[23–25] popularized use of the Borg scale during cardiopulmonary exercise testing in various patient populations and demonstrated its value in mechanistic studies of exertional dyspnea.

Theory of Length-Tension Inappropriateness

Using sensory detection methods for externally imposed mechanical loads, Campbell and colleagues[26] demonstrated that detection of briefly applied, small resistive and elastic mechanical loads in healthy participants required perception of a disparity in the relation of effort to tidal volume, rather than a change in the magnitude of the individual components, in absolute terms. Accordingly, these investigators advanced the theory of length-tension inappropriateness to account for the origin of altered respiratory sensation during these sensory detection studies. They proposed that muscle spindles, which are abundant in respiratory muscles (except the diaphragm), were ideally placed to sense disparities between tension (muscle force) and length (volume) during active muscle contraction, thus providing a proximate source of load detection. This theory, and its extrapolation to dyspnea perception in general, remains popular to this day but is difficult to test or verify in the clinical arena. Most would agree that the respiratory muscles are not the exclusive locus of sensory afferent inputs that modulate dyspnea during physical activity. Indeed, Campbell and Howell[27] later acknowledged that the conscious recognition of "inappropriateness" was pervasive and included the example of the disparity between the prevailing neurochemical demand and breathing achieved.

CURRENT NEUROPHYSIOLOGICAL CONSTRUCTS OF DYSPNEA CAUSATION
Efferent-Afferent Dissociation

Ultimately, respiratory muscle "tension-volume disparity" reflects imbalance between demand and capacity of the respiratory system. This imbalance represents a dissociation between efferent output from regulatory control centers in the brain and afferent inputs from the respiratory muscles and other anatomic structures disrupted by extrinsic or intrinsic (eg, lung diseases) mechanical loading. There is now general agreement that an abundance of sensory receptors in the airways, lung tissue, chest wall, and respiratory muscles can provide precise instantaneous feedback to the somatosensory cortex about the "real-time" dynamic state of the respiratory system. In this context, the popular construct of generalized efferent-afferent dissociation to explain the origins of dyspnea has been bolstered by several mechanistic studies in healthy volunteers.[7,28–33] These have shown that when the spontaneous increase in tidal volume (V_T) is constrained (either volitionally or by external imposition) in the face of increased (or constant) chemostimulation, unpleasant respiratory sensations are provoked (eg, "sense of air hunger" or "unsatisfied inspiration").

Central Corollary Discharge

Normally during spontaneous breathing, there is near perfect matching of IND from command centers in the brain (medulla and cortex), and simultaneous breath-by-breath afferent feedback from abundant sensory receptors throughout the respiratory system.[24,34] Based on animal studies, it is thought that information on the amplitude of motor command output from cortical and medullary centers in the brain is relayed to the somatosensory cortex via central corollary discharge or efferent copy.[34–36] Increased motor command output from cortical centers may be consciously perceived as increased respiratory effort. Simultaneously, diverse afferent inputs from throughout the respiratory apparatus are relayed to regulatory control centers in the brain and to the somatosensory cortex where respiratory sensation is perceived. The collective sensory information from both central (brain) and peripheral (respiratory apparatus) sources is centrally integrated, and any abnormal respiratory sensations are interpreted in the light of past experience and learning (further discussion in the topic is provided in Respiratory Muscle assessment in Clinical Practice).[34–36]

Affective Distress and Dyspnea

In healthy individuals, spontaneous breathing is unimpeded and neuromechanical harmony of the respiratory system is in place: there is normally no conscious awareness of tidal breathing in the absence of focused cognitive attention.[37] During combined chemical and mechanical loading experiments, neuromechanical disharmony (mismatching or dissociation) is introduced and the natural compensatory strategies to minimize breathing discomfort (eg, breathing pattern adjustments) often become insufficient to mitigate unpleasant respiratory sensation.[24,38–41] Beyond a certain threshold, breathing discomfort is consciously registered as a mortal threat or danger. The result is acute fear, anxiety, distress, and respiratory panic, which incidentally is a major component of dyspnea in patients with advanced cardiopulmonary disease.[29,42]

Of interest, recent studies using functional MRI (fMRI) of the brain have shown that when a dissociation between increased reflex chemical drive and the normal mechanical response of the respiratory system is experimentally introduced, there is increased activation of limbic and paralimbic centers in the brain which, together with sympathetic nervous system overactivation, are associated with distressing unpleasantness of breathing and "air hunger," a perceived urgent need to breathe.[42] The same areas of the brain are activated during the anticipation of dyspnea when assessed using fMRI.[43] The activation of these areas both in anticipation of dyspnea and during provoked dyspnea likely contribute to behavioral changes in patients with chronic lung disease that contribute to activity avoidance, further promoting deconditioning and frailty.

Another important development highlighted in the latest ATS statement[1] has been the recognition that measurement of dyspnea should ideally encompass: (1) sensory-perceptual experience (what breathing feels like in terms of intensity and quality); (2) affective distress (how distressing breathing feels) (**Fig. 1**)[44]; and (3) symptom impact or burden (how dyspnea affects function or health status). It is now apparent that in COPD certain therapeutic interventions can favorably affect some dimensions of dyspnea (eg, affective unpleasantness) while having little impact on others (eg, intensity), suggesting that intensity, quality, and affective domains of dyspnea have different pathophysiologic underpinnings.[45–48]

> Increased motor command output from cortical centers is relayed to the somatosensory cortex. Concurrently, multiple afferent inputs are transmitted to the somatosensory cortex where respiratory sensations are perceived. Collective sensory information is then centrally integrated and neuromechanical dissociation can produce profound breathing discomfort in patients with chronic lung disease.

EXERCISE AS THE DYSPNEA-PROVOKING STIMULUS
Exercise Studies in Healthy Subjects

It can be argued that psychophysical studies that use external mechanical and chemical loads to simulate pathologic dyspnea in healthy young volunteers poorly mimic perceived respiratory difficulty in patients. Nonetheless, this traditional methodologic approach has facilitated new

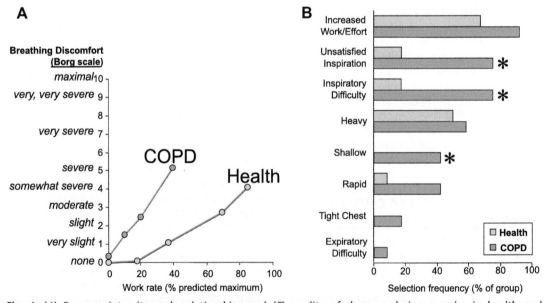

Fig. 1. (A) Dyspnea intensity-work relationships and (B) quality of dyspnea during exercise in health and disease. *P<.05, COPD versus health. (*Reprinted* with permission of the American Thoracic Society. Copyright © 2019 American Thoracic Society. O'Donnell DE, Hong H, Webb KA. Qualitative aspects of exertional breathlessness in chronic airflow limitation: pathophysiologic mechanisms. Am J Resp Crit Care Med 1997;155(1):109–15. The American Journal of Respiratory and Critical Care Medicine is an official journal of the American Thoracic Society.)

theories of causation that can formally be tested in patient populations. For example, the idea that neuromechanical dissociation (here used interchangeably with efferent-afferent dissociation) of the respiratory system is an important mechanism of dyspnea intensity was bolstered by a study in healthy volunteers during exercise under conditions of (in random order): (1) unloaded control (no intervention); (2) dead space (0.6 L) loading; (3) chest wall strapping (to reduce vital capacity to 60% of its baseline value); and (4) the combination of both mechanical and chemical loading (**Fig. 2**).[31] Compared with control, dead space loading was consistently associated with increased V_T and V_E but with minimal increase in dyspnea intensity during exercise. Chest wall strapping constrained the normal V_T response and had negative effects on dyspnea; however, combined chemical and mechanical loading amplified dyspnea intensity and exercise intolerance and introduced new distressing qualitative dimensions of dyspnea that alluded to inspiratory difficulty such as "unsatisfied inspiration." Incidentally, this latter descriptor ("can't get enough air in") has been reported as a commonly selected choice in both chronic restrictive and obstructive lung diseases[49,50] (see later discussion).

Exercise Studies in Chronic Obstructive Pulmonary Disease Patients

Since the late 1980s there has been considerable interest in both research and clinical settings of using standardized exercise tests as the provocative stimulus for dyspnea in patients with various cardiopulmonary diseases (see also Unraveling the Causes of Unexplained Dyspnea: The Value of Exercise Testing for illustrative cases). This approach encompasses measurement of dyspnea intensity (Borg scale) and quality[28,51,52] during and after bouts of exercise (treadmill or cycle ergometry), in conjunction with a panel of relevant physiologic variables (see **Fig. 1**; **Fig. 3**). The Borg scale

has now been validated in large multinational clinical trials and is both reproducible and responsive to interventions.[53] Common physiologic variables that are measured during exercise include: ventilatory output, breathing pattern, operating lung volumes, pulmonary gas exchange, dynamic respiratory mechanics (esophageal manometry), and IND to the diaphragm (electromyography). Associations between dyspnea intensity and independent physiologic variables are identified by correlative analysis, and their validity and strength are subsequently tested by selective manipulations of the independent variables. Therapeutic interventions known to alleviate exertional dyspnea in patients with lung disease provide another unique opportunity to identify the main physiologic mechanisms contributing to dyspnea. Placebo-controlled, double-blind, crossover trials using constant work-rate endurance tests to provoke dyspnea permit rigorous evaluation of clinical efficacy in the form of dyspnea relief of various treatments as well as the underlying mechanisms of benefit.[54]

DEMAND/CAPACITY IMBALANCE DURING EXERCISE

Quoting the renowned Canadian physiologist, Norman Jones,[55] "breathlessness can be seen to result from the imbalance between the demand for breathing and the ability to achieve the demand." As gathered from the preceding sections, this central idea of "imbalance," "inappropriateness," or "dissociation" is pervasive across the scientific literature on dyspnea. Indeed, support for the demand/capacity imbalance theory of dyspnea during physical activity in COPD has come from numerous studies that show strong statistical correlations between the increase in dyspnea intensity during exercise and increase in each of the following physiologic ratios: ventilation/maximal ventilatory capacity (V_E/MVC)[56,57]; tidal esophageal pressure/maximal inspiratory pressure

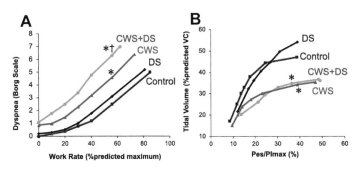

Fig. 2. Dyspnea intensity (A) and tidal volume to Pes/Pimax ratio (B) during control, dead space loading of 0.6 L (DS), chest wall strapping to 60% of control VC (CWS), and a combination of dead space loading and chest wall strapping (CWS + DS). *$P<.05$, intervention versus control at HEWR; †$P<.05$, CWS + DS versus CWS alone at HEWR. CWS, chest wall strapping; DS, dead space; HEWR, highest equivalent work rate; Pes, esophageal pressure; Pimax, maximum inspiratory pressure; VC, vital capacity. (*Adapted from* O'Donnell DE, Hong HH, Webb KA. Respiratory sensation during chest wall restriction and dead space loading in exercising men. J Appl Physiol 2000;88(5):1859–69.)

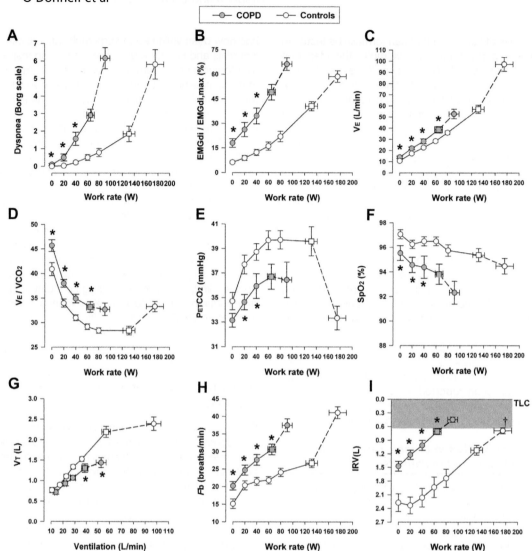

Fig. 3. Dyspnea intensity (Borg units) (*A*), diaphragm electromyography (EMGdi) (*B*), and selected ventilatory and indirect gas exchange responses (*C–I*) to incremental cycle exercise test in patients with moderate COPD and age-matched healthy controls. Values are mean ± SEM. Square symbols represent tidal volume-ventilation inflection points. *$P < .04$ for CODP versus control subjects at rest, at standardized work rates, at peak exercise, at tidal volume-ventilation infection point. COPD, chronic obstructive pulmonary disease; EMGdi/EMGdi,max, index of inspiratory neural drive to the crural diaphragm; Fb, breathing frequency; IRV, inspiratory reserve volume; P_{ETCO_2}, partial pressure of end-tidal carbon dioxide; SEM, standard error of the mean; Sp_{O_2}, oxygen saturation by pulse oximetry; TLC, total lung capacity; V_E, minute ventilation; V_E/V_{CO_2}, ventilatory equivalent for carbon dioxide; V_T, tidal volume. (*Reprinted* with permission of the American Thoracic Society. Copyright © 2019 American Thoracic Society. Faisal A, Alghamdi B, Ciavaglia CE, et al. Common mechanisms of dyspnea in chronic interstitial and obstructive lung disorders. Am J Respir Crit Care Med 2016;193(3):299–309. The American Journal of Respiratory and Critical Care Medicine is an official journal of the American Thoracic Society.)

(Pes/MIP)[24,58]; tidal volume/inspiratory capacity (V_T/IC)[59–61]; and IND to the diaphragm/maximal voluntary diaphragmatic activation (EMGdi/EMGdi,max).[62,63] In other words, exertional dyspnea intensifies as respiratory effort reaches its maximal possible value as mechanical constraints on tidal volume critically worsen and inspiratory reserve volume (IRV) disappears, and as diaphragmatic activation approaches its maximum.

Fundamentally, multiple psychophysical studies in healthy volunteers and various patient populations endorse the proposal that dyspnea worsens as IND (from bulbopontine and cortical motor centers in the brain) progressively increases in the face of an ever-reducing capacity of the respiratory system to respond appropriately, because of excessive mechanical loading and functional weakness of the respiratory muscles.

Increased Ventilatory Demand in Healthy Subjects

At the onset of exercise, a central motor command feedforward stimulus from the motor cortex and midbrain ensures simultaneous coordinated activation of locomotor and respiratory muscles.[36,64–69] Although central cortical motor command is thought to be the primary stimulus for exercise hyperpnea, the ventilatory response is further optimized in each individual to meet the prevailing metabolic demand by alterations in respiratory CO_2 exchange and afferent feedback from the active locomotor muscles (ergoreceptors).[70–73]

In the healthy human the respiratory system is admirably designed to maintain arterial blood gas homeostasis and acid-base balance in the face of the rapidly increasing energy demands of exercise.[74–78] Moreover, several physiologic adaptations (eg, reduced upper and lower airways resistance, precise regulation of end-expiratory lung volume [EELV], and improved pulmonary gas exchange and ventilation/perfusion matching) ensure minimal increases in the work of breathing and result in successful attenuation of respiratory discomfort as V_E progressively increases (as illustrated in Case # 1 in Unraveling the Causes of Unexplained Dyspnea: The Value of Exercise Testing, however, high ventilatory demands associated with obesity may lead to dyspnea in a subject without underlying cardio-respiratory disease).[31,37,79,80] In healthy aging, respiratory mechanics and gas exchange function of the lungs measurably decline, and these important adaptations to minimize work of breathing are undermined to a variable degree. In many individuals, significant ventilatory constraints and dyspnea are seen during high-intensity exercise, particularly in athletic seniors (compared with healthy young adults) who can undertake strenuous exercise at or beyond predicted peak V_{O_2}.[74,76,81,82]

Increased Ventilatory Demand in Chronic Obstructive Pulmonary Disease Patients

COPD disproportionately affects the elderly population. It is now clear that in older individuals with even mild COPD, the aforementioned natural erosion on ventilatory reserve with aging becomes more pronounced: the aging process seems accelerated. This deterioration reflects the pathophysiologic effects of heterogeneous inflammatory changes in the small airways and lung parenchyma and its vasculature.[46,83–85] Thus, superimposed chemical and mechanical perturbations resulting from the injurious effects of tobacco smoke necessitate further compensatory increases in IND to maintain acid-base homeostasis. Unfortunately, this required increase in IND and V_E has negative sensory consequences.[46,49,82,86–89]

The causes of increased IND during exercise in COPD are well established and include chemical and mechanical factors (**Box 1**). In clinical settings where dyspnea becomes problematic, such as during physical activity, IND to the respiratory muscles is invariably increased.[49,62,63,89,90] This increased motor command output is difficult to quantify, and indirect estimates derived from measurement of overall ventilatory output or respiratory muscular effort (Pes/MIP) can result in significant underestimation of IND amplitude. Thus, concomitant limiting mechanical constraint attenuates an increase in ventilation and intrathoracic esophageal pressure (Pes) excursions. The development of diaphragm electromyography (using an esophageal catheter with multiple paired electrodes) has allowed for the measurement of IND to the crural diaphragm, representing a significant advance in the study of dyspnea.[62,63,91–93] During cycle ergometry, diaphragm activation, relative to the value obtained during maximal volitional effort to total lung capacity (TLC) (EMGdi/EMGdi,max), is increased at rest and at any V_{O_2} and V_E throughout exercise.[49,89,90] Of course, the slope of diaphragmatic activation versus work rate becomes steeper as the mechanical and pulmonary gas exchange abnormalities progress (**Fig. 4**).[49,89,90]

Remarkably, the strong association between dyspnea intensity and IND seems to be consistent in health and various lung diseases. For example, the EMGdi/EMGdi,max dyspnea slope is similar in health, COPD, and interstitial lung disease (ILD) despite marked intergroup differences in

---

Box 1
Mechanisms of increased inspiratory neural drive to the diaphragm

1. Increased V_{CO_2}:
   - Increased physiologic dead space
   - Early metabolic acidosis
   - Increased work of breathing
2. Critical arterial O_2 desaturation
3. Increased respiratory muscle loading/weakness
4. Increased ergoreceptor activation
5. Increased sympathetic system activation
6. Altered cardiovascular afferent activity

Abbreviations: O_2, oxygen; V_{CO_2}, carbon dioxide production.

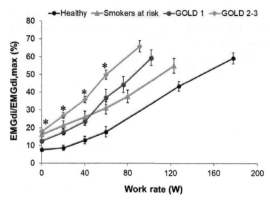

Fig. 4. Inspiratory neural drive during exercise represented by diaphragmatic activation as a percentage of maximal diaphragmatic activation (EMGdi/EMGdi,-max%). Values are means ± SEM. *P<.05, significantly different from healthy controls at a given work rate. EMGdi/EMGdi,max, index of inspiratory neural drive to the crural diaphragm; GOLD, Global Initiative for Chronic Obstructive Lung Disease; SEM, standard error of the mean. (*Data from* Refs.[49,89,90])

relationship between dyspnea intensity and IND is constant across health and lung diseases despite vast intergroup differences in the source and nature of afferent inputs to the brain from an abundance of sensory receptors. Additional evidence of the strength and consistency of the relationship between IND and dyspnea intensity during exercise comes from a study in COPD and mild obesity, tested during cycle and treadmill exercise, and matched for rate of increase in work rate.[94] Despite marked differences in respiratory muscle recruitment patterns, reflecting differences in exercise modality and body position, the close relationship between dyspnea intensity and IND was unaltered within these patients.[94] Collectively, these studies highlight the fact that efforts to alleviate activity-related dyspnea in individuals with COPD must consider the underlying mechanisms of increased IND.

lung compliance, breathing pattern, operating lung volumes, recruitment pattern of respiratory muscle activation, and pulmonary gas exchange abnormalities (**Fig. 5**).[49] This finding suggests that the

> Exertional dyspnea increases as IND progressively increases in the face of an ever-reducing capacity of the respiratory system to respond appropriately.

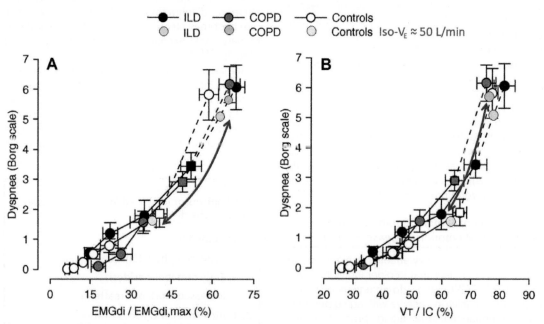

Fig. 5. Exertional dyspnea intensity during incremental cycle exercise in patients with ILD, patients with COPD, and age-matched healthy control subjects. Exertional dyspnea intensity is presented relative to (*A*) indirect measure of inspiratory neural drive (EMGdi/EMGdi,max), and (*B*) V_T/inspiratory capacity (V_T/IC; %). Values are mean ± SEM. Squares represent V_T-ventilation inflection points. COPD, chronic obstructive pulmonary disease; EMGdi/EMGdi,max, index of inspiratory neural drive to the crural diaphragm; IC, inspiratory capacity; ILD, interstitial lung disease; SEM, standard error of the mean; V_T, tidal volume. (*Reprinted* with permission of the American Thoracic Society. Copyright © 2019 American Thoracic Society. Faisal A, Alghamdi B, Ciavaglia CE, et al. Common mechanisms of dyspnea in chronic interstitial and obstructive lung disorders. Am J Respir Crit Care Med 2016;193(3):299–309. The American Journal of Respiratory and Critical Care Medicine is an official journal of the American Thoracic Society.)

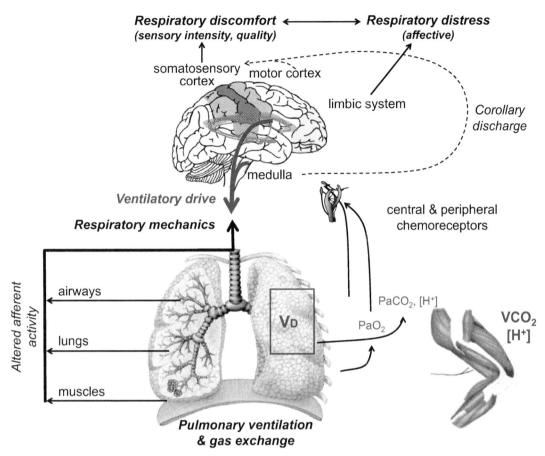

Fig. 6. A neurobiological model of dyspnea in COPD (refer to text for more detail). The somatosensory cortex calibrates and interprets the appropriateness of the mechanical/muscular response of the respiratory system to the prevailing central respiratory motor drive. When the mechanical/muscular response of the respiratory system is constrained below the level dictated or preprogrammed by central respiratory motor drive, the intensity of "respiratory discomfort" (ie, the sense of *unsatisfied inspiration*) increases in proportion to the widening disparity between drive and mechanics; that is, neuromechanical dissociation. Increased activation of limbic structures as a result of neuromechanical dissociation also likely contributes to "respiratory distress." Neural inputs that reach the somatosensory cortex and contribute to dyspnea come from: (1) increased central corollary discharge from brainstem and cortical motor centers; (2) altered afferent information from receptors in the airways (pulmonary stretch receptors, C-fibers), lungs (pulmonary stretch receptors, C-fibers, J-receptors), and from peripheral locomotor and respiratory muscles (muscle spindles, Golgi tendon organs, type III and IV afferents); and (3) feedback from central and peripheral chemoreceptors regarding adequacy of pulmonary ventilation and gas exchange. COPD, chronic obstructive pulmonary disease; [H$^+$], hydrogen ion concentration; Paco$_2$, partial pressure of arterial carbon dioxide; Pao$_2$, partial pressure of arterial oxygen, Vco$_2$, carbon dioxide production. (*Adapted from* O'Donnell DE, Ora J, Webb KA, et al. Mechanisms of activity-related dyspnea in pulmonary diseases. Respir Physiol Neurobiol 2009;167(1):116–32.)

MECHANISMS OF INCREASED INSPIRATORY NEURAL DRIVE IN CHRONIC OBSTRUCTIVE PULMONARY DISEASE
Increased Metabolic and "Pulmonary" Carbon Dioxide Output

In both health and COPD, IND increases as carbon dioxide output (Vco$_2$) increases, reflecting increased metabolic rate during exercise (**Fig. 6**).[95] Exercise hyperpnea is always closely linked to pulmonary CO$_2$ gas exchange. Tobacco-related injury of the lung microvasculature and resultant pulmonary gas exchange abnormalities occur across the severity spectrum of COPD.[46,96] Recent imaging techniques such as MRI using gadolinium have confirmed reduced pulmonary blood flow even in smokers with mild COPD.[97] The extensive vascular attenuation of destructive emphysema is well known, but the physiologic effects and sensory consequences of smaller reductions in perfusion in mild COPD (often with minimal emphysema) may be underestimated. Across the continuum of COPD severity, the ventilatory equivalent for CO_2 (V_E/V_{CO_2}), which is a measure of ventilatory efficiency, is elevated and indicates reduced efficiency compared with healthy controls (see **Fig. 3**D).[96] This observation is accounted for mainly by increased physiologic dead space to V_T ratio (V_D/V_T), reflecting wasted ventilation and the presence of alveolar units with high ventilation/perfusion ratios that do not participate in gas exchange (see also Incorporating Lung Diffusing Capacity for Carbon Monoxide to Clinical Decision Making in Chest Medicine). In mild COPD during exercise, physiologic dead space, V_E/V_{CO_2}, and V_A/V_{CO_2} are elevated compared with healthy controls[46]; this helps to maintain (or actually increase) arterial O_2 hemoglobin saturation during exercise. However, the high V_E in the setting of expiratory flow limitation (EFL) leads to worsening dynamic mechanics at relatively low V_E (see below) (An illustrative case (# 3) is also provided in Unraveling the Causes of Unexplained Dyspnea: The Value of Exercise Testing).[46,82,87] With advancing COPD, the amount of wasted ventilation increases and is particularly marked in the presence of extensive emphysema, and amplified further by characteristic tachypnea and shallow breathing pattern (see **Fig. 3**G–I). In this circumstance the V_E/V_{CO_2} slope may underestimate the size of the true physiologic dead space because of the effects of coexisting critical mechanical constraints on further increasing ventilation. In such individuals the V_E/V_{CO_2} nadir during incremental cardiopulmonary exercise testing is likely more relevant as a crude estimation of the V_D/V_T ratio than the slope per se, but this needs further experimental verification.[96]

Metabolic Acidosis

In COPD, skeletal muscle deconditioning resulting from reduced physical activity is very common, resulting in greater reliance on anaerobic glycolysis and early development of metabolic acidosis (low anaerobic threshold) at relatively low work rates, which is an additional powerful stimulus to increase V_E (further discussion in the topic is provided in The Relevance of Limb Muscle Dysfunction In COPD: A Review for Clinicians).[98–101] In some individuals with more advanced COPD, an altered respiratory exchange ratio (from excessive use of carbohydrate as an energy substrate) and increased work and O_2 cost of breathing (attributable to excessive mechanical loading) may additionally stimulate IND.[102] Arterial hypoxemia (usually <60 mm Hg) resulting from the presence of lung units with low

ventilation/perfusion ratios in the setting of low mixed venous O_2 saturation will stimulate peripheral chemoreceptor activation (intimately integrated with central chemoreceptor activation) and further increase IND as exercise progresses.[103–106] The degree of ventilatory stimulation by arterial hypoxemia during exercise will depend on the individual sensitivity of carotid chemoreceptors and will vary with concomitant arterial Pa_{CO_2}.

Altered Arterial Carbon Dioxide Set Point

The rate of elevation of IND during exercise is also strongly influenced by the regulated level of arterial CO_2 or CO_2 set point. The respiratory system adjusts to maintain Pa_{CO_2} within a narrow range during rest and exercise: the lower the set point, the higher the IND and V_E during exercise.[106,107] This phenomenon is exemplified in COPD patients with coexistent cardiovascular disease, in whom the CO_2 set point may be lower (because of chemohypersensitization and excess sympathetic system excitation) with subsequent high ventilatory demands and alveolar hyperventilation (further discussion in the topic is provided in Update on Chemoreception: Influence on Cardiorespiratory Regulation and Patho-Physiology).[108,109] In a recent study in COPD patients with coexistent congestive heart failure (CHF), Rocha and colleagues[108] confirmed a lower resting end-tidal CO_2 and high V_E/V_{CO_2} nadir in patients with COPD and CHF compared with COPD alone, suggesting an additional source of stimulation of IND. Interestingly this low CO_2 set point amplified respiratory mechanical abnormalities of COPD (ie, increased pulmonary gas trapping) and in this way provoked earlier onset of intolerable dyspnea and premature exercise termination (see also Clinical and Physiological Implications of Negative Cardiopulmonary Interactions in Coexisting COPD-Heart Failure).

Excessive Ergoreceptor Activation

Exercise hyperpnea is also influenced by ascending sensory inputs from thinly myelinated afferents in the active locomotor muscles (further discussion in the topic is provided in Respiratory Determinants of Exercise Limitation: Focus on Phrenic Afferents and The Lung Vasculature).[105] These afferents (metaboreceptors and ergoreceptors) are activated by mechanical distortion and pulmonary and metabolic CO_2 output during exercise and stimulate ventilation via ascending spinal pathways directly relayed to the central respiratory control center in the medulla. In COPD, Gagnon and colleagues[110] have shown that intrathecal fentanyl blockade of these ascending afferents reduced breathing frequency and lowered V_E/V_{CO_2} with corresponding delay in onset of limiting mechanical constraints and intolerable dyspnea.

IND on exertion in COPD is expected to increase as follows: (a) the higher the CO_2 production; (b) the larger the physiologic dead space; (c) the lower the level at which CO_2 is centrally regulated; (d) the higher the afferent stimuli from metabolic (eg, lactic acidosis) and neural (eg, ergoreceptors) sources.

THERAPEUTIC MANIPULATION OF INSPIRATORY NEURAL DRIVE TO REDUCE EXERTIONAL DYSPNEA IN CHRONIC OBSTRUCTIVE PULMONARY DISEASE

To the extent that increased IND is strongly linked to dyspnea intensity during exercise in COPD, therapeutic interventions that reduce IND (without compromising alveolar ventilation) should relieve dyspnea and exercise intolerance. However, few if any interventions selectively inhibit IND in isolation. For example, opiates, O_2 supplementation, and delayed metabolic acidosis from exercise training can all potentially reduce IND. However, these interventions may also influence central processing of dyspnea and its affective component through other mechanisms. Reduction in IND, which usually manifests as reduction in breathing frequency, has favorable downstream effects on dynamic respiratory mechanics (eg, reduced pulmonary gas trapping[106,111]). It has become clear that reduction of IND is not obligatory for dyspnea amelioration in all cases: improved muscular/mechanical responses of the respiratory system for a given IND can favorably influence intensity and qualitative domains of dyspnea by partially restoring more harmonious neuromuscular coupling.[112]

As discussed earlier, reduced ventilatory efficiency is an important source of increased IND and exertional dyspnea in COPD. Physiologic dead space is high at rest and does not decline normally during exercise. Unfortunately, high physiologic dead space is virtually immutable in COPD especially when it represents the destruction of the pulmonary vascular bed. First-line dyspnea-relieving therapies such as bronchodilators, which reduce regional lung hyperinflation and improve breathing pattern and cardiovascular function, result in only small increases in alveolar ventilation with essentially no change in dead

space ventilation.[112] Unfortunately, pharmacotherapy cannot effectively reduce the chemostimulation accorded to high physiologic dead space to a degree that will alleviate exertional dyspnea in COPD. Lung volume reduction surgery has demonstrated a significant improvement in exercise capacity (peak V_{O_2}) and a nonsignificant trend toward a decrease in V_D/V_T following surgery in highly selected COPD patients,[113] and may represent an avenue to improving ventilatory efficiency in this population.

Supplemental Oxygen

The effects of supplemental O_2 on dyspnea during activity in COPD is variable and difficult to predict because many patients remain breathless despite ensuring that Pa_{O_2} levels are within the normal range. Thus, residual sources of increased IND and dyspnea not amenable to O_2 still persist, such as severely impaired respiratory mechanics and altered muscle function necessitating high motor command output. Hyperoxia directly inhibits carotid chemoreceptor stimulation of V_E during exercise (at oxygen flow rates of approximately 3–6 L/min) mainly by reducing breathing frequency (Bf). In addition, improved O_2 delivery to the active locomotor muscles delays lactate accumulation and further contributes to reduced IND during exercise (Fig. 7). The effects of O_2 on IND and V_E are more pronounced in patients with significant baseline arterial hypoxemia; however, those with milder arterial O_2 desaturation during exercise can also benefit.[104,114–116] Other established benefits of supplemental O_2 include: reduced pulmonary gas trapping secondary to reduced Bf; alterations in cognitive function and in central processing of dyspneogenic signals; improved cardiovascular function (eg, reduced pulmonary artery pressure); delayed skeletal muscle fatigue; and altered sensory inputs from ergoreceptors.[105] The relative contribution of these physiologic variables to dyspnea relief will vary across individuals (further discussion in the topic is provided in Physiologic Effects of O_2 Supplementation during Exercise in Chronic Obstructive Pulmonary Disease).

Opiates

There is evidence that elaboration of endogenous opiates can ameliorate unpleasant respiratory sensation during mechanical loading or the stress of exercise in patients with COPD.[117–120] Opiate therapy is widely used for the management of refractory dyspnea in COPD, but the mechanisms of benefit are still unclear. Overt respiratory depression is a well-recognized complication of

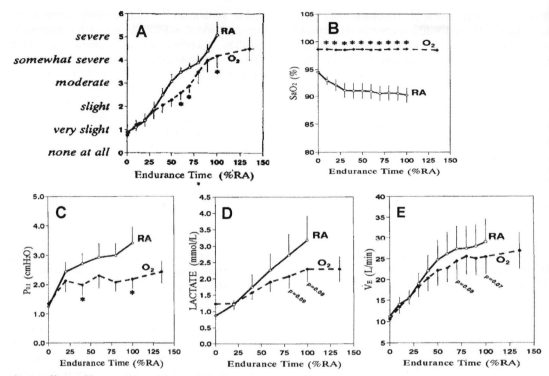

Fig. 7. Effects of hyperoxia on (*A*) breathlessness, (*B*) oxygen saturation, (*C*) P0.1 score, (*D*) lactate, and (*E*) ventilation during exercise compared with room air. *$P<.05$, reduction in slopes with 50% oxygen versus room air. P0.1, occluded airway pressure in first 100 milliseconds of inspiration; Sao_2, oxygen saturation; V_E, minute ventilation. (*Reprinted* with permission of the American Thoracic Society. Copyright © 2019 American Thoracic Society. O'Donnell DE, Bain DJ, Webb KA. Factors contributing to relief of exertional breathlessness during hyperoxia in chronic airflow limitation. Am J Respir Crit Care Med 1997;155(2):530–5. The American Journal of Respiratory and Critical Care Medicine is an official journal of the American Thoracic Society.)

opioid therapy in susceptible older patients with more advanced COPD, and recent epidemiologic studies have raised concerns about the overuse of these medications and increased mortality risk.[121–123] For patients with advanced refractory dyspnea, episodes of severe breakthrough dyspnea are particularly distressing, and administration of fast-acting opiates offers one possible solution. However, recent mechanistic studies on the effects of fast-acting inhaled or oral opiates on dyspnea and exercise tolerance in symptomatic patients with COPD have shown variable responses.[124–127] Abdallah and colleagues[45] have recently shown that a single dose of fast-acting, oral morphine in dyspneic patients with COPD was associated with improvements in dyspnea (intensity and unpleasantness) and exercise tolerance but with considerable variation in response between subjects. Of interest, this subjective improvement occurred in the absence of significant decreases in IND (EMGdi/EMGdi,max) and with only minor reductions in Bf and V_E. The investigators speculated that opiates may alter the central processing of sensory signaling related to

dyspnea and may address the affective dimension by reducing activity in corticolimbic centers by blockade of abundant opioid receptors in these brain regions.

Exercise Training

In their seminal study, Casaburi and colleagues[98] showed that in patients with mainly moderate COPD, a high-intensity exercise training (EXT) program was associated with consistent physiologic training effects such as reduced lactic acid, V_E, Vo_2, and heart rate. Reduced V_E after training was likely explained by altered central and peripheral chemoreflex activation as a result of increased oxidative capacity and reduced hydrogen ion generation in the reconditioned peripheral muscles. Improved breathing pattern (manifested as reduced Bf) improves ventilatory efficiency and reduces pulmonary gas trapping, with consequent delay of intolerable dyspnea.[128–131] It is now clear from recent studies that important improvement in activity-related and anticipatory dyspnea, quality of life, and perceived self-efficacy can occur in the absence of consistent physiologic training effects.[48] Thus in many patients, particularly those with more advanced COPD, supervised multicomponent pulmonary rehabilitation programs modify behavior and the important affective component of dyspnea. This finding is corroborated by a recent study, which demonstrated that pulmonary rehabilitation in COPD consistently altered brain activity measured by fMRI in stimulus valuation networks.[132]

> Although lessening IND (eg, supplemental O_2, opiates, exercise training) is likely to positively affect exertional dyspnea, improved muscular/mechanical responses of the respiratory system for a given drive can also favorably influence intensity and qualitative domains of dyspnea.

REDUCED VENTILATORY CAPACITY IN CHRONIC OBSTRUCTIVE PULMONARY DISEASE

Although EFL is the main physiologic abnormality in COPD, lung hyperinflation is an important consequence that has profound negative sensory implications. Lung hyperinflation in many patients results from emphysematous destruction of lung tissue with changes in lung elasticity (increased lung compliance) that resets the balance of forces between inward lung recoil pressure and outward chest wall recoil at end-expiration. Thus, the relaxation volume of the respiratory system (ie, EELV) is increased compared with healthy individuals. In patients with EFL, EELV is also dynamically determined and is a continuous variable that is influenced by the prevailing breathing pattern. If breathing frequency increases abruptly (and expiratory time decreases and V_T increases), air trapping is inevitable given the slow mechanical time constants for lung emptying in COPD. During exercise or other conditions whereby there is a sudden increase in ventilatory demand (eg, anxiety, acute hypoxemia, infective exacerbation, or voluntary hyperventilation), EELV increases temporarily and variably higher than its resting value: this is termed dynamic lung hyperinflation.[133–135] The resting inspiratory capacity provides an indirect measure of lung hyperinflation: the lower the IC, the higher the EELV, provided the inspiratory muscles are not weak and maximal volitional inspiratory effort to TLC is expended during IC maneuvers. Serial IC measured at intervals (eg, 2-minute) during exercise can track the rate of dynamic hyperinflation on the assumption that TLC remains constant.[135,136] This method of assessing behavior of operating lung volumes has been shown in

multinational studies to be both reproducible and responsive to various volume deflation interventions.[53,137,138]

IC is a simple and useful mechanical measurement that indicates the operating position of tidal volume (V_T) relative to TLC and thus the proximity to the upper curvilinear extreme of the relaxed respiratory system's sigmoidal pressure-volume relation (**Fig. 8**).[139] Breathing close to TLC means that the inspiratory muscles are shortened, functionally weakened, and must contend with increased elastic and inspiratory threshold loading to overcome autopositive end-expiratory pressure (auto-PEEP). The distance between end-inspiratory lung volume and TLC (IRV = IC − V_T) dictates the relation between IND and the mechanical/muscular response of the dynamic respiratory system. In other words, the IRV provides crucial information about the extent of neuromechanical coupling or dissociation of the respiratory system

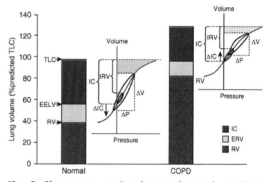

Fig. 8. Shown are resting lung volumes in patients with COPD and in age-matched healthy normal individuals. Pressure-volume (P-V) curves of the respiratory system are shown with tidal P-V curves during rest (filled area) and exercise (open area). In COPD, because of resting and dynamic hyperinflation (a further increase in EELV), exercise V_T encroaches on the upper, nonlinear extreme of the respiratory system P-V curve, where there is increased elastic loading. In COPD, IRV is diminished and the ability to further expand V_T is reduced. COPD, chronic obstructive pulmonary disease; EELV, end-expiratory lung volume; ERV, expiratory reserve volume; IC, inspiratory capacity; IRV, inspiratory reserve volume; RV, residual volume; TLC, total lung capacity; V_T, tidal volume; ΔIC, change in IC from rest to during exercise; ΔP, change in pleural pressure during a tidal breath during exercise; ΔV, change in tidal volume during exercise. (*Reprinted* with permission of the American Thoracic Society. Copyright © 2019 American Thoracic Society. O'Donnell DE, Elbehairy AF, Webb KA, et al. The link between reduced inspiratory capacity and exercise intolerance in chronic obstructive pulmonary disease. Annals ATS 2017;14: S30–39. The Annals of the American Thoracic Society is an official journal of the American Thoracic Society.)

and, hence, the extent of exertional dyspnea. The IC is determined by the FRC/TLC ratio, the strength of the inspiratory muscles, the extent of EFL, and the breathing pattern, which together all importantly influence exercise performance. The lower the resting IC (the greater the increase in EELV), the earlier the point during exercise when V_T reaches an inflection or plateau. Thus, when the V_T/IC ratio reaches approximately 0.7 or the IRV reaches less than 0.5 to 1.0 L below TLC, this marks an important mechanical event. At this point there is widening disparity between IND, which continues to increase, and the V_T response, which becomes progressively constrained and eventually fixed: this represents the onset of neuromechanical dissociation (**Fig. 9**).[140] Under these conditions, asynchrony is present between IND and the mechanical response. In other words, because of the presence of auto-PEEP, inspired flow is absent at the onset of neural activation until the inspiratory threshold load is overcome.[141,142] Moreover, when V_T and IRV become

fixed, afferent inputs from the respiratory system and multiple chest wall mechanoreceptors (and possibly inhibitory vagal receptors) are disrupted, and this information is conveyed to the somatosensory cortex (see **Fig. 3G–I**).

Several studies have shown that the V_T threshold coincides with more abrupt escalation of dyspnea to intolerable levels, and in each individual this is ultimately influenced by the magnitude of the resting IC. Of interest, when qualitative descriptors (effort, inspiratory and expiratory difficulty) are serially rated throughout exercise in COPD, unsatisfied inspiration displaces respiratory effort as the dominant qualitative descriptor of dyspnea at and beyond the V_T plateau[47] (**Fig. 10**). Furthermore, studies have shown that the increase in dyspnea during exercise in COPD correlates strongly with the increases in V_T/IC ratio or the decrease in IRV.[89] It is noteworthy that the IRV reduction is more closely associated with increasing dyspnea than the increase in EELV (dynamic hyperinflation)

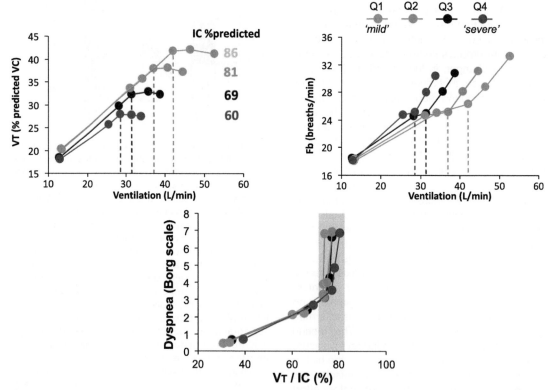

Fig. 9. Interrelationships are shown among ventilation, tidal volume, breathing frequency, exertional dyspnea intensity, and the V_T/IC ratio. After V_T/IC plateaus (ie, the V_T inflection point), dyspnea rises steeply to intolerable levels. Data plotted are mean values at steady-state rest, isotime (ie, 2 minutes, 4 minutes), the V_T/V_E inflection point, and peak exercise. Fb, breathing frequency; IC, inspiratory capacity; V_E, minute ventilation; V_T, tidal volume. (*Adapted from* O'Donnell DE, Guenette JA, Maltais F, et al. Decline of resting inspiratory capacity in COPD: the impact on breathing pattern, dyspnea, and ventilatory capacity during exercise. Chest 2012;141(3):753–62.)

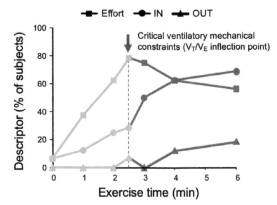

Fig. 10. Selection frequency of 3 descriptor phrases evolution during constant work-rate exercise in COPD patients: "my breathing requires more effort" (Effort), "I cannot get enough air in" (IN), "I cannot get enough air out" (OUT). Arrow indicates the point corresponding to the inflection point of the tidal volume-ventilation relation during exercise. V_E, minute ventilation; V_T, tidal volume. (*Reprinted* with permission of the American Thoracic Society. Copyright © 2019 American Thoracic Society. Laveneziana P, Webb KA, Ora J, et al. Evolution of dyspnea during exercise in chronic obstructive pulmonary disease: impact of critical volume constraints. Am J Respir Crit Care Med 2011;184(12):1367–73. The American Journal of Respiratory and Critical Care Medicine is an official journal of the American Thoracic Society.)

alone. "Acute-on-chronic" lung hyperinflation results in a relatively rapid and shallow breathing pattern: the attendant increased velocity of shortening of the inspiratory muscles is linked to their functional muscle weakness, decreased dynamic lung compliance, worsened pulmonary gas exchange (higher V_D/V_T), and negative cardiopulmonary interactions (reduced venous return and reduced left ventricular ejection fraction).[143–146] As already mentioned, all of these factors together demand a significant increase in IND and attendant respiratory discomfort to sustain higher ventilation during physical activity.

What is not generally appreciated is that significant mechanical respiratory impairment and exertional dyspnea often exist at relatively low exercise levels in patients with ostensibly mild airway obstruction.[82,84,87,90] This finding partly explains the habitually reduced physical activity that is now well documented in this subpopulation with mild COPD.[147–152] The mechanisms of reduced physical activity in this group are multifactorial, although abnormal respiratory mechanics may play a role (see **Fig. 3**). For example, the presence of ventilatory limitation was confirmed during exercise in patients with mild COPD by an experiment that compared V_T changes with responses of age-

matched healthy controls after external dead space loading (0.6 L). CO_2 rebreathing during the added dead space in controls led to the expected increase in V_T but no corresponding increase in dyspnea ratings. By contrast, identical dead space loading in mild COPD resulted in severely attenuated V_T expansion (caused in part by the effects of EFL and dynamic hyperinflation) with a subsequent increase in respiratory discomfort at relatively low exercise levels, confirming the presence of true ventilatory limitation in this group.[82,153] With progressive mechanical impairment across the continuum of COPD, ventilatory limitation and respiratory discomfort become evident at progressively lower exercise levels.

> The onset of neuromechanical dissociation is marked by a plateau in tidal volume during exercise, which becomes progressively constrained. At this point there is widening disparity between IND, which continues to increase, and the muscular/mechanical response of the respiratory system.

THE EFFECT OF IMPROVING RESPIRATORY MECHANICS AND MUSCLE FUNCTION ON EXERTIONAL DYSPNEA

Several intervention studies have shown that therapies that reduce EELV (resting and dynamic) or counterbalance its negative effects on the inspiratory muscles are associated with reduced dyspnea and improved exercise tolerance. These include bronchodilators of every class,[60,61,154–156] bullectomy,[157,158] surgical or endoscopic lung volume reduction, and continuous positive airway pressure or inspiratory pressure assist.[141,142] Bronchodilators, inspiratory muscle training, and combined interventions are reviewed here.

Bronchodilators

Bronchodilators relax airway smooth muscle tone by improving airway conductance and accelerating the time constant for lung emptying. In this way bronchodilators reduce airway resistance and the dynamically determined EELV. This process is linked to increasing IC, and allows greater V_T expansion during exercise and a delay in reaching the critical minimal IRV. Exercise tolerance is therefore increased. Lung deflation improves the strength and endurance of the inspiratory muscles, reducing auto-PEEP. Increased IC means that V_T occupies a lower position relative to TLC on the sigmoidal pressure-volume relation of the relaxed respiratory system

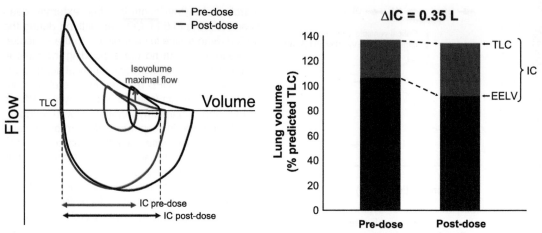

Fig. 11. Pharmacologic lung volume reduction. EELV, end-expiratory lung volume; IC, inspiratory capacity; TLC, total lung capacity.

(**Fig. 11**). The net effect of EELV deflation is therefore reduced elastic and inspiratory threshold loading (auto-PEEP) of the inspiratory muscles together with an increase in their functional strength. Ultimately, lung deflation partially restores a more harmonious relationship between IND and V_T displacement: less effort is now required for a given V_T[79] (**Fig. 12**). Of interest, some studies have shown that the common qualitative descriptor "unsatisfied inspiration" is selected less frequently after bronchodilators in comparison with placebo.[60,61]

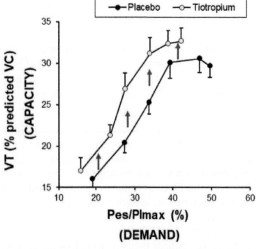

Fig. 12. Demand-capacity relationship in patients with COPD treated with placebo versus bronchodilator. Treatment with bronchodilator increased capacity for work with reduced demand at a given work rate. COPD, chronic obstructive pulmonary disease; Pes, esophageal pressure; Pimax, maximum inspiratory pressure; V_T, tidal volume.

Inspiratory Muscle Training

Although there is evidence that inspiratory muscles favorably adapt to chronic thoracic hyperinflation, this compensation may quickly be overwhelmed during exercise in the setting of acute increases in ventilatory demand and dynamic hyperinflation.[136] In a recent study, Langer and colleagues[159] provided new insights into the mechanisms of relief of dyspnea following inspiratory muscle training (IMT) in COPD. Supervised IMT in patients with severe COPD was associated with increased inspiratory muscle strength (including the diaphragm),

---

Box 2
Management of dyspnea in COPD

1. Increased inspiratory capacity:
   - Bronchodilators
   - Surgical/endoscopic lung volume resection
   - Oxygen/heliox/exercise training

2. Reduce IND:
   - Oxygen
   - Exercise training
   - Opiates/anxiolytics

3. Increase ventilatory muscle strength:
   - Exercise training
   - Specific inspiratory muscle training

4. Alter affective dimension:
   - Opiates/anxiolytics/oxygen/exercise training/counseling/behavioral modification

Abbreviation: IND, inspiratory neural drive.

reduced dyspnea, and improved exercise tolerance compared with control (sham training). In the IMT group IND decreased significantly over the prolonged exercise endurance time (>3 minutes) during which V_E was sustained at approximately 30 L/min. Of interest, IND (EMGdi/EMGdi,max) was diminished after IMT in a setting where there was no change in V_E, breathing pattern, or operating lung volumes. This study, therefore, supports the notion that when the inspiratory muscles are weakened, IND increases, reflecting increasing motor command output from cortical centers to maintain force generation commensurate with the ventilatory demand. The increased IND under these conditions contributes to exertional dyspnea.

Combined Interventions

In reality, dyspnea amelioration in the clinical setting will require multiple interventions with different mechanisms of benefit (**Box 2**). As expected, studies that have used at least 2 different combined interventions have shown additive effects on dyspnea amelioration and exercise tolerance (**Fig. 13**).

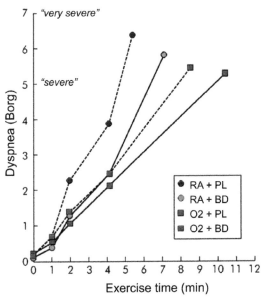

Fig. 13. Mean Borg ratings of dyspnea over time during constant load cycle exercise at 75% peak work rate. Dyspnea/time slopes decreased significantly (*P*<.05) with bronchodilators (BD) and 50% oxygen (O₂), alone and in combination; the combination of O₂ + BD resulted in greater (*P*<.05) dyspnea relief than either BD or O₂ alone. BD, bronchodilator; PL, placebo; RA, room air. (*Adapted from* Peters MM, Webb KA, O'Donnell DE, et al. Combined physiologic effects of bronchodilators and hyperoxia on exertional dyspnea in normoxic COPD. Thorax 2006;61(7):559–67.)

Examples include exercise training and bronchodilators, bronchodilators and oxygen,[115] and helium and oxygen.[160] Collectively these therapeutic intervention studies in COPD have taught us that effective dyspnea relief can be achieved by reducing IND drive by improving respiratory mechanics and by strengthening the inspiratory muscles. Fundamentally, a common final pathway underlying dyspnea relief and improved exercise tolerance across the range of therapeutic intervention is reduced neuromechanical dissociation of the respiratory system.

> Interventions aimed at restoring more harmonious neuromuscular coupling can alleviate exertional dyspnea. Further beneficial effects can be obtained if interventions are combined (eg, exercise training and bronchodilators, bronchodilators and oxygen).

SUMMARY

Current constructs on the origins of activity-related dyspnea in COPD generally endorse the classical demand/capacity imbalance theory. Thus, it is thought that pathophysiologic disruption of integrated central and peripheral sensory inputs, under conditions of neuromechanical dissociation, fundamentally shape the expression of respiratory discomfort in COPD. The anatomic and neurophysiologic components of the "dyspnea matrix" still need to be elucidated with greater precision, although steady progress is being made in this respect. A significant limitation is our inability to measure afferent activity from vagal and diverse peripheral mechanoreceptors to determine their contribution to multicomponent dyspnea. The evolution of respiratory discomfort during incremental exercise in COPD involves: (1) awareness of increased breathing effort reflecting the increased cortical motor command output and force generation of the respiratory muscles—increased contractile effort is required to sustain hyperpnea under conditions of respiratory muscle overload and functional weakness; (2) further IND increases because of the effects of worsening pulmonary gas exchange and acid-base derangements together with progressive dynamic respiratory mechanical abnormalities—this ultimately creates serious neuromechanical dissociation and with it a sense of inspiratory difficulty ("unsatisfied inspiration"), which at this point becomes the dominant qualitative descriptor of dyspnea; and (3) when respiratory discomfort escalates beyond a certain level (which likely varies between individuals), the limbic and paralimbic systems become overactivated—thus the patient is overcome by feelings of fear, anxiety, distress, and even panic, and the physical task must be abandoned. The symptom of exertional dyspnea cannot be effectively eliminated in patients with relatively fixed pathophysiologic impairment. However, there is evidence that combined therapeutic interventions can provide some palliation of severe dyspnea by partially reversing neuromechanical dissociation of the respiratory system and by addressing the affective component of the symptom.

CASE EXAMPLE

By way of an example, let us consider the simple scenario of a patient with severe COPD climbing a short flight of 7 stairs (**Fig. 14**). As the patient contemplates the task ahead, cortical and midbrain motor command centers initiate anticipatory hyperpnea. As ascent begins, feedforward stimuli from these brain centers ensure synchronous activation of the respiratory and locomotor muscles. The cortical motor command output to the respiratory muscles progressively increases to maintain ventilation in pace with metabolic demand of this task in the face of mechanical overloading and functional weakness of the respiratory muscles. This process gives rise to increased sense of effort or work, which continues to escalate (see **Fig. 14**A). On the demand side, the metabolic cost of the task is Vo_2 1.0 L/min. Because of the increasing metabolic Vco_2 and pulmonary Vco_2 (caused by high physiologic dead space), central chemoreceptors are stimulated, and reflex chemostimulation of medullary centers increases linearly as stair climbing continues. Arterial O_2 saturation decreases with progressive exertion (the result of alveolar units with low ventilation/perfusion ratios) and stimulation of carotid chemoreceptors adds to chemoreflex-induced IND increase. Owing to the reduced

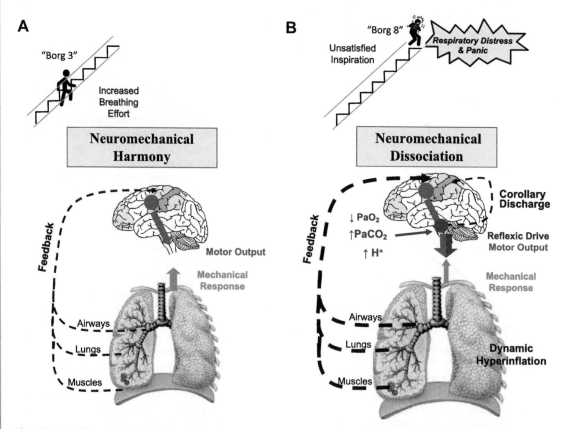

Fig. 14. Initial neuromechanical harmony and progressive dissociation in a patient with COPD during exertion. (*A*) Synchronous activation of the respiratory and locomotor muscles with motor command output progressively increases to maintain ventilation with stair climbing. (*B*) Arterial oxygen desaturation, increased [H+], and increased Vco_2 with corresponding chemostimulation of medullary centers and increased IND. Resting and dynamic hyperinflation and resulting mechanical constraints lead to neuromechanical dissociation and distressing unsatisfied inspiration experienced by the patient. COPD, chronic obstructive pulmonary disease; [H+], hydrogen ion concentration; IND, inspiratory neural drive; $Paco_2$, arterial partial pressure of carbon dioxide; Pao_2, arterial partial pressure of oxygen; Vco_2, carbon dioxide production.

oxidative capacity of chronically deconditioned locomotor muscles an early anaerobic threshold is reached, and increased hydrogen ion release detected by chemoreceptors further augments IND. Changes in the metabolic milieu in the active peripheral muscles, caused by reduced O_2 delivery and use, activates leg muscle metaboreceptors that also stimulate IND (see **Fig. 14**B). The net result of all these factors is that IND to the diaphragm with each breath reaches greater than 60% of maximal diaphragmatic activation at this low exercise intensity.

Examining the capacity side, the ventilatory response to increasing IND is severely blunted because of the combined effects of resting and dynamic lung hyperinflation: inspiratory and expiratory flow limitation is in place and breathing reserve disappears. The inspiratory muscles are overburdened and functionally weakened, and mechanical restrictive constraints are invariable when breathing so close to TLC. At the limits of tolerance peak V_E is 30 L/min, IRV is 95% of TLC, and V_T is 80% of IC, esophageal pressure (effort) is 50% of the maximal value, and IND is 80% of maximum. The severe neuromechanical dissociation after the V_T plateau is associated with the distressing sensation of unsatisfied inspiration: despite almost maximal IND, very little air enters the lung with each breath. This, in turn, provokes a programmed affective response sensed as extreme respiratory distress (see **Fig. 14**B).

REFERENCES

1. Parshall MB, Schwartzstein RM, Adams L, et al. An official American Thoracic Society statement: update on the mechanisms, assessment, and management of dyspnea. Am J Respir Crit Care Med 2012;185(4):435–52.

2. Elkington H, White P, Addington-Hall J, et al. The last year of life of COPD: a qualitative study of symptoms and services. Respir Med 2004;98(5):439–45.

3. Pumar MI, Gray CR, Walsh JR, et al. Anxiety and depression-Important psychological comorbidities of COPD. J Thorac Dis 2014;6(11):1615–31.

4. Maltais F, Decramer M, Casaburi R, et al. An official American Thoracic Society/European Respiratory Society statement: update on limb muscle dysfunction in chronic obstructive pulmonary disease. Am J Respir Crit Care Med 2014;189(9):e15–62.

5. Breuer J, Hering E. Self-steering of the respiration through the nervous vagus (originally published 1868). In: Comroe J, editor. Pulmonary and respiratory physiology Part II. Stroudsbourg (PA): Dowden, Hutchinson & Ross; 1976. p. 108–13.

6. LeGallois CJJ. Experiments on the principle of life, and particularly on the principle of the notions of the heart, and on the seat of this principle (originally published 1813). In: Comroe J, editor. Pulmonary and respiratory physiology Part II. Stroudsbourg (PA): Dowden, Hutchinson & Ross; 1976. p. 12–6.

7. Wright GW, Branscomb BV. The origin of the sensation of dyspnea. Trans Am Clin Climatol Assoc 1955;66:116–25.

8. Kimoff RJ, Cheong TH, Cosio MG, et al. Pulmonary denervation in humans. Effects on dyspnea and ventilatory pattern during exercise. Am Rev Respir Dis 1990;142:1034–40.

9. Paintal AS. Mechanism of stimulation of type J pulmonary receptors. J Physiol 1969;203(3):511–32.

10. Guz A, Noble MI, Widdicombe JG, et al. The role of vagal and glossopharyngeal afferent nerves in respiratory sensation, control of breathing and arterial pressure regulation in conscious man. Clin Sci 1966;30(1):161–70.

11. Haldane JS, Smith JL. Carbon dioxide and regulation of breathing. J Pathol Bacteriol 1893;1(168):318.

12. Fowler WS. Breaking point of breath-holding. J Appl Physiol 1954;6:539–45.

13. Flume PA, Eldridge FL, Edwards LJ, et al. The Fowler breathholding study revisited: continuous rating of respiratory sensation. Respir Physiol 1994;95:53–66.

14. Gandevia SC, Killian K, McKenzie DK, et al. Respiratory sensations, cardiovascular control, kinaesthesia and transcranial stimulation during paralysis in humans. J Physiol 1993;470(Oct):85–107.

15. Stevens SS. The psychophysics of sensory function. Am Sci 1960;48:226–53.

16. Stevens SS. Neural events and the psychophysical law. Science 1970;170:1043–50.

17. Campbell EJ, Freedman S, Smith PS, et al. The ability of man to detect added elastic loads to breathing. Clin Sci 1961;20:223–31.

18. Bennett ED, Jayson MIV, Rubenstein D, et al. The ability of man to detect added non-elastic loads to breathing. Clin Sci 1962;23:155–62.

19. Bakers JHCM, Tenney SM. The perception of some sensations associated with breathing. Respir Physiol 1970;10:85–92.

20. Borg GA. Physical performance and perceived exertion. Lund (Sweden): CWK Gleerup; 1962.

21. Borg G. Perceived exertion as an indicator of somatic stress. Scand J Rehabil Med 1970;2:92–8.

22. Borg GA. Psychophysical bases of perceived exertion. Med Sci Sports Exerc 1982;14(5):377–81.

23. Killian KJ, Jones NL. The use of exercise testing and other methods in the investigation of dyspnea. Clin Chest Med 1984;5(1):99–108.

24. Killian KJ, Gandevia SC, Summers E, et al. Effect of increased lung volume on perception of

breathlessness, effort, and tension. J Appl Physiol 1984;57(3):686–91.

25. Jones NL, Killian KJ. Exercise limitations in health and disease. N Engl J Med 2000;343(9):632–49.

26. Campbell EJ, Dickinson CJ, Dinnick OP, et al. The immediate effects of threshold loads on breathing of men and dogs. Clin Sci 1961;20:223–31.

27. Campbell EJ, Howell JBL. The sensation of breathlessness. Br Med Bull 1963;19:36–40.

28. Schwartzstein RM, Simon PM, Weiss JW, et al. Breathlessness induced by dissociation between ventilation and chemical drive. Am Rev Respir Dis 1989;139(5):1231–7.

29. Manning HL, Shea SA, Schwartzstein RM, et al. Reduced tidal volume increases 'air hunger' at fixed PCO2 in ventilated quadriplegics. Respir Physiol 1992;90(1):19–30.

30. Harty HR, Corfield DR, Schwartzstein RM, et al. External thoracic restriction, respiratory sensation, and ventilation during exercise in men. J Appl Physiol 1999;86(4):1142–50.

31. O'Donnell DE, Hong HH, Webb KA. Respiratory sensation during chest wall restriction and dead space loading in exercising men. J Appl Physiol (1985) 2000;88(5):1859–69.

32. Evans KC, Banzett RB, Adams L, et al. BOLD fMRI identifies limbic, paralimbic, and cerebellar activation during air hunger. J Neurophysiol 2002;88(3):1500–11.

33. Banzett RB, Pedersen SH, Schwartzstein RM, et al. The affective dimension of laboratory dyspnea: air hunger is more unpleasant than work/effort. Am J Respir Crit Care Med 2008;177(12):1384–90.

34. Chen Z, Eldridge FL, Wagner PG. Respiratory-associated thalamic activity is related to level of respiratory drive. Respir Physiol 1992;90(1):99–113.

35. Chen Z, Eldridge FL, Wagner PG. Respiratory-associated rhythmic firing of midbrain neurones in cats: relation to level of respiratory drive. J Physiol 1991;437:305–25.

36. Eldridge FL, Millhorn DE, Waldrop TG. Exercise hyperpnea and locomotion: parallel activation from the hypothalamus. Science 1981;211(4484):844–6.

37. Jensen D, Ofir D, O'Donnell DE. Effects of pregnancy, obesity and aging on the intensity of perceived breathlessness during exercise in healthy humans. Respir Physiol Neurobiol 2009;167:87–100.

38. el-Manshawi A, Killian KJ, Summers E, et al. Breathlessness during exercise with and without resistive loading. J Appl Physiol (1985) 1986;61(3):896–905.

39. Lane R, Adams L, Guz A. Is low-level respiratory resistive loading during exercise perceived as breathlessness? Clin Sci 1987;73:627–34.

40. Campbell EJ, Gandevia SC, Killian KJ, et al. Changes in the perception of inspiratory resistive loads during partial curarization. J Physiol 1980; 309:93–100.

41. Moosavi SH, Topulos GP, Hafter A, et al. Acute partial paralysis alters perceptions of air hunger, work and effort at constant P(CO(2)) and V(E). Respir Physiol 2000;122:45–60.

42. von Leupoldt A, Sommer T, Kegat S, et al. The unpleasantness of perceived dyspnea is processed in the anterior insula and amygdala. Am J Respir Crit Care Med 2008;177(9):1026–32.

43. Stoeckel MC, Esser RW, Gamer M, et al. Brain responses during the anticipation of dyspnea. Neural Plast 2016;2016:6434987.

44. O'Donnell DE, Bertley JC, Chau LK, et al. Qualitative aspects of exertional breathlessness in chronic airflow limitation: pathophysiologic mechanisms. Am J Respir Crit Care Med 1997;155(1):109–15.

45. Abdallah SJ, Wilkinson-Maitland C, Saad N, et al. Effect of morphine on breathlessness and exercise endurance in advanced COPD: a randomised crossover study. Eur Respir J 2017;50(4). https://doi.org/10.1183/13993003.01235-2017.

46. Elbehairy AF, Ciavaglia CE, Webb KA, et al. Pulmonary gas exchange abnormalities in mild chronic obstructive pulmonary disease. Implications for dyspnea and exercise intolerance. Am J Respir Crit Care Med 2015;191(12):1384–94.

47. Laveneziana P, Webb KA, Ora J, et al. Evolution of dyspnea during exercise in chronic obstructive pulmonary disease: impact of critical volume constraints. Am J Respir Crit Care Med 2011;184(12):1367–73.

48. Wadell K, Webb KA, Preston ME, et al. Impact of pulmonary rehabilitation on the major dimensions of dyspnea in COPD. COPD 2013;10(4):425–35.

49. Faisal A, Alghamdi BJ, Ciavaglia CE, et al. Common mechanisms of dyspnea in chronic interstitial and obstructive lung disorders. Am J Respir Crit Care Med 2016;193(3):299–309.

50. O'Donnell DE, Neder JA, Harle I, et al. Chronic breathlessness in patients with idiopathic pulmonary fibrosis: a major challenge for caregivers. Expert Rev Respir Med 2016;10(12):1295–303.

51. Simon PM, Schwartzstein RM, Weiss JW, et al. Distinguishable sensations of breathlessness induced in normal volunteers. Am Rev Respir Dis 1989;140(4):1021–7.

52. Simon PM, Schwartzstein RM, Weiss JW, et al. Distinguishable types of dyspnea in patients with shortness of breath. Am Rev Respir Dis 1990; 142(5):1009–14.

53. O'Donnell DE, Travers J, Webb KA, et al. Reliability of ventilatory parameters during cycle ergometry in multicentre trials in COPD. Eur Respir J 2009;34(4):866–74.

54. O'Donnell DE, Elbehairy AF, Berton D, et al. Exercise testing in the evaluation of pharmacotherapy in COPD. In: Palange P, Laveneziana P, Neder JA, et al, editors. ERS monographs, vol. 80. Sheffield (United Kingdom): European Respiratory Society; 2018. p. 235–50.

55. Jones NL. The Ins and Outs of Breathing: how we learnt about the body's most vital function. Bloomington (IN): iUniverse; 2011.

56. Means JH. Dyspnea. Medical monographs, vol. 5. Baltimore (MD): Williams & Wilkins; 1924. p. 309–416.

57. Cournand A, Richards DW. Pulmonary insufficiency, part IL. Discussion of a physiological classification and presentation of clinical tests. Am Rev Tuberc 1941;44:26–41.

58. Bradley TD, Chartrand DA, Fitting JW, et al. The relation of inspiratory effort sensation to fatiguing patterns of the diaphragm. Am Rev Respir Dis 1986;134(6):1119–24.

59. O'Donnell DE, Revill SM, Webb KA. Dynamic hyperinflation and exercise intolerance in chronic obstructive pulmonary disease. Am J Respir Crit Care Med 2001;164(5):770–7.

60. O'Donnell DE, Voduc N, Fitzpatrick M, et al. Effect of salmeterol on the ventilatory response to exercise in chronic obstructive pulmonary disease. Eur Respir J 2004;24(1):86–94.

61. O'Donnell DE, Sciurba F, Celli B, et al. Effect of fluticasone propionate/salmeterol on lung hyperinflation and exercise endurance in COPD. Chest 2006;130(3):647–56.

62. Jolley CJ, Luo YM, Steier J, et al. Neural respiratory drive in healthy subjects and in COPD. Eur Respir J 2009;33(2):289–97.

63. Jolley CJ, Luo YM, Steier J, et al. Neural respiratory drive and breathlessness in COPD. Eur Respir J 2015;45(2):355–64.

64. Krogh A, Linhard J. The regulation of respiration and circulation during the initial stages of muscular work. J Physiol 1913;47:112–36.

65. Thorton JM, Guz A, Murphy K, et al. Identification of higher brain centres that may encode the cardiorespiratory response to exercise in humans. J Physiol 2001;533:823–36.

66. Gandevia SC, Rothwell JC. Activation of the human diaphragm from the motor cortex. J Physiol 1987; 384(1):109–18.

67. Iwamoto GA, Wappel SM, Fox GM, et al. Identification of diencephalic and brainstem cardiorespiratory areas activated during exercise. Brain Res 1996;726(1–2):109–22.

68. Forster HV, Haouzi P, Dempsey JA. Control of breathing during exercise. Compr Physiol 2012; 2(1):743–77.

69. Paterson DH. Defining the neurocircuitry of exercise hyperpnoea. J Physiol 2013;592(3).

70. Haouzi P, Chenuel B, Huszczuk A. Sensing vascular distention in skeletal muscle by slow conducting afferent fibres: neurophysiological basis and implication for respiratory control. J Appl Physiol 2004;96(2):407–18.

71. Amann M, Proctor LT, Sebranek JJ, et al. Somatosensory feedback from the limbs exerts inhibitory influences on central neural drive during whole body endurance exercise. J Appl Physiol 2008; 105(6):1714–24.

72. Amann M, Proctor LT, Sebranek JJ, et al. Opioid-mediated muscle afferents inhibit central motor drive and limit peripheral muscle fatigue development in humans. J Physiol 2009;587(1):271–83.

73. Dempsey JA. New perspectives concerning feedback influences on cardiorespiratory control during rhythmic exercise and on exercise performance. J Physiol 2012;590(17):4129–44.

74. Johnson BD, Reddan WG, Seow KC, et al. Mechanical constraints on exercise hyperpnea in a fit aging population. Am Rev Respir Dis 1991; 143(5 Pt 1):968–77.

75. Johnson BD, Reddan WG, Pegelow DF, et al. Flow limitation and regulation of functional residual capacity during exercise in a physically active aging population. Am Rev Respir Dis 1991;143(5 Pt 1):960–7.

76. Aaron EA, Seow KC, Johnson BD, et al. Oxygen cost of exercise hyperpnea: implications for performance. J Appl Physiol (1985) 1992;72(5):1818–25.

77. Johnson BD, Badr MS, Dempsey JA. Impact of the aging pulmonary system on the response to exercise. Clin Chest Med 1994;15(2):229–46.

78. Johnson BD, Weisman IM, Zeballos RJ, et al. Emerging concepts in the evaluation of ventilatory limitation during exercise: the exercise tidal flow-volume loop. Chest 1999;116(2):488–503.

79. O'Donnell DE, Hamilton AL, Webb KA. Sensory-mechanical relationships during high-intensity, constant-work-rate exercise in COPD. J Appl Physiol (1985) 2006;101(4):1025–35.

80. Jensen D, Webb KA, Davies GAL, et al. Mechanical ventilatory constraints during incremental cycle exercise in human pregnancy: implications for respiratory sensation. J Physiol 2008;586(19):4735–50.

81. Faisal A, Webb KA, Guenette JA, et al. Effect of age-related ventilatory inefficiency on respiratory sensation during exercise. Respir Physiol Neurobiol 2015;205:129–39.

82. Chin RC, Guenette JA, Cheng S, et al. Does the respiratory system limit exercise in mild chronic obstructive pulmonary disease? Am J Respir Crit Care Med 2013;187(12):1315–23.

83. Elbehairy AF, Webb KA, Neder JA, et al. Should mild COPD be treated? Evidence for early pharmacological intervention. Drugs 2013;73(18):1991–2001.

84. Elbehairy AF, Faisal A, Guenette JA, et al. Resting physiological correlates of reduced exercise

capacity in smokers with mild airway obstruction. COPD 2017;14(3):267–75.

85. Elbehairy AF, Parraga G, Webb KA, et al. Mild chronic obstructive pulmonary disease: why spirometry is not sufficient! Expert Rev Respir Med 2017; 11(7):549–63.

86. Cabanski M, Fields B, Boue S, et al. Transcriptional profiling and targeted proteomics reveals common molecular changes associated with cigarette smoke-induced lung emphysema development in five susceptible mouse strains. Inflamm Res 2015;64(7):471–86.

87. Ofir D, Laveneziana P, Webb KA, et al. Mechanisms of dyspnea during cycle exercise in symptomatic patients with GOLD stage I chronic obstructive pulmonary disease. Am J Respir Crit Care Med 2008;177(6):622–9.

88. Guenette JA, Chin RC, Cory JM, et al. Inspiratory capacity during exercise: measurement, analysis, and interpretation. Pulm Med 2013;2013:956081.

89. Guenette JA, Chin RC, Cheng S, et al. Mechanisms of exercise intolerance in global initiative for chronic obstructive lung disease grade 1 COPD. Eur Respir J 2014;44(5):1177–87.

90. Elbehairy AF, Guenette JA, Faisal A, et al. Mechanisms of exertional dyspnoea in symptomatic smokers without COPD. Eur Respir J 2016;48(3): 694–705.

91. Lou YM, Lyall RA, Harris ML, et al. Effect of lung volume on the oesophageal diaphragm EMG assessed by magnetic phrenic nerve stimulation. Eur Respir J 2000;15(6):1033–8.

92. Lou YM, Hart N, Mustfa N, et al. Effect of diaphragm fatigue on neural respiratory drive. J Appl Physiol 2001;90(5):1691–9.

93. Lou YM, Moxham J. Measurement of neural respiratory drive in patients with COPD. Respir Physiol Neurobiol 2005;146(2–3):165–74.

94. Ciavaglia CE, Guenette JA, Langer D, et al. Differences in respiratory muscle activity during cycling and walking do not influence dyspnea perception in obese patients with COPD. J Appl Physiol (1985) 2014;117(11):1292–301.

95. O'Donnell DE, Ora J, Webb KA, et al. Mechanisms of activity-related dyspnea in pulmonary diseases. Respir Physiol Neurobiol 2009;167(1):116–32.

96. Neder JA, Berton DC, Muller PT, et al. Ventilatory inefficiency and exertional dyspnea in early chronic obstructive pulmonary disease. Ann Am Thorac Soc 2017;14(Supplement_1):S22–9.

97. Hueper K, Vogel-Claussen J, Parikh MA, et al. Pulmonary microvascular blood flow in mild chronic obstructive pulmonary disease and emphysema. The MESA COPD Study. Am J Respir Crit Care Med 2015;192(5):570–80.

98. Casaburi R, Patessio A, Ioli F, et al. Reductions in exercise lactic acidosis and ventilation as a result of exercise training in patients with obstructive lung disease. Am Rev Respir Dis 1991;143(1): 9–18.

99. Patessio A, Casaburi R, Carone M, et al. Comparison of gas exchange, lactate, and lactic acidosis thresholds in patients with chronic obstructive pulmonary disease. Am Rev Respir Dis 1993;148(3): 622–6.

100. Maltais F, Leblanc P, Simard C, et al. Skeletal muscle adaptation to endurance training in patients with chronic obstructive pulmonary disease. Am J Respir Crit Care Med 1996;154(2):442–7.

101. Maltais F, Simard AA, Simard C, et al. Oxidative capacity of the skeletal muscle and lactic acid kinetics during exercise in normal subjects and in patients with COPD. Am J Respir Crit Care Med 1996;153(1):288–93.

102. Sue DY, Chung MM, Grosvenor M, et al. Effect of altering the proportion of dietary fat and carbohydrate on exercise gas exchange in normal subjects. Am Rev Respir Dis 1989;139(6): 1430–4.

103. Amann M, Regan MS, Kobitary M, et al. Impact of pulmonary system limitations on locomotor muscle fatigue in patients with COPD. Am J Physiol Regul Integr Comp Physiol 2010;299(1):314–24.

104. O'Donnell DE, D'Arsigny C, Webb KA. Effects of hyperoxia on ventilatory limitation during exercise in advanced chronic obstructive pulmonary disease. Am J Respir Crit Care Med 2001;163(4): 892–8.

105. Ponikowski PP, Chua TP, Francis DP, et al. Muscle ergoreceptor overactivity reflects deterioration in clinical status and cardiorespiratory reflex control in chronic heart failure. Circulation 2001;104(19): 2324–30.

106. Porszasz J, Emtner M, Goto S, et al. Exercise training decreases ventilatory requirements and exercise-induced hyperinflation at submaximal intensities in patients with COPD. Chest 2005; 128(4):2025–34.

107. Ward SA, Whipp BJ. Kinetics of the ventilatory and metabolic responses to moderate-intensity exercise in humans following prior exercise-induced metabolic acidaemia. Adv Exp Med Biol 2009; 669:323–6.

108. Rocha A, Arbex FF, Sperandio PA, et al. Excess ventilation in chronic obstructive pulmonary disease-heart failure overlap. Implications for dyspnea and exercise intolerance. Am J Respir Crit Care Med 2017;196(10):1264.

109. Neder JA, Rocha A, Alencar MC, et al. Current challenges in managing comorbid heart failure and COPD. Expert Rev Cardiovasc Ther 2018; 16(9):653–73.

110. Gagnon P, Bussieres JS, Ribeiro F, et al. Influences of spinal anesthesia on exercise tolerance in

patients with chronic obstructive pulmonary disease. Am J Respir Crit Care Med 2012;186(7):606–15.

111. Puente-Maestu L, Abad YM, Pedraza F, et al. A controlled trial of the effects of leg training on breathing pattern and dynamic hyperinflation in severe COPD. Lung 2006;184(3):159–67.

112. Elbehairy AF, Webb KA, Laveneziana P, et al. Acute bronchodilator therapy does not reduce wasted ventilation during exercise in COPD. Respir Physiol Neurobiol 2018;252-253:64–71.

113. Keller CA, Ruppel G, Hibbett A, et al. Thoracoscopic lung volume reduction surgery reduces dyspnea and improves exercise capacity in patients with emphysema. Am J Respir Crit Care Med 1997;156(1):60–7.

114. O'Donnell DE, Bain DJ, Webb KA. Factors contributing to relief of exertional breathlessness during hyperoxia in chronic airflow limitation. Am J Respir Crit Care Med 1997;155(2):530–5.

115. Peters MM, Webb KA, O'Donnell DE. Combined physiological effects of bronchodilators and hyperoxia on exertional dyspnoea in normoxic COPD. Thorax 2006;61(7):559–67.

116. Ekström M, Ahmadi Z, Bornefalk-Hermansson A, et al. Oxygen for breathlessness in patients with chronic obstructive pulmonary disease who do not qualify for home oxygen therapy. Cochrane Database Syst Rev 2016;(11):CD006429.

117. Santiago TV, Remolina C, Scoles V, et al. Endorphins and the control of breathing. N Engl J Med 1981;304(20):1190–5.

118. Santiago TV, Edelman NH. Opioids and breathing. J Appl Physiol (1985) 1985;59(6):1675–85.

119. Scardella AT, Parisi RP, Phair DK, et al. The role of endogenous opioids in the ventilatory response to acute flow-resistive loads. Am Rev Respir Dis 1986;133(1):26–31.

120. Mahler DA, Murray JA, Waterman LA, et al. Endogenous opioids modify dyspnoea during treadmill exercise in patients with COPD. Eur Respir J 2009;33(4):771–7.

121. Vozoris NT, Wang X, Austin PC, et al. Adverse cardiac events associated with incident opioid drug use among older adults with COPD. Eur J Clin Pharmacol 2017;73(10):1287–95.

122. Vozoris NT, Wang X, Fischer HD, et al. Incident opioid drug use and adverse respiratory outcomes among older adults with COPD. Eur Respir J 2016;48(3):683–93.

123. Vozoris NT, Wang X, Fischer HD, et al. Incident opioid drug use among older adults with chronic obstructive pulmonary disease: a population-based cohort study. Br J Clin Pharmacol 2016;81(1):161–70.

124. Jensen D, Alsuhail A, Viola R, et al. Inhaled fentanyl citrate improves exercise endurance during high-intensity constant work rate cycle exercise in chronic obstructive pulmonary disease. J Pain Symptom Manage 2012;43(4):706–19.

125. Johnson MJ, Bland JM, Oxberry SG, et al. Opioids for chronic refractory breathlessness: patient predictors of beneficial response. Eur Respir J 2013;42(3):758–66.

126. Rocker GM, Simpson AC, Horton R, et al. Opioid therapy for refractory dyspnea in patients with advanced chronic obstructive pulmonary disease: patients' experiences and outcomes. CMAJ Open 2013;1(1):E27–36.

127. Ekstrom M, Nilsson F, Abernethy AA, et al. Effects of opioids on breathlessness and exercise capacity in chronic obstructive pulmonary disease. A systematic review. Ann Am Thorac Soc 2015;12(7):1079–92.

128. O'Donnell DE, Webb KA. Exertional breathlessness in patients with chronic airflow limitation. The role of lung hyperinflation. Am Rev Respir Dis 1993;148(5):1351–7.

129. Somfay A, Porszasz J, Lee SM, et al. Dose-response effect of oxygen on hyperinflation and exercise endurance in nonhypoxaemic COPD patients. Eur Respir J 2001;18(1):77–84.

130. O'Donnell DE, D'Arsigny C, Fitzpatrick M, et al. Exercise hypercapnia in advanced chronic obstructive pulmonary disease: the role of lung hyperinflation. Am J Respir Crit Care Med 2002;166(5):663–8.

131. Laveneziana P, Webb KA, Wadell K, et al. Does expiratory muscle activity influence dynamic hyperinflation and exertional dyspnea in COPD? Respir Physiol Neurobiol 2014;199:24–33.

132. Herigstad M, Faull OK, Hayen A, et al. Treating breathlessness via the brain: changes in brain activity over a course of pulmonary rehabilitation. Eur Respir J 2017;50(3):1701029.

133. Olafsson S, Hyatt RE. Ventilatory mechanics and expiratory flow limitation during exercise in normal subjects. J Clin Invest 1969;48(3):564–73.

134. Dodd DS, Brancatisano T, Engel LA. Chest wall mechanics during exercise in patients with severe chronic air-flow obstruction. Am Rev Respir Dis 1984;129(1):33–8.

135. Stubbing DG, Pengelly LD, Morse JLC, et al. Pulmonary mechanics during exercise in subjects with chronic airflow obstruction. J Appl Physiol 1980;49:511–5.

136. Similowski T, Yan S, Gauthier AP, et al. Contractile properties of the human diaphragm during chronic hyperinflation. N Engl J Med 1991;325(13):917–23.

137. Puente-Maestu L, Palange P, Casaburi R, et al. Use of exercise testing in the evaluation of interventional efficacy: an official ERS statement. Eur Respir J 2016;47(2):429–60.

138. Palange P, Ward SA, Carlsen KH, et al. Recommendations on the use of exercise testing in clinical practice. Eur Respir J 2007;29(1):185–209.

139. O'Donnell DE, Elbehairy AF, Webb KA, et al. The link between reduced inspiratory capacity and exercise intolerance in chronic obstructive pulmonary disease. Ann Am Thorac Soc 2017; 14(Supplement_1). S30–s39.

140. O'Donnell DE, Guenette JA, Maltais F, et al. Decline of resting inspiratory capacity in COPD: the impact on breathing pattern, dyspnea, and ventilatory capacity during exercise. Chest 2012;141(3):753–62.

141. O'Donnell DE, Sanii R, Giesbrecht G, et al. Effect of continuous positive airway pressure on respiratory sensation in patients with chronic obstructive pulmonary disease during submaximal exercise. Am Rev Respir Dis 1988;138(5):1185–91.

142. O'Donnell DE, Sanii R, Younes M. Improvement in exercise endurance in patients with chronic airflow limitation using continuous positive airway pressure. Am Rev Respir Dis 1988;138:1510–4.

143. Laveneziana P, Palange P, Ora J, et al. Bronchodilator effect on ventilatory, pulmonary gas exchange, and heart rate kinetics during high-intensity exercise in COPD. Eur J Appl Physiol 2009;107(6): 633–43.

144. Laveneziana P, Valli G, Onorati P, et al. Effect of heliox on heart rate kinetics and dynamic hyperinflation during high-intensity exercise in COPD. Eur J Appl Physiol 2011;111(2):225–34.

145. Chiappa GR, Borghi-Silva A, Ferreira LF, et al. Kinetics of muscle deoxygenation are accelerated at the onset of heavy-intensity exercise in patients with COPD: relationship to central cardiovascular dynamics. J Appl Physiol (1985) 2008;104(5): 1341–50.

146. Berton DC, Barbosa PB, Takara LS, et al. Bronchodilators accelerate the dynamics of muscle O2 delivery and utilisation during exercise in COPD. Thorax 2010;65(7):588–93.

147. Pitta F, Troosters T, Spruit MA, et al. Characteristics of physical activities in daily life in chronic obstructive pulmonary disease. Am J Respir Crit Care Med 2005;171:972–7.

148. Watz H, Waschki B, Boehme C, et al. Extrapulmonary effects of chronic obstructive pulmonary disease on physical activity: a cross-sectional study. Am J Respir Crit Care Med 2008;177:743–51.

149. Watz H, Troosters T, Beeh KM, et al. ACTIVATE: the effect of aclidinium/formoterol on hyperinflation, exercise capacity, and physical activity in patients with COPD. Int J Chron Obstruct Pulmon Dis 2017;12:2545–58.

150. Troosters T, Maltais F, Leidy N, et al. Effect of bronchodilation and exercise training with behavior modification on exercise tolerance and downstream effects on symptoms and physical activity in COPD. Am J Respir Crit Care Med 2018; 198(8):1021–32.

151. Troosters T, Sciurba F, Battaglia S, et al. Physical inactivity in patients with COPD, a controlled multicenter pilot-study. Respir Med 2010;104(7):1005–11.

152. Troosters T, van der Molen T, Polkey M, et al. Improving physical activity in COPD: towards a new paradigm. Respir Res 2013;14:115.

153. Dempsey JA. Limits to ventilation (for sure!) and exercise (maybe?) in mild chronic obstructive pulmonary disease. Am J Respir Crit Care Med 2013;187(12):1282–3.

154. Donohue JF, van Noord JA, Bateman ED, et al. A 6-month, placebo-controlled study comparing lung function and health status changes in COPD patients treated with tiotropium or salmeterol. Chest 2002;122(1):47–55.

155. Buhl R, Maltais F, Abrahams R, et al. Tiotropium and olodaterol fixed-dose combination versus mono-components in COPD (GOLD 2-4). Eur Respir J 2015;45(4):969–79.

156. Fuhr R, Magnussen H, Sarem K, et al. Efficacy of aclidinium bromide 400 mug twice daily compared with placebo and tiotropium in patients with moderate to severe COPD. Chest 2012; 141(3):745–52.

157. O'Donnell DE, Webb KA, Bertley JC, et al. Mechanisms of relief of exertional breathlessness following unilateral bullectomy and lung volume reduction surgery in emphysema. Chest 1996; 110(1):18–27.

158. Elbehairy AF, Faisal A, Ciavaglia CE, et al. Severe exertional dyspnea in an ex-smoker with a large apical bulla. Ann Am Thorac Soc 2018;15(10): 1221–8.

159. Langer D, Ciavaglia CE, Faisal A, et al. Inspiratory muscle training reduces diaphragm activation and dyspnea during exercise in COPD. J Appl Physiol (1985) 2018;125(2):381–92.

160. Eves ND, Sandmeyer LC, Wong EY, et al. Helium-hyperoxia: a novel intervention to improve the benefits of pulmonary rehabilitation for patients with COPD. Chest 2009;135(3):609–18.

The Relevance of Limb Muscle Dysfunction in Chronic Obstructive Pulmonary Disease
A Review For Clinicians

Kim-Ly Bui, MPT[a], André Nyberg, RPT, PhD[b],
Roberto Rabinovich, PhD[c,d], Didier Saey, PT, PhD[a],
François Maltais, MD[a,*]

KEYWORDS

- Chronic obstructive pulmonary disease • Quadriceps • Muscle atrophy • Muscle weakness
- Muscle • Exercise

KEY POINTS

- Limb muscle dysfunction is frequent in chronic obstructive pulmonary disease (COPD) and it contributes to its morbidity and even mortality.
- Limb muscle dysfunction in COPD is characterized by atrophy, weakness, and reduced oxidative capacity. The extent of these muscle abnormalities is heterogeneous across the COPD population.
- Chronic physical inactivity certainly plays an important role in explaining the development of limb muscle dysfunction in COPD but is probably not the sole factor involved.
- Limb muscle atrophy and strength can be measured with simple and valid tools.
- Limb muscle dysfunction in COPD, is amenable to therapy, notably with exercise training.

INTRODUCTION
Limb Muscle Dysfunction in Patients with Chronic Obstructive Pulmonary Disease; a Clinically Relevant Problem

The term "limb muscle dysfunction" encompasses a variety of morphologic and structural abnormalities within the muscle that compromise its function. Depending on the criteria used, up to a third of patients with COPD express some form of muscle dysfunction, including atrophy and weakness.[1] Although the extent of muscle atrophy and weakness is greater in more advanced disease, muscle dysfunction may also occur in early disease.[1,2] Importantly, limb muscle dysfunction can be reversible, at least partially, with interventions such as exercise training.[3–5]

Arguably, the most perverse consequence of muscle dysfunction is its negative effect on life expectancy. Reduced mid-thigh cross-sectional

Disclosure Statement: This work was supported by the GSK/CIHR Chair on COPD at Université Laval.
[a] Centre de Recherche, Institut Universitaire de Cardiologie et de Pneumologie de Québec, 2725 chemin Ste-Foy, Université Laval, Québec G1V4G5, Canada; [b] Department of Community Medicine and Rehabilitation, Section of Physiotherapy. Umeå University, Umeå, Sweden; [c] ELEGI and COLT Laboratories, Queen's Medical Research Institute, The University of Edinburgh, 47 Little France Crescent, Edinburgh EH16 4TJ, UK; [d] Department of Respiratory Medicine, Royal Infirmary of Edinburgh, 51 Little France Crescent, Edinburgh EH 16 4SA, UK
* Corresponding author.
E-mail address: Francois.maltais@med.ulaval.ca

Clin Chest Med 40 (2019) 367–383
https://doi.org/10.1016/j.ccm.2019.02.013

area[6] and fat-free mass,[7] lower quadriceps strength,[8] and vastus lateralis fiber-type shift[9] are predictors of mortality in COPD. Limb muscle dysfunction also contributes to exercise intolerance. The links that exist between limb muscles and relevant clinical outcomes in COPD stress out the importance for clinicians to monitor body composition and muscle strength.

Features of Limb Muscle Dysfunction in Chronic Obstructive Pulmonary Disease

This section focuses on the quadriceps, because it is the most commonly investigated limb muscle in COPD and also because of its relevance of activities of daily living. The features of quadriceps dysfunction in COPD are summarized in **Fig. 1**. These include atrophy, fiber-type shift toward the glycolytic type II fibers, reduced oxidative capacity, and impaired mitochondrial function. The functional consequences of these morphologic and structural changes are muscle atrophy, weakness and reduced endurance. The *true* prevalence of muscle dysfunction in COPD is uncertain. Estimation varies according to the population being investigated and the criteria used to define dysfunction. In a population-based study consisting mostly of subjects with mild airflow limitation, investigators used bioelectrical impedance to report that 15% of patients with COPD exhibits low whole-body fat-free mass index.[10] In more advanced disease, fat-free mass, quadriceps atrophy, and weakness may occur in up to a third of patients with COPD.[1,11,12] One muscle biopsy study reported fiber-type shift in approximately one-third of patients and fiber atrophy in 20%.[13] Importantly, the process is heterogeneous across patients and quadriceps atrophy and weakness may also occur in mild disease.[2,10] Last, a preserved body mass index (BMI) does not exclude muscle atrophy and weakness.[2,10,12] Accordingly,

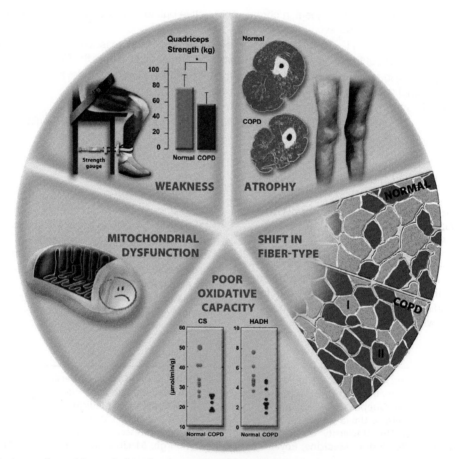

Fig. 1. Features of quadriceps dysfunction in COPD. (*Courtesy of* The American Thoracic Society, Copyright © 2018; with permission; and *Data from* Maltais F, Decramer M, Casaburi R, et al. An official American Thoracic Society/European Respiratory Society statement: update on limb muscle dysfunction in chronic obstructive pulmonary disease. Am J Respir Crit Care Med 2014;189:e15–62.)

one should not rely solely on BMI to predict muscle mass in patients with COPD. Lower limb muscles are particularly affected by the atrophying process in COPD. In 2 studies, mid-thigh cross-sectional area was reduced by 15% to 20% in patients with moderate COPD when compared with age-matched controls.[14]

Limb muscle endurance, defined as the ability to sustain a specific task over time is also common in COPD[15] and it has relevance to tasks of daily living.[16] Importantly, the impairment in muscle endurance cannot be predicted from muscle strength, highlighting that both aspects of muscle function should be evaluated.[17]

A shift in skeletal muscle fiber-type proportion of the quadriceps is one of the most constant features of limb muscle in COPD. In contrast to the decrease in type II fiber proportion typically seen with aging,[18] patients with COPD exhibit a reduction in type I fiber proportion in favor of type II in the quadriceps.[19] This fiber-type profile in COPD contributes to muscle susceptibility to fatigue[20] and it has been associated with mortality.[9] Consistent with this shift in fiber-type proportion, the activity of oxidative enzymes such as 3-hydroxyacyl-CoA dehydrogenase, essential for β-oxidation of the lipids, and citrate synthase, a rate-limiting enzyme of the citric acid cycle, is reduced in the COPD quadriceps,[21,22] whereas an increased activity of glycolytic enzymes has been reported in the same muscle.[22–24] Thus, these patients are likely to use less-effective metabolic pathways to produce ATP because Krebs cycle and β-oxidation pathways are downregulated in favor of the glycolytic metabolism in their quadriceps, a situation contributing to deterioration in exercise performance during endurance tasks.[24,25]

When compared with healthy controls, reduced mitochondrial density and function are seen in the limb muscle of patients with COPD.[26–31] Specific alterations in mitochondrial respiration independent of density also have been reported.[27,29–31] Besides their contribution to impaired oxidative metabolism, these mitochondrial alterations have been associated with enhanced skeletal muscle oxidative stress[27,31] that can lead to muscle protein breakdown and apoptosis,[32] mechanical inefficiency,[33] and exercise intolerance.[30,34]

Adequate oxygen delivery at the muscle cell level is essential for optimal muscle and exercise performance. In COPD, muscle blood flow and oxygen delivery may be compromised upstream from the muscles, in relation to possible impairment in cardiac output or to a blood flow redistribution phenomenon redirecting blood flow toward the respiratory muscles at the expense of lower limb muscles (further discussion in the topic is provided in Respiratory Determinants of Exercise Limitation: Focus on Phrenic Afferents and The Lung Vasculature).[35] Muscle microcirculation may also be affected in patients with COPD, as evidenced by a lower number of muscle capillaries and by the reduction of capillary contacts with oxidative fibers.[36,37] Near-infrared spectroscopy, which provides a noninvasive assessment of the microcirculation in contracting muscles,[38] has been used to document enhanced muscle extraction during exercise compatible with impaired microvascular function in COPD.[39]

> Atrophy, fiber-type shift toward the glycolytic type II fibers, reduced oxidative capacity, and impaired mitochondrial function are translated into muscle atrophy, weakness, and reduced endurance in patients with COPD with lower limb muscle dysfunction.

Limb Muscle Dysfunction and Exercise Intolerance in Chronic Obstructive Pulmonary Disease

Limb muscle dysfunction exerts a negative influence on important clinical outcomes such as mortality and exercise intolerance (**Fig. 2**). Despite the central role of the abnormal breathing mechanics (as discussed in The Pathophysiology of Dyspnea and Exercise Intolerance in COPD), clinical and research evidence support a contributing role of limb muscle dysfunction to exercise intolerance in COPD. In the early 1990s, it was noted that exercise intolerance could persist in double lung transplant recipients, despite normalization of lung function.[40] Furthermore, the degree of impairment in lung function is not a strong predictor of the severity of exercise intolerance[41] and leg fatigue, rather than dyspnea, is the exercise-limiting symptom in a proportion of patients with COPD.[42–44] Beyond the perceptual response, objective evidence of quadriceps fatigue, defined as a postexercise fall muscle force that recovers with rest, has been documented during exercise in patients with COPD.[43,45] Major supporting evidence for the role of limb muscle dysfunction in exercise intolerance is that the exercise response to acute bronchodilation is modulated by the presence of contractile fatigue of the quadriceps; when fatigue is present, the bronchodilator-induced improvement in lung function does not translate into better exercise capacity.[43] The occurrence of contractile fatigue after exercise is not in itself abnormal, but the problem in COPD

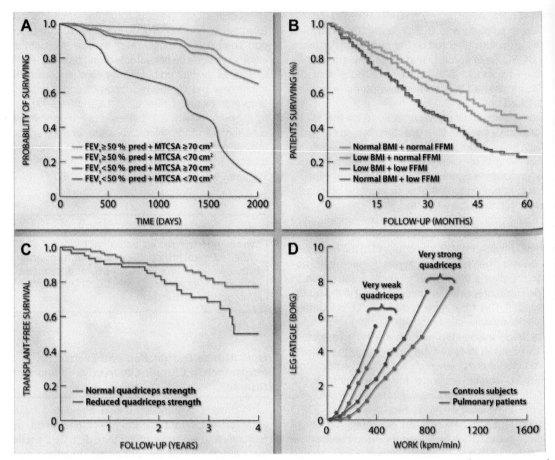

Fig. 2. The impact of limb muscle dysfunction in patients with COPD. Marquis and colleagues[6] (*A*), Schols and colleagues[7] (*B*), Swallow and colleagues[8] (*C*), and Hamilton and colleagues[56] (*D*). FEV1, forced expiratory volume in 1 second; FFMI, fat-free mass index; MTCSA, mid-thigh muscle cross sectional area. (*Courtesy of* The American Thoracic Society, Copyright © 2018; with permission; and *Data from* Maltais F, Decramer M, Casaburi R, et al. An official American Thoracic Society/European Respiratory Society statement: update on limb muscle dysfunction in chronic obstructive pulmonary disease. Am J Respir Crit Care Med 2014;189:e15–62.)

is that it occurs at a much lower exercise intensity than in healthy individuals.[46] Patients with COPD are therefore disadvantaged while performing daily activities because they are vulnerable to fatigue, even during mildly intense exercise (further discussion in the topic is provided in Strategies to Increase Physical Activity in Chronic Respiratory Diseases).

Susceptibility to muscle fatigue in COPD is assumed to be related to the reduction in the proportion of fatigue-resistant muscle fibers and in oxidative enzyme activity.[30,34,36] These phenotypic and enzymatic muscle changes modify muscle energy metabolism during exercise, resulting in a higher reliance on carbohydrate utilization, premature muscle acidosis, lactate accumulation, and fatigue.[34,47,48] The idea of a competition for blood flow between limb and respiratory muscles

has been set forward as an important cause of peripheral muscle fatigue in COPD.[35] However, unloading the respiratory muscles with noninvasive ventilatory support, presumably reducing their blood flow requirement to the benefit of the contracting leg muscles, only partially reduces quadriceps fatigue (by approximately one-third) supporting the view that susceptibility to fatigue in COPD is largely related to intrinsic muscle alterations.[35]

A remarkable observation is that the degree of muscle fatigue reached during exercise may not be simply a mere consequence of exercise but rather a tightly regulated variable.[49] The nature and location of the "fatigue controller" is still a matter of dispute.[50,51] One theory supports the existence of a line of communication between the contracting muscles and the brain. According to this theory, afferent feedback signals, originating from mechanosensitive and metabosensitive receptors within the contracting muscles and traveling to the central nervous system via metaboreceptive A-δ (group III) and C fibers (group IV), lead to the inhibition the central motor drive thus preventing subsequent locomotor recruitment and the development of dangerous and potentially irreversible fatigue.[49,52] Importantly, this neural pathway is also involved in orchestrating the ventilatory and circulatory responses to exercise, an observation that might have special relevance to patients with COPD who are ventilatory limited and in whom this pathway may even be more activated than in healthy individuals (further discussion in the topic is provided in Respiratory Determinants of Exercise Limitation: Focus on Phrenic Afferents and The Lung Vasculature).[53] An elegant way to document how feedback information from the lower limbs modulates central motor output is to interrupt the communication between the contracting muscles and the central command with spinal (L3-L4) anesthesia with intrathecal fentanyl injection. This drug attenuates the activity of the nociceptive group III/IV sensory afferent signalization without inducing motor blockade. In athletes, this methodology does not affect overall performance because of an initial overshoot in the central command that could not be maintained throughout exercise.[54] However, the degree of muscle fatigue achieved is increased by 40% under spinal anesthesia, providing a clear indication of the importance of the feedback originating within the contracting muscles in the regulation of muscle fatigue. Using a similar approach, the influences of the sensory afferent signals from the lower limb muscles on exercise performance in patients with COPD were documented.[55] In COPD, spinal anesthesia attenuates the ventilatory response during exercise in COPD as well as the perception of dyspnea and leg fatigue.[55] As a result, the central inhibition of exercise is unlocked and central motor output to the contracting muscles is increased, allowing patients to exercise for longer and to develop a deeper degree of fatigue. Exercise limitation in COPD should be considered from an integrative perspective in which lower limb muscles contribute to poor exercise tolerance via several mechanisms, including enhanced perception of fatigue[56] and the stimulation of group III/IV sensory afferents that in turn enhance ventilatory requirements, dynamic hyperinflation, and dyspnea. This vicious circle is further promoted by reduced limb muscle oxidative capacity,[24,57] which is likely to enhance the degree of stimulation from metaboreceptors.

> Exercise limitation in COPD should be considered from an integrative perspective in which lower limb muscles contribute to poor exercise tolerance via several mechanisms, including enhanced perception of fatigue and the stimulation of group III/IV sensory afferents that in turn enhance ventilatory requirements, dynamic hyperinflation, and dyspnea.

Mechanisms of Muscle Dysfunction in Patients with Chronic Obstructive Pulmonary Disease

The origin of limb muscle dysfunction is most likely multifactorial, with possible contribution from malnutrition, chronic inactivity, hypoxemia, oxidative stress, and systemic inflammation. However, none of these mechanisms is fully satisfactory[58] and their relative contribution is likely to vary according to the clinical context. The molecular mechanisms involved in the loss of muscle tissue is intensely investigated,[59] hoping that this will lead to new treatments specific for this condition.[60]

Despite cigarette smoking being the main risk factor for COPD, its impact on limb muscle has received little attention. The available information suggests that smoking tobacco is associated with reduced muscle mass,[61] increased oxidative stress,[62] and a shift toward type II fibers.[63] An interesting debate is whether chronic inactivity is the sole culprit of limb muscle dysfunction in COPD or if a specific form of muscle disease exists in this condition. Proponents of the chronic inactivity theory contend that reduced physical activity is ubiquitous in COPD,[64,65] and that limb muscle adaptation seen in COPD is typical of what is seen in sedentary individuals (further discussion in the topic is provided in Strategies to Increase Physical Activity in Chronic Respiratory Diseases).[66,67] Another line of argument is that limb muscle function improves with exercise training (see later in this article). On the other hand, several observations favor the existence of a specific muscle disease in COPD. For example, muscle impairment in COPD is poorly related to the degree of physical activity,[13,31,34] and differences in muscle structure and function persist between patients with COPD and healthy controls even when controlling for physical activity.[31,68] Furthermore, exercise training does not fully restore limb muscle structure and function[3,14]; some investigators even argue that the COPD limb muscle may not respond normally to exercise training.[69–71] Despite the attempt for controlling the level of physical activities in human investigations, there are obvious methodological limits of this experimental approach. For example, although matching patients with COPD and healthy controls for the level of physical activity at a specific moment in their life is likely feasible, it is uncertain whether the same could be done with lifelong physical activity profile. In one animal investigation in which physical activity was tightly matched between emphysematous and healthy hamsters reported a decreased muscle oxidative capacity in the former animals, supporting that factors other than physical inactivity play a role in limb muscle dysfunction in COPD.[72] In summary, the debate surrounding physical inactivity and limb muscle dysfunction in COPD is not fully resolved. The thinking is nevertheless evolving,[31,73] with accumulating evidence supporting the view that this consequence of COPD is unlikely to be the sole consequence of physical inactivity.

Muscle dysfunction may be aggravated during episodes of COPD exacerbation[74,75] during which inflammatory bursts, reduction in physical activity, and exposure to systemic corticosteroids all concur to further loss in muscle mass and strength,[74–77] and consequently in functional status. This should not be neglected considering that muscle weakness[78] and atrophy[79] and low functional status are predictors of readmission in COPD.[77]

> The origin of limb muscle dysfunction is most likely multifactorial with possible contribution from malnutrition, chronic inactivity, hypoxemia, oxidative stress, and systemic inflammation. The relative contribution of these underlying mechanisms is likely to vary according to the clinical context.

HOW TO ASSESS LIMB MUSCLES IN CLINICAL PRACTICE
Body Composition

Beyond weight loss, a 2-compartment model of body composition, provides a more accurate approach to assess the impact of chronic conditions such as COPD on muscle mass. This model divides the body mass into fat-free mass and fat mass. In clinical practice, 2 methods are available to measure body composition with reasonable accuracy. Bioelectrical impedance analysis is based on the higher conductivity of an electric current through fat-free mass than fat mass.[80] Bioelectrical impedance measures a voltage drop between 2 electrodes, enabling the determination of total body water, and subsequently fat-free

mass. When longitudinal assessments are needed, it is therefore recommended to the measurements under the same fluid balance conditions, at the same time of the day. Although multifrequency analyzers exist, most bioelectrical impedance equipment use a single frequency current of 50 kHz. Bioelectrical impedance is low-cost, noninvasive, quick, and does not require patient's collaboration. This technique has been validated against total body water assessed by deuterium dilution in COPD.[81] When estimating fat-free mass from bioelectrical impedance, equations that have been validated in the population studied should be used instead of built-in equations provided by manufacturers.[82,83] Dual-energy X-ray absorptiometry (DEXA) scan is based on the comparison of X-ray attenuations of 2 different energies measuring total body composition and fat content. Similar to bioelectrical impedance, this method does not require patient collaboration and is considered valid and reliable to assess fat-free mass in COPD.[58,84] The method is more expensive and less accessible than bioelectrical impedance. DEXA provides systematically higher values for fat-free mass compared with other techniques such as deuterium dilution[85] and bioelectrical impedance.[82–84] DEXA results may differ between different commercial devices; this is particularly important when longitudinal assessments are made.

Muscle Strength

Volitional muscle strength can be measured with numerous devices, including strain gauge, hand-held dynamometer, and more complex systems, such as computerized dynamometers, weight machines, or manual muscle testing[86] (**Table 1**). Muscle strength can be assessed independently from a patient's motivation and effort with electrical or magnetic stimulations of the muscle or its motor nerve[87]; these techniques are usually in the realm of clinical research.

When choosing how to assess muscle strength in COPD, clinicians must consider the advantages and limitations of the different standardized protocols (number of trials, rest periods), devices, and techniques (static or dynamic).[88,89] During static testing (isometric), the tested limb is fixed and there is no change in muscle length throughout the contraction. Measuring isometric quadriceps strength has been recommended by the 2014 joint statement of the American Thoracic Society and European Respiratory Society[58] because it is related to mortality[8] and responsive to intervention, such as exercise training.[90] However, this parameter is less informative about the ability to

Table 1
Devices and protocols used to assess limb muscle strength and endurance in patients with COPD

Measuring equipment	1. Strain gauge or fixed handheld systems	2. Computerized dynamometers	3. Repetition maximum	4. Handgrip gauges
Type of contraction	Isometric (static)	Isometric (static) and isokinetic (dynamic)	Isotonic (dynamic)	Isometric (static)
Picture of measurement/ device				
Positioning of tested limbs in COPD studies	Knee and hip flexed at 90°; Elbow and/or shoulder flexed at 90°.	Isometric: Elbow flexed at 90° Knee flexed 60° - 120°. Isokinetic: Knee flexed at 90° to full knee extension.	Not well described in COPD studies.	Elbow flexed at 90° with arm unsupported.
Measurements of muscle strength in COPD studies	Perform 3–5 MVC, each lasting 3–5 s with at least 30-s rest between attempts. Highest value used as measurement of strength.	Isometric: Perform 3–5 MVC and 1–2 min rest between attempts (hold each contraction for 3–5 s). Highest value used as measurement of strength. Isokinetic: Perform MVC over the joint range of motion at the preset velocity (usually 60 or 90/s for quadriceps and 30, 90 or 120/s for elbow flexion), for 1 set of 3–5 contractions. Peak torque determined as the highest average value reached over 250 ms during the test.	Not well described in COPD studies. Follow ACSM recommendations + use metronome and control start and stop positions.	Perform 3 MVC with each lasting at least 3 s and 30–60 s of rest between attempts. Highest value used as measurement of strength.

Measurements of muscle endurance in COPD studies	Measure the time during which a contraction at 60%–80% of MVC can be maintained in one set, until exhaustion. Audio or visual feedback is allowed to control targeted range of MVC.	*Isometric:* Measure the time during which a submaximal contraction (60% ± 5% of MVC) is maintained, until exhaustion. *Isokinetic:* Measure the total amount of work performed from 1 set of 30 MVC at 60° or 90°/s.	Number of repetitions performed. One set of dynamic contractions at 30%–40% of MVC until exhaustion + use metronome and control start and stop positions.	Measure the time during which a contraction at 50% ± 5% can be maintained until exhaustion. Audio or visual feedback is allowed to control targeted range of MVC.
Advantages	Results are valid, reliable and reproducible when dynamometers are fixed. Easy to use, portable, time efficient and inexpensive.	Results are valid, reliable and reproducible. Easy to standardize. Different speeds and angles could be tested.	Assesses muscle function in the whole range of motion. Can be executed using available equipment (eg, elastic bands, free weights, pulley systems).	No familiarization, easy to use, easy to standardize. Part of frailty and sarcopenia screening assessments.
Limitations	Measures only in one angle. Standardization is crucial for validity and reliability.	Low availability. Requires expensive equipment. Needs familiarization session.	Time-consuming and more difficult to standardize than isometric measurements. Underestimation of strength is possible (induced fatigue) if many attempts are needed.	Measures only handgrip strength.

Abbreviations: ACSM, American College of Sports Medicine; COPD, chronic obstructive pulmonary disease; MVC, maximal voluntary contraction.
Courtesy of The American Thoracic Society. Copyright © 2018; with permission; and *Data from* Nyberg A, Saey D, Maltais F. Why and how limb muscle mass and function should be measured in patients with chronic obstructive pulmonary disease. Ann Am Thorac Soc 2015;12:1269–77.

perform functional tasks as a part of daily living. Handgrip isometric strength is also commonly assessed in COPD studies because of its ease of use,[86] but its clinical purpose is yet unclear in COPD, where it does not appear to be decreased more than in the general older population nor associated with disease severity.[91] However, handgrip strength testing is part of frailty assessment and sarcopenia screening that are closely associated with muscle function and functional status.[92,93]

Assessing strength dynamically with isokinetic (fixed speed of movement) and isotonic (fixed resistance applied to the muscle during the movement) tests might more accurately reflect functional activities. Computerized dynamometers are considered to be the gold standard instrument and provide reliable measures of muscle strength in COPD,[94,95] but are mostly used in research settings because they are more expensive and require more space. Simpler and less costly instruments that nevertheless provide valid and reliable results such as fixed handheld dynamometers are more likely to be implemented in clinical practice. Isometric and isotonic muscle strength reference values using different devices are available, even though not yet widely used.[96–99]

How to Measure Muscle Strength

Standardization of limb position, performing ≥3 maximal voluntary contractions (MVC) held for 4 to 5 seconds, spaced with 1-minute rest periods are important to obtain valid and reproducible results.[86,98,100,101] Underestimation of muscle strength is possible if the clinician is unsuccessful in opposing sufficient force to keep the tested limb in the static position[102]; this is particularly true for strong muscles such as the quadriceps. Fixing the portable dynamometer on a rigid support thus becomes an interesting way to avoid this evaluator-based bias, and was recently shown to be reliable and valid in COPD.[103,104] Strong continuous verbal encouragements should be given and familiarization should be performed with warm-up trials to diminish any possible learning bias or underestimation of one's strength.[105] The peak torque recorded is usually the highest value from 2 to 3 reproducible maneuvers.[58,103,104]

Isokinetic strength assessment is usually performed at a fixed angular velocity of 60° to 90° per second for quadriceps strength assessment in COPD studies.[86,106] Isotonic muscle strength can be assessed with hydraulic resistance devices, force transducer platforms adapted to weight machines, or with 1-repetition

maximum (1-RM) tests.[86] The latter requires little material (from simple elastic bands and free weights to more complex pulley systems and computerized dynamometers), is easily conductible in clinical settings with patients with COPD, and represents the highest load that can be lifted once throughout the whole range of motion.[86,88] We advise clinicians to strictly follow the standardized procedure from the American College of Sports Medicine,[99] even if information on crucial elements, such as positioning, warm-up, number of trials, velocity of the movement, rest period, and familiarization, often lack in COPD studies.[86] 1-RM strength testing is safe and well tolerated by patients with COPD,[107] but this measurement can be time-consuming and it may induce fatigue if it takes too many attempts to find the optimal load for testing. Familiarization with the procedure is necessary to prevent learning bias from neural adaptations.[86,108]

> Volitional muscle strength can be measured with numerous devices, including strain gauge, handheld dynamometer, and more complex systems, such as computerized dynamometers, weight machines, or manual muscle testing.

Muscle Endurance

Limb muscle endurance refers to a muscle's ability to sustain or repeat a specific task over time.[99] It reflects the ability to perform tasks requiring a small number of submaximal contractions, such as climbing a set of stairs as well as tasks requiring a multitude of submaximal contractions such as bicycling or walking over a long distance. Even though both types of tasks involve the endurance quality of the muscle, it is obvious that the same assessment method cannot be used to evaluate muscle performance in both situations and that no single test can evaluate all aspects of limb muscle endurance.[15,99] Limb muscle endurance can be reliably measured using static (isometric) or dynamic strategies (isokinetic, isotonic) and by using either sustained or repeated contractions performed at a specific intensity. Irrespective of the selected strategy, subjects should be familiarized with the procedures and the measuring conditions should be standardized.[109]

How to Measure Muscle Endurance

Static measurements of limb muscle endurance are performed by asking the subject to maintain a muscle contraction at an intensity corresponding to a prespecified intensity of their MVC (typically between 50% and 80% MVC), until exhaustion[15,20] (see **Table 1**). Isokinetic endurance and fatigue assessment protocols are performed at a fixed angular velocity during maximal contraction(s) and throughout the whole joint range of motion. An angular velocity of 90° per second is recommended for assessment of isokinetic muscle endurance and fatigue in patients with COPD.[95] Results of such assessments can be expressed as either the total work developed during the procedure, as a fatigue index, for example, the ratio of work performed during the last 10 repetitions to the work performed during the first 10 repetitions,[95] or as the rate of decline in muscle work over time.[95] Isotonic endurance protocols are performed with a constant external loading and by controlling the range of motion and speed of movement (eg, using a metronome) to minimize variation in testing.[88] In COPD, external loads corresponding to 10% up to 50% of the individual MVC have been used during repeated contractions performed until failure.[17,110] Results are quantified by reporting the time or number of repetitions performed.[15,110] An advantage of isotonic muscle testing over isometric and isokinetic techniques is that it could be performed using simple equipment, such as elastic bands,[110] exercise platforms/benches,[17] or pulley systems.[111]

> Limb muscle endurance refers to a muscle's ability to sustain or repeat a specific task over time. It is an important muscle characteristic, as it affects the patient's ability to perform tasks requiring a small number of submaximal contractions, such as climbing a set of stairs, as well as tasks requiring a multitude of submaximal contractions, such as bicycling or walking over a long distance.

Treatment of Limb Muscle Dysfunction

Exercise training, nutritional supplementation alone, or in combination with an anabolic stimulus have been shown to improve at various aspects of muscle function, resulting in better quality of life and enhanced exercise tolerance in COPD.[58] In this article, we focus on exercise training, the most effective and available treatment for this condition. The "conventional" training modalities include aerobic/endurance training and strength/resistive exercises or a combination of these 2 training modalities.[58,112] Continuous or interval aerobic training improves muscle oxidative capacity,[5] whereas specific resistance training has a greater potential to improve muscle mass, strength, and endurance than whole-body aerobic training.[113]

The optimal characteristics of continuous and interval endurance aerobic training are summarized in **Table 2**. The main objective of this training modality is to improve aerobic exercise capacity. Determination of adequate frequency, duration, and intensity of training are all thought to be important. It is generally recommended that aerobic training include 3 weekly 20-minute to 30-minute exercise sessions for 8 to 12 weeks. Even though the optimal intensity is still debatable in COPD, greater physiologic and muscle training responses and larger improvements in submaximal exercise tolerance have been obtained when training at high intensity (>60% of maximal work rate) compared with low intensity (below 50% of maximal work rate).[48,114] However, additional physiologic benefits of a high-intensity training program, do not necessarily translate into additional gains in quality of life[114] and high-intensity training cannot be achieved in all patients.[115] Therefore, interval training, in which 2 to 3 minutes of high-intensity exercise are interspersed with lower intensity exercise or even rest periods may allow the most disabled patient to reach an adequate training stimulus.[116,117] Portioning exercise training is another strategy that can be used to improve tolerance to whole-body aerobic exercise[118]

The main physiologic response to aerobic training consists of structural changes in the cardiovascular and limb muscle systems; these account for improvements in the capacity to transport and use oxygen and in exercise capacity.[119] Increases in muscle oxidative capacity and cross-sectional area of all muscle fiber types,[5,36,120,121] as well as reduction in proportion of type IIx fibers[5,121] and in exercise-induced lactate production are usually reported after aerobic training in patients with COPD.[5,58,121] Functionally, improved muscle strength and endurance are consistently observed after aerobic training in patients with COPD.[3,4,112,113,122,123] These positive muscle adaptations contribute to improve exercise tolerance, reduce dyspnea and leg fatigue perception leading to better quality of life.[124]

It is important to tailor the muscle training intervention to the specific needs of the patient. Greater effects on muscle mass and strength are expected with resistance training protocols that use relatively large weights (80%–100% of 1RM) and a low number of repetitions (often 1–12 repetitions).[125] In contrast, limb muscle endurance and resistance to muscle fatigue will be most improved by training strategies using lower weights (30%–80% of 1RM) with a high number of repetitions (often 15–25 repetitions). The suggested optimal

Table 2
Characteristics of specific resistance training regimens and continuous/interval endurance aerobic training

	Muscle Training			Aerobic Training
Modalities/Exercise selection	Upper and lower limb exercises Weight machine, pulley systems, exercise platforms/benches free weight, body weight, elastic band			Large muscle mass Walking, cycling, stair, steps, rowing, and so forth
Loading	*Strength* 80%–100% of 1RM	*Strength-endurance* 70%–85% of 1RM	*Endurance* 30%–80% of 1RM	*High Intensity* (60%–80% maximal work rate or RPE of 12–14) *Low intensity* (<50% maximal work rate) or RPE of 10–12)
Volume/duration	1–3 sets of 1–12 repetitions	3 sets of 8–12 repetitions	1–3 sets of 10–15 repetitions	*Interval training:* At least 20 min per session (2 or 3 min of high intensity interspersed with 1 or 2 min of lower intensity or rest)
Frequency	4–5 d wk^{-1} (maintenance 1–2 d wk^{-1})	2–4 d wk^{-1} (maintenance 2 d wk^{-1})	2–4 d wk^{-1} (maintenance 1–2 d wk^{-1})	3 d wk^{-1}
Progression	Increase number of repetitions before loading 2%–10% increase			Increase duration before intensity
Duration program	8–12 wk Minimum 20 training sessions			8–12 wk Minimum 20 training sessions

Abbreviations: D wk^{-1}, days a week; RM, maximal repetition; RPE, rating of perceived exertion; RPE, rating of perceived exertion on a 6 to 20 Borg rating of perceived exertion scale.

characteristics of resistance training programs are summarized in **Table 2**.[126]

The effects of resistance training on muscle structure include increases in type II fiber size, enhanced expression of muscle IGF-1,[127,128] as well as increases in mid-thigh cross-sectional area, diminished inflammation and stimulation of satellite cells (which maintain muscle mass and contribute in muscle fibers regeneration).[129] Rigorous resistance muscle training is also feasible for people with COPD as evidenced by high levels of adherence and few or any adverse events. The tolerability of resistance training is considered to be superior to aerobic training because it results in less dyspnea, allowing more patients to reach targeted exercise intensities, thus optimizing the training effects. Greater effects on muscle strength are obtained with resistance training in comparison with aerobic training alone or when resistance training is added to an aerobic training protocol.[123,130] Interestingly, the improvement in muscle function induced by resistance training may translate into better performance of some daily activities[131] and to larger improvement in health-related quality of life than aerobic training.[132]

Because limb muscle function is likely to be impaired during exacerbation and hospitalization, several interventions to prevent or counteract muscle impairment during these episodes have been successfully considered.[74,75] Resistance training initiated during hospitalization may prevent further deterioration in limb muscle function.

Exercise training, nutritional supplementation alone, or in combination with anabolic stimulation have been shown to improve various aspects of muscle function, resulting in better quality of life and enhanced exercise tolerance in COPD.

SUMMARY

Limb muscle dysfunction is a clinically relevant manifestation of COPD, influencing important clinical outcomes, such as exercise capacity, health-related quality of life, and even survival. Although not currently routinely performed in clinical practice, simple and valid measuring tools exist to quantify muscle strength and mass. Clinicians are therefore encouraged to use them to assess limb muscle function in patients with COPD. Doing so may attract the attention of the medical team toward a potentially treatable cause of exercise intolerance and disability.

REFERENCES

1. Seymour JM, Spruit MA, Hopkinson NS, et al. The prevalence of quadriceps weakness in COPD and the relationship with disease severity. Eur Respir J 2010;36:81–8.
2. Shrikrishna D, Patel M, Tanner RJ, et al. Quadriceps wasting and physical inactivity in patients with COPD. Eur Respir J 2012;40:1115–22.
3. Bernard S, Whittom F, Leblanc P, et al. Aerobic and strength training in patients with COPD. Am J Respir Crit Care Med 1999;159:896–901.
4. Ortega F, Toral J, Cejudo P, et al. Comparison of effects of strength and endurance training in patients with chronic obstructive pulmonary disease. Am J Respir Crit Care Med 2002;166:669–74.
5. Vogiatzis I, Terzis G, Nanas S, et al. Skeletal muscle adaptations to interval training in patients with advanced COPD. Chest 2005;128:3838–45.
6. Marquis K, Debigaré R, LeBlanc P, et al. Mid-thigh muscle cross-sectional area is a better predictor of mortality than body mass index in patients with COPD. Am J Respir Crit Care Med 2002;166:809–13.
7. Schols AM, Broekhuizen R, Weling-Scheepers CA, et al. Body composition and mortality in chronic obstructive pulmonary disease. Am J Clin Nutr 2005;82:53–9.
8. Swallow EB, Reyes D, Hopkinson NS, et al. Quadriceps strength predicts mortality in patients with moderate to severe chronic obstructive pulmonary disease. Thorax 2007;62:115–20.
9. Patel MS, Natanek SA, Stratakos G, et al. Vastus lateralis fiber shift is an independent predictor of mortality in chronic obstructive pulmonary disease. Am J Respir Crit Care Med 2014;190:350–2.
10. Vestbo J, Prescott E, Almdal T, et al. Body mass, fat-free body mass, and prognosis in patients with chronic obstructive pulmonary disease from a random population sample: findings from the Copenhagen City Heart Study. Am J Respir Crit Care Med 2006;173:79–83.
11. Engelen MPKJ, Schols AMWJ, Baken WC, et al. Nutritional depletion in relation to respiratory and peripheral skeletal muscle function in out-patients with COPD. Eur Respir J 1994;7:1793–7.
12. Schols AMWJ, Soeters PB, Dingemans MC, et al. Prevalence and characteristics of nutritional depletion in patients with stable COPD eligible for pulmonary rehabilitation. Am Rev Respir Dis 1993;147:1151–6.
13. Natanek SA, Gosker HR, Slot IG, et al. Heterogeneity of quadriceps muscle phenotype in chronic obstructive pulmonary disease (COPD); implications for stratified medicine? Muscle Nerve 2013;48(4):488–97.

14. Bernard S, Leblanc P, Whittom F, et al. Peripheral muscle weakness in patients with chronic obstructive pulmonary disease. Am J Respir Crit Care Med 1998;158:629–34.

15. Evans RA, Kaplovitch E, Beauchamp MK, et al. Is quadriceps endurance reduced in COPD? Chest 2015;147:673–84.

16. Nyberg A, Tornberg A, Wadell K. Correlation between limb muscle endurance, strength, and functional capacity in people with chronic obstructive pulmonary disease. Physiother Can 2016;68:46–53.

17. Coronell C, Orozco-Levi M, Mendez R, et al. Relevance of assessing quadriceps endurance in patients with COPD. Eur Respir J 2004;24:129–36.

18. Larsson L. Histochemical characteristics of human skeletal muscle during aging. Acta Physiol Scand 1983;117:469–71.

19. Gosker HR, Zeegers MP, Wouters EF, et al. Muscle fibre type shifting in the vastus lateralis of patients with COPD is associated with disease severity: a systematic review and meta-analysis. Thorax 2007;62:944–9.

20. Allaire J, Maltais F, Doyon JF, et al. Peripheral muscle endurance and the oxidative profile of the quadriceps in patients with COPD. Thorax 2004;59:673–8.

21. Maltais F, Leblanc P, Whittom F, et al. Oxidative enzyme activities of the vastus lateralis muscle and the functional status in patients with COPD. Thorax 2000;55:848–53.

22. Green HJ, Bombardier E, Burnett M, et al. Organization of metabolic pathways in vastus lateralis of patients with chronic obstructive pulmonary disease. Am J Physiol Regul Integr Comp Physiol 2008;295:R935–41.

23. Jakobsson P, Jorfeldt L, Henriksson J. Metabolic enzyme activity in the quadriceps femoris muscle in patients with severe chronic obstructive pulmonary disease. Am J Respir Crit Care Med 1995;151:374–7.

24. Saey D, Lemire BB, Gagnon P, et al. Quadriceps metabolism during constant workrate cycling exercise in chronic obstructive pulmonary disease. J Appl Physiol 2011;110:116–24.

25. Saey D, Michaud A, Couillard A, et al. Contractile fatigue, muscle morphometry, and blood lactate in chronic obstructive pulmonary disease. Am J Respir Crit Care Med 2005;171:1109–15.

26. Gosker HR, Hesselink MK, Duimel H, et al. Reduced mitochondrial density in the vastus lateralis muscle of patients with COPD. Eur Respir J 2007;30:73–9.

27. Puente-Maestu L, Perez-Parra J, Godoy R, et al. Abnormal mitochondrial function in locomotor and respiratory muscles of COPD patients. Eur Respir J 2009;33:1045–52.

28. Picard M, Godin R, Sinnreich M, et al. The mitochondrial phenotype of peripheral muscle in chronic obstructive pulmonary disease: disuse or dysfunction? Am J Respir Crit Care Med 2008;178:1040–7.

29. Naimi AI, Bourbeau J, Perrault H, et al. Altered mitochondrial regulation in quadriceps muscles of patients with COPD. Clin Physiol Funct Imaging 2011;31:124–31.

30. Gifford JR, Trinity JD, Layec G, et al. Quadriceps exercise intolerance in patients with chronic obstructive pulmonary disease: the potential role of altered skeletal muscle mitochondrial respiration. J Appl Physiol 2015;119:882–8.

31. Gifford JR, Trinity JD, Kwon OS, et al. Altered skeletal muscle mitochondrial phenotype in COPD: disease vs. disuse. J Appl Physiol 2018;124:1045–53.

32. Taivassalo T, Hussain SN. Contribution of the mitochondria to locomotor muscle dysfunction in patients with COPD. Chest 2016;149:1302–12.

33. Layec G, Haseler LJ, Hoff J, et al. Evidence that a higher ATP cost of muscular contraction contributes to the lower mechanical efficiency associated with COPD: preliminary findings. Am J Physiol Regul Integr Comp Physiol 2011;300:R1142–7.

34. van den Borst B, Slot IG, Hellwig VA, et al. Loss of quadriceps muscle oxidative phenotype and decreased endurance in patients with mild-to-moderate COPD. J Appl Physiol 2013;114:1319–28.

35. Amann M, Regan MS, Kobitary M, et al. Impact of pulmonary system limitations on locomotor muscle fatigue in patients with COPD. Am J Physiol Regul Integr Comp Physiol 2010;299:R314–24.

36. Whittom F, Jobin J, Simard PM, et al. Histochemical and morphological characteristics of the vastus lateralis muscle in COPD patients. Comparison with normal subjects and effects of exercise training. Med Sci Sports Exerc 1998;30:1467–74.

37. Eliason G, Abdel-Halim SM, Piehl-Aulin K, et al. Alterations in the muscle-to-capillary interface in patients with different degrees of chronic obstructive pulmonary disease. Respir Res 2010;11:97.

38. Mancini D. Application of near infrared spectroscopy to the evaluation of exercise performance and limitations in patients with heart failure. J Biomed Opt 1997;2:22–30.

39. Chiappa GR, Borghi-Silva A, Ferreira LF, et al. Kinetics of muscle deoxygenation are accelerated at the onset of heavy-intensity exercise in patients with COPD: relationship to central cardiovascular dynamics. J Appl Physiol 2008;104:1341–50.

40. Williams TJ, Patterson GA, McClean PA, et al. Maximal exercise testing in single and double lung transplant recipients. Am Rev Respir Dis 1992;145:101–5.

41. Jones NL, Killian KJ, Cherniack NS. Limitation of exercise in chronic airway obstruction. Chronic obstructive pulmonary disease. Philadelphia: W.B. Saunders; 1991. p. 196–206.

42. Killian KJ, Leblanc P, Martin DH, et al. Exercise capacity and ventilatory, circulatory, and symptom limitation in patients with airflow limitation. Am Rev Respir Dis 1992;146:935–40.

43. Saey D, Debigaré R, LeBlanc P, et al. Contractile leg fatigue after cycle exercise: a factor limiting exercise in patients with COPD. Am J Respir Crit Care Med 2003;168:425–30.

44. Ofir D, Laveneziana P, Webb KA, et al. Mechanisms of dyspnea during cycle exercise in symptomatic patients with gold stage i chronic obstructive pulmonary disease. Am J Respir Crit Care Med 2008;177:622–9.

45. Mador MJ, Kufel TJ, Pineda L. Quadriceps fatigue following cycle exercise in patients with COPD. Am J Respir Crit Care Med 2000;161:447–53.

46. Mador MJ, Bozkanat E, Kufel TJ. Quadriceps fatigue after cycle exercise in patients with COPD compared with healthy control subjects. Chest 2003;123:1104–11.

47. Maltais F, Simard AA, Simard C, et al. Oxidative capacity of the skeletal muscle and lactic acid kinetics during exercise in normal subjects and in patients with COPD. Am J Respir Crit Care Med 1996;153:288–93.

48. Casaburi R, Patessio A, Ioli F, et al. Reductions in exercise lactic acidosis and ventilation as a result of exercise training in patients with obstructive lung disease. Am Rev Respir Dis 1991;143:9–18.

49. Amann M, Dempsey JA. Locomotor muscle fatigue modifies central motor drive in healthy humans and imposes a limitation to exercise performance. J Physiol 2008;586:161–73.

50. Marcora S. Is peripheral locomotor muscle fatigue during endurance exercise a variable carefully regulated by a negative feedback system? J Physiol 2008;586:2027–8 [author reply: 2029–30].

51. Hureau TJ, Romer LM, Amann M. The 'sensory tolerance limit': a hypothetical construct determining exercise performance? Eur J Sport Sci 2018;18:13–24.

52. Gandevia SC. Spinal and supraspinal factors in human muscle fatigue. Physiol Rev 2001;81:1725–89.

53. Bruce RM, Turner A, White MJ. Ventilatory responses to muscle metaboreflex activation in chronic obstructive pulmonary disease. J Physiol 2016;594:6025–35.

54. Amann M, Proctor LT, Sebranek JJ, et al. Opioid-mediated muscle afferents inhibit central motor drive and limit peripheral muscle fatigue development in humans. J Physiol 2009;587:271–83.

55. Gagnon P, Bussieres JS, Ribeiro F, et al. Influences of spinal anesthesia on exercise tolerance in patients with chronic obstructive pulmonary disease. Am J Respir Crit Care Med 2012;186:606–15.

56. Hamilton AL, Killian KJ, Summers E, et al. Muscle strength, symptom intensity and exercise capacity in patients with cardiorespiratory disorders. Am J Respir Crit Care Med 1995;152:2021–31.

57. Maltais F, Jobin J, Sullivan MJ, et al. Metabolic and hemodynamic responses of the lower limb during exercise in patients with COPD. J Appl Physiol 1998;84:1573–80.

58. Maltais F, Decramer M, Casaburi R, et al. An Official American Thoracic Society/European Respiratory Society Statement: update on limb muscle dysfunction in chronic obstructive pulmonary disease. Am J Respir Crit Care Med 2014;189:e15–62.

59. Barreiro E, Jaitovich A. Muscle atrophy in chronic obstructive pulmonary disease: molecular basis and potential therapeutic targets. J Thorac Dis 2018;10:S1415–24.

60. Polkey MI, Praestgaard J, Berwick A, et al. Activin type II receptor blockade for treatment of muscle depletion in COPD: a randomized trial. Am J Respir Crit Care Med 2019;199(3):313–20.

61. van den Borst B, Koster A, Yu B, et al. Is age-related decline in lean mass and physical function accelerated by obstructive lung disease or smoking? Thorax 2011;66:961–9.

62. Barreiro E, Peinado VI, Galdiz JB, et al. Cigarette smoke-induced oxidative stress: a role in COPD skeletal muscle dysfunction. Am J Respir Crit Care Med 2010;182(4):477–88.

63. Montes de Oca M, Loeb E, Torres SH, et al. Peripheral muscle alterations in non-COPD smokers. Chest 2008;133:13–8.

64. Pitta F, Troosters T, Spruit MA, et al. Characteristics of physical activities in daily life in chronic obstructive pulmonary disease. Am J Respir Crit Care Med 2005;171:972–7.

65. Troosters T, Sciurba F, Battaglia S, et al. Physical inactivity in patients with COPD, a controlled multi-center pilot-study. Respir Med 2010;104:1005–11.

66. Franssen FM, Wouters EF, Schols AM. The contribution of starvation, deconditioning and ageing to the observed alterations in peripheral skeletal muscle in chronic organ diseases. Clin Nutr 2002;21:1–14.

67. Remels AH, Schrauwen P, Broekhuizen R, et al. Peroxisome proliferator-activated receptor expression is reduced in skeletal muscle in COPD. Eur Respir J 2007;30:245–52.

68. Couillard A, Prefaut C. From muscle disuse to myopathy in COPD: potential contribution of oxidative stress. Eur Respir J 2005;26:703–19.

69. Rabinovich RA, Ardite E, Troosters T, et al. Reduced muscle redox capacity after endurance training in patients with chronic obstructive pulmonary disease. Am J Respir Crit Care Med 2001;164:1114–8.

70. Radom-Aizik S, Kaminski N, Hayek S, et al. Effects of exercise training on quadriceps muscle gene

expression in chronic obstructive pulmonary disease. J Appl Physiol 2007;102:1976–84.

71. Gouzi F, Préfaut C, Abdellaoui A, et al. Blunted muscle angiogenic training-response in COPD patients versus sedentary controls. Eur Respir J 2013; 41:806–14.

72. Mattson JP, Poole DC. Pulmonary emphysema decreases hamster skeletal muscle oxidative enzyme capacity. J Appl Physiol 1998;85:210–4.

73. Richardson RS. Skeletal muscle dysfunction vs. muscle disuse in patients with COPD. J Appl Physiol 1999;86:1751–3.

74. Troosters T, Probst VS, Crul T, et al. Resistance training prevents deterioration in quadriceps muscle function during acute exacerbations of chronic obstructive pulmonary disease. Am J Respir Crit Care Med 2010;181:1072–7.

75. Abdulai RM, Jensen TJ, Patel NR, et al. Deterioration of limb muscle function during acute exacerbation of chronic obstructive pulmonary disease. Am J Respir Crit Care Med 2018;197:433–49.

76. Decramer M, Lacquet LM, Fagard R, et al. Corticosteroids contribute to muscle weakness in chronic airflow obstruction. Am Rev Respir Dis 1994;150: 11–6.

77. Pitta F, Troosters T, Probst VS, et al. Physical activity and hospitalization for exacerbation of COPD. Chest 2006;129:536–44.

78. Decramer M, Gosselink R, Troosters T, et al. Muscle weakness is related to utilization of health care resources in COPD patients. Eur Respir J 1997;10: 417–23.

79. Greening NJ, Harvey-Dunstan TC, Chaplin EJ, et al. Bedside assessment of quadriceps muscle by ultrasound after admission for acute exacerbations of chronic respiratory disease. Am J Respir Crit Care Med 2015;192:810–6.

80. Lukaski HC, Johnson PE, Bolonchuk WW, et al. Assessment of fat-free mass using bioelectrical impedance measurements of the human body. Am J Clin Nutr 1985;41:810–7.

81. Schols AMWJ, Wouters EFM, Soeters PB, et al. Body composition by bioelectrical-impedance analysis compared with deuterium dilution and skinfold anthropometry in patients with chronic obstructive pulmonary disease. Am J Clin Nutr 1991;53:421–4.

82. Steiner MC, Barton RL, Singh SJ, et al. Bedside methods versus dual energy x-ray absorptiometry for body composition measurement in COPD. Eur Respir J 2002;19:626–31.

83. Rutten EP, Spruit MA, Wouters EF. Critical view on diagnosing muscle wasting by single-frequency bio-electrical impedance in COPD. Respir Med 2010;104:91–8.

84. Lerario MC, Sachs A, Lazaretti-Castro M, et al. Body composition in patients with chronic

obstructive pulmonary disease: which method to use in clinical practice? Br J Nutr 2006;96:86–92.

85. Engelen MP, Schols AM, Heidendal GA, et al. Dual-energy x-ray absorptiometry in the clinical evaluation of body composition and bone mineral density in patients with chronic obstructive pulmonary disease. Am J Clin Nutr 1998;68:1298–303.

86. Robles PG, Mathur S, Janaudis-Fereira T, et al. Measurement of peripheral muscle strength in individuals with chronic obstructive pulmonary disease: a systematic review. J Cardiopulm Rehabil Prev 2011;31:11–24.

87. Man WDc, Moxham J, Polkey MI. Magnetic stimulation for the measurement of respiratory and skeletal muscle function. Eur Respir J 2004;24:846–60.

88. Nyberg A, Saey D, Maltais F. Why and how limb muscle mass and function should be measured in patients with COPD. Ann Am Thorac Soc 2015; 12:1269–77.

89. Saey D, Troosters T. Measuring skeletal muscle strength and endurance, from bench to bedside. Clin Invest Med 2008;31:307–11.

90. Vaidya T, Beaumont M, de Bisschop C, et al. Determining the minimally important difference in quadriceps strength in individuals with COPD using a fixed dynamometer. Int J Chron Obstruct Pulmon Dis 2018;13:2685–93.

91. Jeong M, Kang HK, Song P, et al. Hand grip strength in patients with chronic obstructive pulmonary disease. Int J Chron Obstruct Pulmon Dis 2017;12:2385–90.

92. Marengoni A, Vetrano DL, Manes-Gravina E, et al. The relationship between chronic obstructive pulmonary disease and frailty: a systematic review and meta-analysis of observational studies. Chest 2018;154:21–40.

93. Jones SE, Maddocks M, Kon SS, et al. Sarcopenia in COPD: prevalence, clinical correlates and response to pulmonary rehabilitation. Thorax 2015;70:213–8.

94. Taylor N, Sanders R, Howick E, et al. Static and dynamic assessment of the Biodex dynamometer. Eur J Appl Physiol Occup Physiol 1991; 62:180–8.

95. Ribeiro F, Lepine PA, Garceau-Bolduc C, et al. Test-retest reliability of lower limb isokinetic endurance in COPD: a comparison of angular velocities. Int J Chron Obstruct Pulmon Dis 2015; 10:1163–72.

96. Meldrum D, Cahalane E, Conroy R, et al. Maximum voluntary isometric contraction: reference values and clinical application. Amyotroph Lateral Scler 2007;8:47–55.

97. Andrews AW, Thomas MW, Bohannon RW. Normative values for isometric muscle force measurements obtained with hand-held dynamometers. Phys Ther 1996;76:248–59.

98. Danneskiold-Samsøe B, Bartels EM, Bülow PM, et al. Isokinetic and isometric muscle strength in a healthy population with special reference to age and gender. Acta Physiol (Oxf) 2009; 197:1–68.

99. Thompson WR, Gordon NF, Linda S. ACSM's guidelines for exercise testing and prescription. Philadelphia: Wolters Kluwer/Lippincott Williams & Wilkins; 2010.

100. Bachasson D, Villiot-Danger E, Verges S, et al. Maximal isometric voluntary quadriceps strength assessment in COPD. Rev Mal Respir 2014;31: 765–70.

101. Brown L, Weir JP. ASEP procedures recommendation I: accurate assessment of muscular strength and power. J Exerc Physiol Online 2001;4:1–21.

102. Visser J, Mans E, De Visser M, et al. Comparison of maximal voluntary isometric contraction and hand-held dynamometry in measuring muscle strength of patients with progressive lower motor neuron syndrome. Neuromuscul Disord 2003;13: 744–50.

103. Beaumont M, Kerautret G, Peran L, et al. Reproductibilité de la mesure de la force et de l'endurance du quadriceps dans la BPCO. Rev Mal Respir 2017;34:1000–6.

104. Bui K-L, Mathur S, Dechman G, et al. Fixed hand-held dynamometry provides reliable and valid values for quadriceps isometric strength in patients with COPD: a multicenter study. Phys Ther, in press.

105. Levinger I, Goodman C, Hare DL, et al. The reliability of the 1rm strength test for untrained middle-aged individuals. J Sci Med Sport 2009; 12:310–6.

106. Vieira L, Bottaro M, Celes R, et al. Isokinetic muscle evaluation of quadriceps in patients with chronic obstructive pulmonary disease. Rev Port Pneumol 2010;16:717–36.

107. Kealin ME, Swank AM, Adams KJ, et al. Cardiopulmonary responses, muscle soreness, and injury during the one repetition maximum assessment in pulmonary rehabilitation patients. J Cardiopulm Rehabil 1999;19:366–72.

108. Zanini A, Aiello M, Cherubino F, et al. The one repetition maximum test and the sit-to-stand test in the assessment of a specific pulmonary rehabilitation program on peripheral muscle strength in COPD patients. Int J Chron Obstruct Pulmon Dis 2015; 10:2423–30.

109. Wallerstein LF, Barroso R, Tricoli V, et al. The influence of familiarization sessions on the stability of ramp and ballistic isometric torque in older adults. J Aging Phys Act 2010;18:390–400.

110. Nyberg A, Saey D, Martin M, et al. Acute effects of low-load/high-repetition single-limb resistance training in COPD. Med Sci Sports Exerc 2016;48: 2353–61.

111. Clark CJ, Cochrane L, Mackay E. Low intensity peripheral muscle conditioning improves exercise tolerance and breathlessness in COPD. Eur Respir J 1996;9:2590–6.

112. Troosters T, Gosselink R, Janssens W, et al. Exercise training and pulmonary rehabilitation: new insights and remaining challenges. Eur Respir Rev 2010;19:24–9.

113. Spruit MA, Gosselink R, Troosters T, et al. Resistance versus endurance training in patients with COPD and peripheral muscle weakness. Eur Respir J 2002;19:1072–8.

114. Puente-Maestu L, Sanz ML, Sanz P, et al. Comparison of effects of supervised versus self-monitored training programmes in patients with chronic obstructive pulmonary disease. Eur Respir J 2000;15:517–25.

115. Maltais F, Leblanc P, Jobin J, et al. Intensity of training and physiologic adaptation in patients with chronic obstructive pulmonary disease. Am J Respir Crit Care Med 1997;155:555–61.

116. Coppoolse R, Schols AMWJ, Baarends EM, et al. Interval versus continuous training in patients with severe COPD: a randomized clinical trial. Eur Respir J 1999;14:258–63.

117. Vogiatzis I, Nanas S, Roussos C. Interval training as an alternative modality to continuous exercise in patients with COPD. Eur Respir J 2002;20:12–9.

118. Dolmage TE, Goldstein RS. Effects of one-legged exercise training of patients with COPD. Chest 2008;133:370–6.

119. O'Donnell DE, McGuire M, Samis L, et al. General exercise training improves ventilatory and peripheral muscle strength and endurance in chronic airflow limitation. Am J Respir Crit Care Med 1998;157:1489–97.

120. Maltais F, Leblanc P, Simard C, et al. Skeletal muscle adaptation to endurance training in patients with chronic obstructive pulmonary disease. Am J Respir Crit Care Med 1996;154:442–7.

121. Vogiatzis I, Stratakos G, Simoes DC, et al. Effects of rehabilitative exercise on peripheral muscle tnfalpha, IL-6, IGF-I and MyoD expression in patients with COPD. Thorax 2007;62: 950–6.

122. Mador MJ, Kufel TJ, Pineda LA, et al. Effect of pulmonary rehabilitation on quadriceps fatiguability during exercise. Am J Respir Crit Care Med 2001;163:930–5.

123. Vonbank K, Strasser B, Mondrzyk J, et al. Strength training increases maximum working capacity in patients with COPD–randomized clinical trial comparing three training modalities. Respir Med 2012;106:557–63.

124. Spruit MA, Troosters T, Trappenburg JC, et al. Exercise training during rehabilitation of patients with COPD: a current perspective. Patient Educ Couns 2004;52:243–8.

125. O'Shea SD, Taylor NF, Paratz JD. Progressive resistance exercise improves muscle strength and may improve elements of performance of daily activities for people with COPD: a systematic review. Chest 2009;136:1269–83.

126. Kraemer WJ, Adams K, Cafarelli E, et al. American college of sports medicine position stand. Progression models in resistance training for healthy adults. Med Sci Sports Exerc 2002;34:364–80.

127. Lewis MI, Fournier M, Storer TW, et al. Skeletal muscle adaptations to testosterone and resistance training in men with COPD. J Appl Physiol 2007;103:1299–310.

128. De Brandt J, Spruit MA, Derave W, et al. Changes in structural and metabolic muscle characteristics following exercise-based interventions in patients with COPD: a systematic review. Expert Rev Respir Med 2016;10:521–45.

129. Menon MK, Houchen L, Singh SJ, et al. Inflammatory and satellite cells in the quadriceps of patients with COPD and response to resistance training. Chest 2012;142:1134–42.

130. Lepsen UW, Jorgensen KJ, Ringbaek T, et al. A systematic review of resistance training versus endurance training in COPD. J Cardiopulm Rehabil Prev 2015;35:163–72.

131. O'Shea SD, Taylor NF, Paratz J. Peripheral muscle strength training in COPD: a systematic review. Chest 2004;126:903–14.

132. Normandin EA, McCusker C, Connors M, et al. An evaluation of two approaches to exercise conditioning in pulmonary rehabilitation. Chest 2002;121:1085–91.

Physiologic Effects of Oxygen Supplementation During Exercise in Chronic Obstructive Pulmonary Disease

Asli Gorek Dilektasli, MD[a,b], Janos Porszasz, MD, PhD[a],
William W. Stringer, MD[a], Richard Casaburi, PhD, MD[a,*]

KEYWORDS

• Oxygen supplementation • Exercise-induced hypoxemia • COPD

KEY POINTS

• Supplemental long-term O_2 therapy (LTOT) is a well-established therapy with evidence for prolonged survival in patients with COPD with resting hypoxemia.
• There is evidence suggesting that exertional desaturation is a significant prognostic factor in patients with COPD who do not have severe resting hypoxemia.
• Research shows that O_2 supplementation during exercise improves exercise endurance, breathlessness, and patient-centered outcomes in patients with COPD who are not hypoxemic at rest but have exertional desaturation.
• However, studies failing to show long-term benefits of O_2 supplementation in patients with exertional desaturation are available in the literature, including the latest randomized multi-center long-term O_2 therapy trial.
• Multifactorial mechanisms, such as reduced ventilatory drive, improved limb muscle function, reduced dynamic hyperinflation, and improved pulmonary hemodynamics are suggested to contribute to improvements in exercise tolerance by supplemental O_2 therapy during exercise in COPD.

Supplemental long-term oxygen (O_2) therapy (LTOT) is a well-established therapy with evidence for prolongation of survival in patients with chronic obstructive pulmonary disease (COPD) with resting arterial O_2 partial pressure (PaO_2) consistently less than 55 mm Hg or resting PaO_2 of 55 to 59 mm Hg with evidence of right heart failure.[1,2] Current practice prescribing long-term O_2 treatment is mainly based on 2 randomized controlled trials involving a total of approximately 300 severely hypoxemic patients with COPD reported in the early 1980s: the NOTT (Nocturnal Oxygen Therapy Trial) and the MRC (Medical Research Council) trial.[1,2] The dose-response relationship between the number of hours of O_2 use per day and the magnitude of the survival benefit was observed for hypoxemic patients with COPD in MRC and NOTT studies and in a separate analysis that combined both study results.[3] LTOT was also shown to be associated with reductions in days spent in hospital and readmission rates compared with the study patients' pre-LTOT initiation period in hypoxemic patients with compliant with O_2 therapy (defined by using at least 15 h/d) by Ringbaek and colleagues.[4] Current evidence suggests that LTOT improves survival, right heart failure,

Disclosure Statement: None to declare (A.G. Dilektasli, J. Porszasz, W.W. Stringer, R. Casaburi).
[a] Rehabilitation Clinical Trials Center, Los Angeles Biomedical Research Institute at Harbor-UCLA Medical Center, 1124 W. Carson Street, Building CDCRC, Torrance, CA 90502, USA; [b] Faculty of Medicine, Department of Pulmonary Medicine, Uludağ University, Turkey
* Corresponding author. Rehabilitation Clinical Trials Center, Los Angeles Biomedical Research Institute at Harbor-UCLA Medical Center, 1124 W. Carson Street, Building CDCRC, Torrance, CA 90502.
E-mail address: casaburi@ucla.edu

pulmonary hypertension, and reduces hospitalization rates in hypoxemic patients with COPD.[1,2,4,5]

BENEFITS OF SUPPLEMENTAL OXYGEN THERAPY ON EXERCISE TOLERANCE, QUALITY OF LIFE, AND DYSPNEA IN PATIENTS WITH EXERTIONAL HYPOXEMIA

A significant proportion of patients with COPD do not have resting hypoxemia but develop severe desaturation with exercise.[6] Moreover, the type of exercise being performed (walking versus cycle) is an important factor that may affect occurrence of desaturation and the level of desaturation observed in patients with COPD. A lower occurrence of clinically important O_2 desaturation has been reported during cycling compared with treadmill exercise in COPD.[7–10] This observation may be clinically important when making decisions about O_2 supplementation during exercise. There are potential physiologic mechanisms explaining the differences in exercise desaturation in walking and cycling exercise.[8] Peak oxygen uptake ($\dot{V}O_2$) response is usually higher, and the lactate threshold is higher in treadmill exercise than cycling,[11] possibly because of involvement of a smaller muscle mass during cycling. Pulmonary ventilation ($\dot{V}_E$) and carbon dioxide output ($\dot{V}CO_2$) are similar between cycling and treadmill at low exercise levels, but, at higher $\dot{V}O_2$ levels, progressively greater $\dot{V}_E$ and $\dot{V}CO_2$ are observed during cycling.[8] The finding that, at heavy exercise intensities, $\dot{V}CO_2$ response at a given $\dot{V}O_2$ is higher during cycling is likely to be related to earlier lactic acidosis onset in the cycle ergometer test.[8] Because the lactic acid is buffered by bicarbonate, the byproduct carbon dioxide is exhaled in the breath; the higher $\dot{V}_E$ is related to higher $\dot{V}CO_2$. The higher $\dot{V}_E$ at a given $\dot{V}O_2$ yields a higher Pao_2 (and, thus, a higher O_2 saturation).

> The severity of exertional hypoxemia is less pronounced during cycling compared with walking, in part due to a higher metabolic acidosis and alveolar ventilation at a similar work rate during cycling compared with walking.

Exertional desaturation is an important feature in COPD, with important consequences. Several studies have suggested an association between exertional desaturation and mortality in COPD. Casanova and colleagues[12] reported a 2.63 times increased risk for mortality in patients with COPD demonstrating O_2 desaturation (fall in $Spo_2 \geq 4\%$ or $Spo_2 <90\%$) during a 6-minute walk test in a 3-year follow-up period. Moreover, severity of exercise-induced hypoxemia assessed by Pao_2 slope (rate of change of Pao_2 as a function of Vo_2 from rest to peak exercise) observed during incremental cardio-pulmonary exercise testing was identified as a prognostic factor that determines poor survival in COPD.[13] Pao_2 slope less than -10.7 kPa $L^{-1}.min^{-1}$ was associated with increased mortality (hazard ratio: 3.09, 95% CI: 1.41–6.77, $P = .0046$). A separate analysis, performed in the COPD subgroup without resting hypoxemia, suggested that a steep decrease in Pao_2 slope during exercise is an independent predictor of mortality.[13] On the other hand, a retrospective analysis of National Emphysema Treatment Trial studied emphysema patients who were non-hypoxemic at rest, but hypoxemic during exercise, and demonstrated that use of continuous O_2 was associated with worse disease severity and survival.[14] However, after adjusting the proportional hazards model for body mass index, age, and forced expiratory volume in 1 second (FEV_1), the mortality difference between 2 groups ($Pao_2 > 60$ mm Hg + continuous oxygen versus $Pao_2 > 60$ mm Hg + no oxygen) were no longer significant. One other important observation from this retrospective analysis was that patients with exercise desaturation had similar mortality regardless of whether they were using continuous, intermittent, or no oxygen. Although exertional desaturation is common and has been determined to be a significant prognostic factor in patients with COPD who do not meet the criteria for LTOT, it is an area of interest regarding whether any clinical benefits can be obtained by supplemental O_2 therapy during exercise. A recent randomized multi-center trial, the Long-term Oxygen Treatment Trial (LOTT), interrogated whether supplemental O_2 would result in a survival benefit compared with no use of supplemental O_2 among stable patients with COPD with moderate resting desaturation (Spo_2 89%–93%) or moderate exercise-induced desaturation ($Spo_2 < 90\%$ for ≥ 10 seconds and $Spo_2 \geq 80\%$ for ≥ 5 minutes during a 6-minute walk test) in 732 patients followed for 1 to 6 years.[15] These researchers did not observe differences between the O_2 supplemented and non-O_2 supplemented groups in any of the study outcomes (time to death, time to first hospitalization, hospitalization rates, quality of life, anxiety, depression, lung function, or distance walked in 6 minutes). They concluded that the prescription of long-term supplemental O_2 for patients with stable COPD and either mild resting or exercise-induced moderate desaturation did not provide sustained benefits in the measured outcomes of this study.[15] In contrast with the limitations of the previous LTOT studies (NOTT and MRC),[1,2] the LOTT trial used a large sample size, a broad set of inclusion criteria, and a broad range of participants, allowing for meaningful subgroup analyses.[16] Nevertheless, the LOTT study design still leaves some questions unanswered regarding the adherence to O_2 therapy in subjects randomized to receive O_2. The NOTT and MRC trials showed that the benefit of supplemental O_2 therapy was dependent on daily duration of the therapy. Because LTOT was an intrusive therapy, adherence to O_2 therapy may be poor.[17] Relying on self-report to assess patient adherence may create inaccurate and possibly overestimated assessments.[18] Methods that allow clinicians and researchers to obtain reliable adherence information is of great importance. The LOTT trial did not succeed in obtaining objective adherence monitoring in most participants and relied on self-reported use of supplemental O_2.

Although the accuracy of adherence assessment to O_2 supplementation in the recent long-term oxygen therapy trial (LTOT) remains questionable, its results do not support a survival benefit of ambulatory O_2 supplementation in patients who failed to qualify for O_2 therapy based on resting arterial blood gas criteria.

On the other hand, published evidence shows that supplemental O_2 during exercise enhances exercise endurance and relieves breathlessness in patients with COPD with mild resting hypoxemia.[19–22] O'Donnell and colleagues[22] enrolled 11 patients with severe airflow limitation (mean FEV_1: 0.97 ± 0.13 L) and mildly hypoxemia at rest (mean Pao_2: 74 ± 3 mm Hg) in a randomized double-blind placebo-controlled crossover study. Study patients breathed room air or 60% O_2 during constant work rate cycle exercise tests to determine factors contributing to the relief of exertional dyspnea in response to O_2 supplementation during exercise. Breathing 60% O_2 during exercise resulted in a 2.5 ± 0.8 min ($35\% \pm 11\%$) increase in endurance time. Slopes of perceived breathlessness and leg effort were significantly reduced over time during exercise in patients breathing 60% O_2 (**Fig. 1**). Percent change in endurance time correlated best with percent change in breathlessness-time slope, but did not correlate with leg effort change slope. Accordingly, the authors concluded that improvement in exercise endurance resulting from O_2 supplementation was explained primarily by amelioration of breathlessness. In patients with COPD without resting hypoxemia, but who desaturate with exercise, O_2 supplementation during exercise resulted in improved exercise tolerance.[23]

Despite evidence showing that supplemental O_2 during exercise enhances exercise endurance and relieves breathlessness in COPD, few randomized trials have evaluated the benefits of supplemental O_2 therapy applied during exercise training as part of a pulmonary rehabilitation program.[21,24–26] Emtner and colleagues[21] evaluated whether non-hypoxemic patients with COPD undergoing

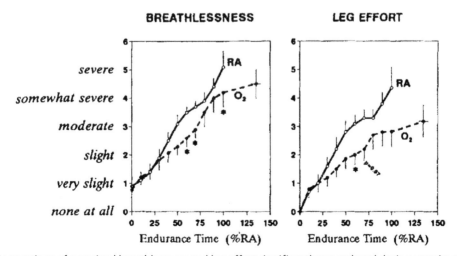

Fig. 1. Borg ratings of perceived breathlessness and leg effort significantly are reduced during exercise with 60% O_2 supplementation compared with 21% O_2 (room air). * Represents comparison of iso-time responses ($P < .05$). RA, room air; O_2, 60% O_2 supplementation. (*Reprinted* with permission of the American Thoracic Society. Copyright © 2019 American Thoracic Society. O'Donnell DE, Bain DJ, Webb KA. Factors contributing to relief of exertional breathlessness during hyperoxia in chronic airflow limitation. Am J Respir Crit Care Med 1997;155(2):530–535. The American Journal of Respiratory and Critical Care Medicine is an official journal of the American Thoracic Society.)

exercise training while breathing supplemental O_2 achieve higher intensity exercise, and therefore improve exercise capacity more than patients breathing room air in a double-blind randomized trial. They showed that, during the last week of the program, the supplemental O_2-trained group achieved a higher training work rate than the air-trained group (62 ± 19 versus 52 ± 22 W, respectively, $P < .005$). Patients with COPD randomized to supplemental O_2 group increased the training work rate more rapidly than the air group (**Fig. 2**). Endurance time significantly increased in both arms, but a 40% greater endurance gain was evident in the O_2-trained group than in the air-trained group. The authors suggested that O_2 supplementation during exercise training is a promising approach for improving the effectiveness of pulmonary rehabilitation. Some other studies evaluating the effect of supplemental O_2 during pulmonary rehabilitation showed no benefits for patients in the supplemental O_2 group.[24–26] Importantly, studies with negative results had substantially different experimental designs, such as lacking of a double-blinding as well as lacking assessment of training intensity and effort-

independent outcomes (eg, iso-time responses), which may explain the differing results.[21]

Significant improvements in health-related quality of life (assessed by the Chronic Respiratory Questionnaire and Short Form-36), as well as the psychological distress assessed by Hospital Anxiety Depression scale with ambulatory O_2 therapy, were observed in a 12-week double-blind, randomized crossover study of domiciliary O_2 (4 L/min) during any activity that provoked dyspnea (vs compressed air) that enrolled patients with COPD with exercise-induced desaturation but without severe resting hypoxemia.[27] Important physiologic responses to O_2 (versus compressed air) were also noted, with significant improvements in 6-minute walking distance (by 40 m, 377 ± 94 m versus 337 ± 113 m) and post-test Borg dyspnea score. On the other hand, in patients with COPD with exertional desaturation, but who were not hypoxemic at rest, there were no gains in quality of life assessed by Chronic Respiratory Disease Questionnaire in a 12-week, double-blind, randomized crossover study of O_2 (versus compressed air).[28] Statistically significant, but small, increments in 6-minute walking distance were

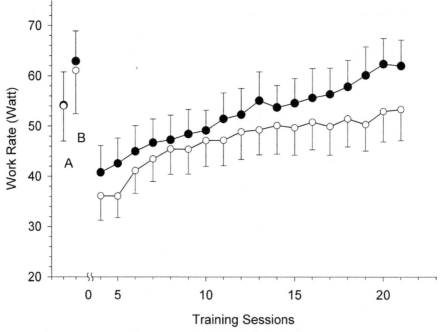

Fig. 2. Training work rate (watts) achieved during the last 6 weeks of exercise training in non-hypoxemic patients with COPD undergoing exercise training while breathing 30% supplemental O_2 (*closed circles*) versus air (*open circles*). Despite similar pre-training exercise tolerance, the 30% supplemental O_2 group was able to exercise at a higher work rate throughout the exercise training program. Values and error bars represent the mean and the SEM. (*Reprinted* with permission of the American Thoracic Society. Copyright © 2019 American Thoracic Society. Emtner M, Porszasz J, Burns M, Somfay A, Casaburi R. Benefits of supplemental O2 in exercise training in nonhypoxemic chronic obstructive pulmonary disease patients. Am J Respir Crit Care Med 2003;168(9):1034–1042. The American Journal of Respiratory and Critical Care Medicine is an official journal of the American Thoracic Society.)

seen after 6 weeks both in subjects randomized to supplemental domiciliary O_2 and those randomized to supplemental air (19 m increase compared with baseline in the domiciliary O_2 group and 20 m increase in domiciliary air group).[28] More recently, in a larger randomized, double-blind placebo-controlled study with a similar study design that enrolled 143 patients with COPD who did not have resting hypoxemia but had severe exertional dyspnea, no significant benefits in quality of life, mood disturbances, or 6-minute walking distance were found between groups receiving cylinder air versus cylinder O_2.[29] A recent meta-analysis that combined results of 4 randomized controlled trials (with a total of 331 patients with COPD who were not hypoxemic at rest) comparing ambulatory O_2 versus placebo (room air)[27–30] identified small improvements in the dyspnea (mean difference 0.28, 95% CI: 0.10–0.45, P = .002) and in the fatigue (mean difference 0.17, 95% CI: 0.04–0.31, P = .009) domains of the Chronic Respiratory Disease Questionnaire in favor of the O_2 group.[31] However, no benefits in survival or 6-minute walking distance were observed.[31] Interpretation of the available studies is difficult because of considerable variability between the designs of the cited studies. Therefore, differences in study design might have contributed to differing results between various studies.

> Despite the sound physiologic rationale for correcting hypoxemia as a strategy to improve exercise tolerance in patients with COPD, there are conflicting results concerning the clinical value of O_2 supplementation in improving outcomes of pulmonary rehabilitation and decreasing dyspnea in daily life.

HOW DOES OXYGEN SUPPLEMENTATION YIELD IMPROVEMENTS DURING EXERCISE IN COPD?

Accumulating evidence supports physiologic benefits of O_2 supplementation during exercise in COPD. There are several, likely multifactorial, mechanisms hypothesized to contribute to improvements in exercise tolerance (endurance, breathlessness, dynamic hyperinflation) by supplemental O_2 therapy in COPD.

Increased Arterial Po_2 Resulting in Depression of Carotid Chemoreceptor and Ventilatory Drive

Hypoxemia is a well-described ventilatory stimulant contributing to breathlessness.[32] Some of the effects of O_2 supplementation are related to the depression of carotid body output. Carotid bodies are active chemoreceptors for sensing hyperoxia, and they are responsible for the prolongation of breath-holding time as alveolar O_2 tension is increased (by increasing Fio_2), resulting in depression of ventilatory drive (further discussion in the topic is provided in Update on Chemoreception: Influence on Cardiorespiratory Regulation and Patho-Physiology).[33] Breathing O_2 reduces the ventilatory requirement during exercise at the same work intensity, and allows the patient with COPD to exercise longer until maximum ventilation is reached at a higher work rate.[23] Stein and colleagues[23] observed a linear correlation (r = 0.63) between minute ventilation and arterial O_2 saturation in patients with severe COPD. Iso-time ventilation was consistently lower in patients with COPD breathing supplemental O_2 at a 0.30 Fio_2 compared with patients breathing air, suggesting that the reduction in ventilation is related to reduced hypoxic drive because of elevated O_2 saturation that supplemental O_2 yields.[23]

Somfay and colleagues[34] aimed to examine whether O_2 supplementation causes a dose-dependent effect on functional and symptomatic improvement during exercise in non-hypoxemic patients with COPD. The authors randomized patients with severe COPD with mild hypoxemia (mean Sao_2 $\geq$92% at rest and $\geq$88% during exercise) and healthy subjects to 5 constant work rate tests (at 75% of peak work rate in a preceding incremental exercise test) while breathing compressed air at a range of Fio_2 values including 0.30, 0.50, 0.75, or 1.00. Compared with compressed air breathing, endurance time increased by 92% $\pm$ 20% with 0.30 Fio_2, and increased by 157% $\pm$ 30% breathing 0.50 Fio_2. Further Fio_2 increases did not result in additional exercise endurance increase. Similar findings, showing a substantial increase in cycling endurance time by increasing Fio_2 to 0.30 and a further but slight increase by increasing Fio_2 to 0.50, were reported by Davidson and colleagues.[20] Accordingly, results of the study by Somfay suggested that improvement in exercise endurance time and symptom perception by O_2 supplementation during exercise is dose dependent in patients with COPD who are not hypoxemic at rest.[34] One possible explanation for the plateauing dose-response relationship observed in both studies[33,34] might be that the depression of ventilation (by carotid chemoreceptor suppression) is maximal at inspired O_2 fractions greater than 0.50 and that hypoxic ventilatory drive is extinguished.[35]

> A decrease in respiratory neural drive secondary to lower ventilation is an important mechanism by which supplemental O_2 may lessen exertional dyspnea.

Reduction of Limb Muscle Dysfunction and Lactic Acid Production in the Exercising Muscles

Morphologic and structural alterations, such as muscle atrophy, muscle weakness, fiber-type shift, mitochondrial dysfunction, and poor oxidative capacity exist in limb muscles of patients with COPD (further discussion in the topic is provided in The Relevance of Limb Muscle Dysfunction In COPD: A Review for Clinicians).[36] Morphologic studies in patients with COPD reveal a shift in the proportion of slow-twitch, more fatigue-resistant oxidative (type I) fibers toward fast-twitch, and more fatigable glycolytic (type II) fibers, which depend more on anaerobic metabolism.[37] Under conditions of chronic hypoxemia, muscle mass and oxidative capacity of muscles are decreased in humans.[38] Chronic hypoxemia is one of the contributing factors to limb muscle dysfunction in COPD.[36] Chronically altered O_2 transport compromises oxidative capacity and facilitates oxidative stress in skeletal muscles.[39–41] Hypoxemia significantly alters muscle energy metabolism,[42] and may also potentiate inflammatory response[41] leading to muscle atrophy.

Both exercise and hypoxemia are conditions that may result in inadequate O_2 delivery to skeletal muscles. Although beneficial effects of supplemental O_2 on exercise performance were observed, effects of acute correction of hypoxemia on peripheral muscle metabolism during exercise in patients with COPD with chronic hypoxemia were examined by Payen and colleagues.[43] The authors reported an improvement in impaired indices of muscular oxidative metabolism and utilization of high-energy phosphate compounds with acute O_2 supplementation in a group of patients with COPD during exercise, suggesting an improvement in oxidative capacity of skeletal muscle, potentially because of increased O_2 delivery.[43] A recent study by Amann and colleagues[44] examined the effects of changes in respiratory muscle work associated with altering arterial O_2 saturation on exercise-induced peripheral muscle fatigue in patients with COPD. Their results showed that increasing O_2 transport by inhaling O_2 at 0.60 Fio_2, significantly reduced exercise-induced leg muscle fatigue assessed by quadriceps twitch compared with patients with COPD with no O_2

supplementation during exercise. Accordingly, the authors suggested that high susceptibility to leg muscle fatigue is a consequence of arterial hypoxemia and excessive respiratory muscle work in patients with COPD, contributing to insufficient O_2 transport to the muscles of ambulation. To quantify the effects of acute O_2 supplementation on lower limb blood flow, O_2 delivery, and O_2 uptake, Maltais and colleagues[45] randomized patients with COPD to O_2 supplementation (Fio_2: 0.75) versus air during symptom-limited incremental cycle tests. They observed a significant increase in the peak exercise capacity when supplemental O_2 was used. Lower limb blood flow, lower limb O_2 delivery, and O_2 uptake were significantly greater at peak exercise with O_2 supplementation than with air. Moreover, the increase in peak work rate correlated ($r = 0.66$) with the increase in peak lower limb O_2 delivery and O_2 uptake. The findings of Maltais and co-workers show that the improvement in peak exercise capacity with O_2 supplementation are accompanied by increases in lower limb O_2 delivery and O_2 uptake, which enables the lower limb muscles to perform more external work.[45]

Patients with COPD develop lactic acidosis at low work rates.[46,47] During exercise, $\dot{V}O_2$ kinetics are slowed in skeletal muscles of patients with COPD.[48] Gas exchange responses following the onset of moderate-intensity constant work rate exercise are characterized by 3 phases. Phase 1 is the fast component that represents the rapid increase in gas exchange mostly related to abrupt increase of pulmonary blood flow at the start of exercise.[49] Phase 2 is a slower phase during which cellular respiration in the working muscles increases with a further increase in cardiac output. Circulatory and tissue stores, as well as phosphocreatine breakdown produce the energy required for the work.[42,50] Phase 3 is either a steady state or, above a certain work rate, a further slow increase that starts 3 to 4 minutes after the onset of exercise. Diminished O_2 delivery to the muscle or intrinsic factors related to the muscle, such as impaired muscle oxidative capacity or inadequate capillarity, were the leading factors suggested to determine the speed of $\dot{V}O_2$ response. Improved skeletal muscle O_2 delivery by supplemental O_2 administration during moderate constant work rate exercise was suggested to enhance oxidative metabolism.[42,51] Patients with COPD, breathing room air and exercising below their lactate threshold, exhibited slow phase 2 kinetics of $\dot{V}O_2$ increase, yielding a large O_2 deficit.[42,52] In these patients, supplemental O_2 (Fio_2 of 30%) resulted in (1) significant reductions in the O_2 deficit and speeding of the

$\dot{V}O_2$ response to moderate exercise onset (approaching those of control subjects breathing room air), presumably because of an increase in muscle O_2 delivery,[42] and (2) significant reductions in steady-state ventilation.[42,51] Finally, peripheral muscle fatigue is a factor-limiting exercise capacity in many patients with COPD.[53] Improved skeletal muscle O_2 delivery by supplemental O_2 was hypothesized to reduce lactic acidosis and, as a result, reduce ventilatory requirement and to reduce perception of fatigue.[51] To better define consequences of O_2 supplementation in COPD on muscle metabolism at the onset of moderate-intensity exercise and whether O_2 supplementation during exercise reduces lactate increase, Somfay and colleagues[51] sampled arterialized venous blood and measured lactate, pH and P_{CO_2} at frequent intervals and compared $\dot{V}O_2$ kinetics while subjects with COPD and a healthy group exercised breathing air or 40% O_2. $\dot{V}O_2$ time courses were slower in patients with COPD, and O_2 supplementation did not result in acceleration of the $\dot{V}O_2$ kinetics in either group (**Fig. 3**). However, $\dot{V}CO_2$ were significantly slower in patients with COPD, and O_2 supplementation resulted in significant prolongation of the $\dot{V}CO_2$ kinetic responses in healthy and COPD groups. The results suggested to the authors that, during moderate exercise, the lower ventilatory requirement induced by O_2 supplementation is primarily caused by direct chemoreceptor inhibition rather than improved muscle function.[51]

> Improvement in O_2 delivery to, and utilization by, the working skeletal muscles may contribute to improved peak exercise performance during exertional O_2 supplementation in patients with COPD.

Effects on Operational Lung Volumes

Dynamic hyperinflation causing dyspnea on exertion is a well-defined feature of COPD (further discussion in the topic is provided in The Pathophysiology of Dyspnea and Exercise Intolerance in COPD).[54,55] The study by Somfay focused on operating lung volumes to understand the effect of O_2 supplementation on dynamic hyperinflation during exercise.[34] As expected, end-expiratory lung volume (EELV) and end-inspiratory lung volume (EILV) increased significantly from rest to end-exercise during constant work rate test in the COPD group while breathing room air. At the end of exercise, EILV was significantly lower in the COPD group compared with healthy subjects. The time course of dynamic lung volume changes throughout constant work rate exercise while breathing compressed air and increasing O_2 concentrations were remarkably different in patients with COPD and healthy subjects (**Fig. 4**).

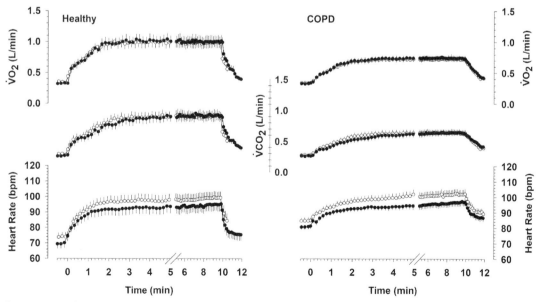

Fig. 3. Gas exchange and cardiorespiratory kinetics during room air (*open circles*) and 40% supplemental O_2 (*closed circles*) breathing in healthy and COPD groups. Each data point represents the 10-second average and SEM. (*From* Somfay A, Porszasz J, Lee SM, et al. Effect of hyperoxia on gas exchange and lactate kinetics following exercise onset in nonhypoxemic COPD patients. Chest 2002;121(2):393–400.)

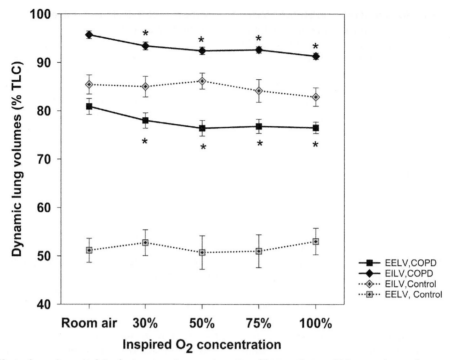

Fig. 4. Effect of supplemental O_2 during exercise on operational lung volumes. Values and error bars represented the iso-time mean and the SEM. Open (□) and closed (■) squares represent end-expiratory lung volume in healthy subjects and patients with COPD, respectively; open (◇) and closed (◆) diamonds represent end-inspiratory lung volume in healthy subjects and patients with with COPD, respectively. *$P < .05$ for comparison of iso-time supplemental O_2 responses compared with room air. TLC, total lung capacity. (*From* Somfay A, Porszasz J, Lee SM, et al. Dose-response effect of oxygen on hyperinflation and exercise endurance in nonhypoxaemic COPD patients. Eur Respir J 2001;18(1):77–84.)

EELV increased markedly and EILV was close to total lung capacity in patients with COPD breathing compressed room air at the end of exercise. Increasing Fio_2 to 30% resulted in significant reductions at iso-time EELV (represented as ■ for the COPD group in **Fig. 4**), EILV (represented as ◆ for the COPD group in **Fig. 4**), minute ventilation, and respiratory frequency compared with room air in patients with COPD. Additional mild reductions were noted by increasing Fio_2 to 50%, but higher Fio_2 did not cause further improvement in operational lung volumes or reductions in respiratory frequency. Significant correlations between the change in operational lung volumes and increasing endurance time were observed in the COPD group. The degree of improvement in exercise endurance caused by O_2 supplementation was correlated with the reduction in ventilatory requirement during exercise. It was suggested that reduced ventilatory requirement enabled a reduction in respiratory rate and a prolonged time for exhalation, yielding less dynamic hyperinflation.[34] Clearly, dynamic hyperinflation occurs even in mild COPD when inspiratory reserve volume reaches a lower limit (the O'Donnell Threshold, the inspiratory reserve volume at which intolerable dyspnea limits exercise).[56] Whether supplemental O_2 therapy alters the O'Donnell Threshold requires further research.

> Lower exercise ventilation (and breathing frequency) with supplemental O_2 is associated with a reduced pulmonary gas trapping during exercise thereby postponing the attainment of critical inspiratory constraints and intolerable dyspnea.

Pulmonary Vasodilation, Increase in Cardiac Output, and Decrease in Pulmonary Artery Pressure

Despite pulmonary blood flow markedly increasing during exercise, only a slight increase (at about 4–6 mm Hg) in pulmonary artery pressure (Ppa) is evident in healthy people.[57,58] In contrast, pulmonary artery pressure shows a greater increase in patients with COPD than in healthy people during exercise.[57,59] The observed increase in Ppa correlates with resting Ppa in COPD (if the resting pulmonary artery pressure is higher, pulmonary artery pressure shows a greater increase during exercise).[57,60,61] Pulmonary vascular hypertension occurs with exercise even in some patients with mild COPD who are not hypoxemic at rest.[57] Hemodynamic catheterization data indicate that exercise causes a greater rise in both pulmonary artery and pulmonary wedge pressures in patients with more severe emphysema than those of patients with minimal or no disease.[57] Several explanations have been proposed for the prominent increase of Ppa in COPD during exercise, including hypoxic pulmonary vasoconstriction, reduction in capillary bed because of lung destruction, reduced distensibility of pulmonary arteries owing to pulmonary vascular remodeling[59] and extramural compression caused by increased alveolar pressure because of air trapping (see also Clinical and Physiological Implications of Negative Cardiopulmonary Interactions in Coexisting COPD-Heart Failure).[62] To evaluate the contributing effects of hypoxic pulmonary vasoconstriction on pulmonary hemodynamics during exercise in patients with COPD, Wright and colleagues[57] used right heart catheterization to measure cardiac output, pulmonary artery and capillary wedge pressures when the subjects were breathing air or 100% O_2 at rest and after 10 minutes of cycle ergometer exercise. These investigators observed that O_2 breathing had no effect at rest but lowered pulmonary artery and pulmonary wedge pressures during exercise.

This review recognizes that there are many limitations in the available studies in the literature that need to be addressed to clarify the effectiveness of supplemental O_2 in patients with COPD who desaturate during exercise and who are normoxemic at rest. First, a uniform definition for exertional desaturation is lacking in the literature. Second, various exercise protocols have been used (from daily activities to maximal incremental cycle ergometry) in studies testing the benefits of acute supplemental O_2 administration.[63] Third, the concentration and mode of supplemental O_2 delivery vary between studies. And fourth, in long-term O_2 administration studies, adherence to the prescribed O_2 is not monitored in most of the studies,[18] or, if monitored, is not measured with precision. This is important, because adherence rates vary largely among subjects and between studies.[64]

REFERENCES

1. Continuous or nocturnal oxygen therapy in hypoxemic chronic obstructive lung disease: a clinical trial. Nocturnal Oxygen Therapy Trial Group. Ann Intern Med 1980;93(3):391–8.

2. Long term domiciliary oxygen therapy in chronic hypoxic cor pulmonale complicating chronic bronchitis and emphysema. Report of the Medical Research Council Working Party. Lancet 1981; 1(8222):681–6.

3. Petty TL. Home oxygen - a revolution in the care of advanced COPD. Med Clin North Am 1990;74(3): 715–29.

4. Ringbaek TJ, Viskum K, Lange P. Does long-term oxygen therapy reduce hospitalisation in hypoxaemic chronic obstructive pulmonary disease? Eur Respir J 2002;20(1):38–42.

5. Buyse B, Demedts M. Long-term oxygen therapy with concentrators and liquid oxygen. Acta Clin Belg 1995;50(3):149–57.

6. Soguel Schenkel N, Burdet L, de Muralt B, et al. Oxygen saturation during daily activities in chronic obstructive pulmonary disease. Eur Respir J 1996; 9(12):2584–9.

7. Cockcroft A, Beaumont A, Adams L, et al. Arterial oxygen desaturation during treadmill and bicycle exercise in patients with chronic obstructive airways disease. Clin Sci 1985;68(3):327–32.

8. Hsia D, Casaburi R, Pradhan A, et al. Physiological responses to linear treadmill and cycle ergometer exercise in COPD. Eur Respir J 2009;34(3):605–15.

9. Palange P, Forte S, Onorati P, et al. Ventilatory and metabolic adaptations to walking and cycling in patients with COPD. J Appl Physiol (1985) 2000;88(5): 1715–20.

10. Poulain M, Durand F, Palomba B, et al. 6-minute walk testing is more sensitive than maximal incremental cycle testing for detecting oxygen desaturation in patients with COPD. Chest 2003;123(5):1401–7.

11. Porszasz J, Casaburi R, Somfay A, et al. A treadmill ramp protocol using simultaneous changes in speed and grade. Med Sci Sports Exerc 2003;35(9): 1596–603.

12. Casanova C, Cote C, Marin JM, et al. Distance and oxygen desaturation during the 6-min walk test as predictors of long-term mortality in patients with COPD. Chest 2008;134(4):746–52.

13. Hiraga T, Maekura R, Okuda Y, et al. Prognostic predictors for survival in patients with COPD using cardiopulmonary exercise testing. Clin Physiol Funct Imaging 2003;23(6):324–31.

14. Drummond MB, Blackford AL, Benditt JO, et al. Continuous oxygen use in nonhypoxemic emphysema patients identifies a high-risk subset of patients: retrospective analysis of the National Emphysema Treatment Trial. Chest 2008;134(3): 497–506.

15. Albert RK, Au DH, Blackford AL, et al. A randomized trial of long-term oxygen for COPD with moderate desaturation. N Engl J Med 2016;375(17):1617–27.

16. Yusen RD, Criner GJ, Sternberg AL, et al. The long-term oxygen treatment trial for chronic obstructive

pulmonary disease: rationale, design, and lessons learned. Ann Am Thorac Soc 2018;15(1):89–101.

17. Katsenos S, Constantopoulos SH. Long-term oxygen therapy in COPD: factors affecting and ways of improving patient compliance. Pulm Med 2011; 2011:325362.

18. Casaburi R. Long-term oxygen therapy: the three big questions. Ann Am Thorac Soc 2018;15(1):14–5.

19. Woodcock AA, Gross ER, Geddes DM. Oxygen relieves breathlessness in "pink puffers". Lancet 1981;1(8226):907–9.

20. Davidson AC, Leach R, George RJ, et al. Supplemental oxygen and exercise ability in chronic obstructive airways disease. Thorax 1988;43(12): 965–71.

21. Emtner M, Porszasz J, Burns M, et al. Benefits of supplemental oxygen in exercise training in nonhypoxemic chronic obstructive pulmonary disease patients. Am J Respir Crit Care Med 2003;168(9): 1034–42.

22. O'Donnell DE, Bain DJ, Webb KA. Factors contributing to relief of exertional breathlessness during hyperoxia in chronic airflow limitation. Am J Respir Crit Care Med 1997;155(2):530–5.

23. Stein DA, Bradley BL, Miller WC. Mechanisms of oxygen effects on exercise in patients with chronic obstructive pulmonary disease. Chest 1982;81(1): 6–10.

24. Rooyackers JM, Dekhuijzen PN, Van Herwaarden CL, et al. Training with supplemental oxygen in patients with COPD and hypoxaemia at peak exercise. Eur Respir J 1997;10(6):1278–84.

25. Wadell K, Henriksson-Larsen K, Lundgren R. Physical training with and without oxygen in patients with chronic obstructive pulmonary disease and exercise-induced hypoxaemia. J Rehabil Med 2001;33(5):200–5.

26. Garrod R, Paul EA, Wedzicha JA. Supplemental oxygen during pulmonary rehabilitation in patients with COPD with exercise hypoxaemia. Thorax 2000; 55(7):539–43.

27. Eaton T, Garrett JE, Young P, et al. Ambulatory oxygen improves quality of life of COPD patients: a randomised controlled study. Eur Respir J 2002; 20(2):306–12.

28. McDonald CF, Blyth CM, Lazarus MD, et al. Exertional oxygen of limited benefit in patients with chronic obstructive pulmonary disease and mild hypoxemia. Am J Respir Crit Care Med 1995; 152(5):1616–9.

29. Moore RP, Berlowitz DJ, Denehy L, et al. A randomised trial of domiciliary, ambulatory oxygen in patients with COPD and dyspnoea but without resting hypoxaemia. Thorax 2011;66(1):32–7.

30. Nonoyama ML, Brooks D, Guyatt GH, et al. Effect of oxygen on health quality of life in patients with chronic obstructive pulmonary disease with transient exertional hypoxemia. Am J Respir Crit Care Med 2007;176(4):343–9.

31. Ameer F, Carson KV, Usmani ZA, et al. Ambulatory oxygen for people with chronic obstructive pulmonary disease who are not hypoxaemic at rest. Cochrane Database Syst Rev 2014;(6): CD000238.

32. Swinburn CR, Wakefield JM, Jones PW. Relationship between ventilation and breathlessness during exercise in chronic obstructive airways disease is not altered by prevention of hypoxaemia. Clin Sci (Lond) 1984;67(5):515–9.

33. Davidson JT, Whipp BJ, Wasserman K, et al. Role of the carotid bodies in breath-holding. N Engl J Med 1974;290(15):819–22.

34. Somfay A, Porszasz J, Lee SM, et al. Dose-response effect of oxygen on hyperinflation and exercise endurance in nonhypoxaemic COPD patients. Eur Respir J 2001;18(1):77–84.

35. Kozlowski S, Rasmussen B, Wilkoff WG. The effect of high oxygen tensions on ventilation during severe exercise. Acta Physiol Scand 1971;81(3): 385–95.

36. Maltais F, Decramer M, Casaburi R, et al. An official American Thoracic Society/European Respiratory Society statement: update on limb muscle dysfunction in chronic obstructive pulmonary disease. Am J Respir Crit Care Med 2014;189(9):15–62.

37. Hughes RL, Katz H, Sahgal V, et al. Fiber size and energy metabolites in five separate muscles from patients with chronic obstructive lung diseases. Respiration 1983;44(5):321–8.

38. Hoppeler H, Kleinert E, Schlegel C, et al. Morphological adaptations of human skeletal muscle to chronic hypoxia. Int J Sports Med 1990;11(Suppl 1):S3–9.

39. Rabinovich RA, Bastos R, Ardite E, et al. Mitochondrial dysfunction in COPD patients with low body mass index. Eur Respir J 2007;29(4):643–50.

40. Puente-Maestu L, Perez-Parra J, Godoy R, et al. Abnormal mitochondrial function in locomotor and respiratory muscles of COPD patients. Eur Respir J 2009;33(5):1045–52.

41. Koechlin C, Couillard A, Simar D, et al. Does oxidative stress alter quadriceps endurance in chronic obstructive pulmonary disease? Am J Respir Crit Care Med 2004;169(9):1022–7.

42. Palange P, Galassetti P, Mannix ET, et al. Oxygen effect on O2 deficit and VO2 kinetics during exercise in obstructive pulmonary disease. J Appl Physiol (1985) 1995;78(6):2228–34.

43. Payen JF, Wuyam B, Levy P, et al. Muscular metabolism during oxygen supplementation in patients with chronic hypoxemia. Am Rev Respir Dis 1993; 147(3):592–8.

44. Amann M, Regan MS, Kobitary M, et al. Impact of pulmonary system limitations on locomotor muscle

fatigue in patients with COPD. Am J Physiol Regul Integr Comp Physiol 2010;299(1):314–24.

45. Maltais F, Simon M, Jobin J, et al. Effects of oxygen on lower limb blood flow and O2 uptake during exercise in COPD. Med Sci Sports Exerc 2001;33(6):916–22.

46. Sue DY, Wasserman K, Moricca RB, et al. Metabolic acidosis during exercise in patients with chronic obstructive pulmonary disease. Use of the V-slope method for anaerobic threshold determination. Chest 1988;94(5):931–8.

47. Casaburi R, Patessio A, Ioli F, et al. Reductions in exercise lactic acidosis and ventilation as a result of exercise training in patients with obstructive lung disease. Am Rev Respir Dis 1991;143(1):9–18.

48. Maltais F, Simard AA, Simard C, et al. Oxidative capacity of the skeletal muscle and lactic acid kinetics during exercise in normal subjects and in patients with COPD. Am J Respir Crit Care Med 1996;153(1):288–93.

49. Casaburi R, Daly J, Hansen JE, et al. Abrupt changes in mixed venous blood gas composition after the onset of exercise. J Appl Physiol (1985) 1989;67(3):1106–12.

50. Nery LE, Wasserman K, Andrews JD, et al. Ventilatory and gas exchange kinetics during exercise in chronic airways obstruction. J Appl Physiol Respir Environ Exerc Physiol 1982;53(6):1594–602.

51. Somfay A, Porszasz J, Lee SM, et al. Effect of hyperoxia on gas exchange and lactate kinetics following exercise onset in nonhypoxemic COPD patients. Chest 2002;121(2):393–400.

52. Casaburi R, Porszasz J, Burns MR, et al. Physiologic benefits of exercise training in rehabilitation of patients with severe chronic obstructive pulmonary disease. Am J Respir Crit Care Med 1997;155(5):1541–51.

53. Gosselink R, Troosters T, Decramer M. Peripheral muscle weakness contributes to exercise limitation in COPD. Am J Respir Crit Care Med 1996;153(3):976–80.

54. O'Donnell DE, Webb KA. Exertional breathlessness in patients with chronic airflow limitation. The role of lung hyperinflation. Am Rev Respir Dis 1993;148(5):1351–7.

55. O'Donnell DE, Bertley JC, Chau LK, et al. Qualitative aspects of exertional breathlessness in chronic airflow limitation: pathophysiologic mechanisms. Am J Respir Crit Care Med 1997;155(1):109–15.

56. Casaburi R, Rennard SI. Exercise limitation in chronic obstructive pulmonary disease. The O'Donnell threshold. Am J Respir Crit Care Med 2015;191(8):873–5.

57. Wright JL, Lawson L, Pare PD, et al. The structure and function of the pulmonary vasculature in mild chronic obstructive pulmonary disease. The effect of oxygen and exercise. Am Rev Respir Dis 1983;128(4):702–7.

58. Slonim NB, Ravin A, Balchum OJ, et al. The effect of mild exercise in the supine position on the pulmonary arterial pressure of five normal human subjects. J Clin Invest 1954;33(7):1022–30.

59. Kubo K, Ge RL, Koizumi T, et al. Pulmonary artery remodeling modifies pulmonary hypertension during exercise in severe emphysema. Respir Physiol 2000;120(1):71–9.

60. Schrijen F, Uffholtz H, Polu JM, et al. Pulmonary and systemic hemodynamic evolution in chronic bronchitis. Am Rev Respir Dis 1978;117(1):25–31.

61. Burrows B, Kettel LJ, Niden AH, et al. Patterns of cardiovascular dysfunction in chronic obstructive lung disease. N Engl J Med 1972;286(17):912–8.

62. Butler J, Schrijen F, Henriquez A, et al. Cause of the raised wedge pressure on exercise in chronic obstructive pulmonary disease. Am Rev Respir Dis 1988;138(2):350–4.

63. Stoller JK, Panos RJ, Krachman S, et al. Oxygen therapy for patients with COPD: current evidence and the long-term oxygen treatment trial. Chest 2010;138(1):179–87.

64. Lacasse Y, Tan AM, Maltais F, et al. Home oxygen in chronic obstructive pulmonary disease. Am J Respir Crit Care Med 2018;197(10):1254–64.

Strategies to Increase Physical Activity in Chronic Respiratory Diseases

Thierry Troosters, PT, PhD[a,b],*, Astrid Blondeel, PT, MSc[a,b],
Fernanda M. Rodrigues, PT, MSc[a,b],
Wim Janssens, MD, PhD[b,c], Heleen Demeyer, PT, PhD[a,b]

KEYWORDS

• COPD • Physical activity • Exercise training • Behavioral intervention

KEY POINTS

- Physical activity and exercise tolerance are 2 distinct concepts. Exercise tolerance relates to the physiologic abilities of a person, physical activity relates to the behavior of the subject.
- Physical activity can be increased but this requires a behavioral intervention.
- In patients who lack the physiologic capacity to engage in physical activity, interventions that try to enhance physical activity are less likely to be successful. Hence, patient selection for these interventions is crucial.

PHYSICAL ACTIVITY, A COMPLEX CONSTRUCT FOR PHYSIOLOGISTS

Physical activity is important in the maintenance of good health, or rather, lack of physical activity leads to the onset of several chronic diseases. This was recently reiterated by the US Department of Health and Human Services.[1] The most frequently used definition of physical activity is any bodily movement produced by skeletal muscles that results in energy expenditure.[2] Exercise or sports activities are therefore only a fraction of structured, planned, and repetitive physical activities. Physical activity entails also bodily movement for work, leisure, or domestic activities.[3] Physical activity is needed to sustain life but the amount of physical activity subjects engage in is largely variable within subjects from day to day

and between subjects. In the paper of Caspersen and colleagues[2] that provided the definition, the emphasis was on the energy expenditure and the proposed metric to quantify physical activity was suggested to be kilojoules. In the assessment of respiratory patients, the emphasis is rather on the bodily movement and metrics to quantify physical activity capture time in activities such as walking, cycling, stair climbing, the number of steps, intensity of physical activity, and so forth. There are 2 main reasons to emphasize movement rather than energy expenditure. First, a lack of skeletal muscle activation (through motion), rather than low whole body energy expenditure per se, causes significant nonrespiratory problems in patients with chronic diseases in general and in patients with respiratory diseases in particular. These problems can be observed as

Disclosure Statement: None of the authors have a relevant financial interest in the present review.
[a] Department of Rehabilitation Sciences, Laboratory of Pneumology, University Hospitals Leuven, KU Leuven–University of Leuven, Herestraat 49, Onderwijs en Navorsing 1, PO Box 706, Leuven 3000, Belgium; [b] Respiratory Division, University Hospitals Leuven, Leuven, Belgium; [c] Department of Chronic Diseases, Metabolism and Aging, Laboratory of Pneumology, University Hospitals Leuven, KU Leuven, Herestraat 49, Onderwijs en Navorsing 1, PO Box 706, Leuven 3000, Belgium
* Corresponding author. Department Rehabilitation Sciences, Laboratory of Pneumology, University Hospitals Leuven, Herestraat 49, Onderwijs en Navorsing 1, PO Box 706, 3000 Leuven, Belgium.
E-mail address: Thierry.troosters@kuleuven.be

cardiovascular, muscular, metabolic, bone, or mental comorbidity. In patients with mild chronic obstructive pulmonary disease (COPD), the lack of physical activity, rather than the underlying COPD, was associated with the development of comorbidities.[4] Second, assessment of energy expenditure is difficult when no direct measures can be made. Resting energy expenditure in patients can be elevated due to the enhanced work of breathing or the presence of a catabolic state in some patients.[5] Energy expenditure during activities is increased due to variable (and often impaired) mechanical efficiency due to metabolic skeletal muscle abnormalities[6] and increased ventilatory requirements. Therefore, any estimate of energy expenditure based on accelerometry (capturing acceleration and deceleration of the body during motion) will at best provide a rough estimate of the true energy expenditure.[7] This article, therefore, refers to physical activity as any voluntary bodily movement executed by skeletal muscles. Physical activity is characterized by 3 features:

1. The type of activity (eg, walking, cycling, and complex tasks such as household activities or errands)
2. The duration of activity, typically summarized per day or per week. Another dimension of time is the duration of a bout of physical activity, reported as the average bout duration of physical activity throughout a day
3. The intensity of physical activity, typically summarized as the time a person has spent above a certain (and approximate) metabolic rate. For the latter, a cutpoint of 1.5 times the resting metabolic rate (ie, 1.5 METS) captures any meaningful activity and an intensity of 3 times the resting metabolic rate (ie, 3 METS) is considered an activity at moderate intensity.

Number of steps, a frequently used metric to capture physical activity in COPD, is considered a proxy for any activity but does not capture time nor intensity, nor does it accurately capture activities that are not walking. Nevertheless, the number of steps is an easily obtained metric that can be assessed with most currently available physical activity monitors. The other dimensions are more difficult to capture, require more advanced processing of physical activity signals, and depend more on the used algorithms. Valid activity monitors exist[7,8] that provide reliable estimates of physical activity when patients are monitored for an appropriate time.[3,9]

> Movement and energy expenditure are not equivalent in patients with chronic respiratory disease: whereas a deficit in motion, rather than low energy expenditure, is associated with nonrespiratory comorbidities (eg, cardiovascular, musculoskeletal, metabolic, mental), total energy expenditure may be preserved or even increased despite the relative lack of movement.

WHAT PATIENTS NEED TO ENGAGE IN PHYSICAL ACTIVITY

The overall amount and intensity of physical activity patients engage in depends on several factors. In the general population, some of the variance in physical activity behavior seems to be explained by genetic factors,[10,11] as well as environmental and societal factors or policy incentives.[12] In patients with chronic diseases, exercise intolerance becomes an increasingly more important limiting factor to engage in physical activity. It can easily be understood that with extreme exercise intolerance, physical activity, particularly at higher intensity, becomes almost impossible. **Fig. 1** shows the relationship between functional exercise tolerance as assessed by the 6-minute walking distance (6MWD) and physical activity with the proxy of the number of steps per day. It is clear that when the 6MWD is less than 300 to 350 m, physical activity levels are generally low. Therefore, a minimum exercise tolerance seems a prerequisite to enable physical activity.

Once a critical threshold of exercise tolerance and stamina is reached, it is likely that other factors related to motivation, habits, genetics, and self-efficacy become gradually more important.

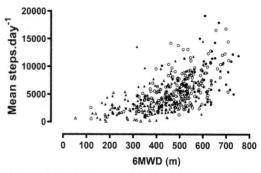

Fig. 1. Relationship between functional exercise tolerance (assessed as 6-minute walking distance [6MWD]) and physical activity as assessed by steps per day in patients with mild (●), moderate (○), severe (▲), and very severe (△) COPD tested at the authors' center.

Several reports have shown that whereas there is a relationship between exercise tolerance and physical activity in cross-sectional studies, the link between changes in exercise tolerance and changes in physical activity is not linear. In fact, the authors' group recently demonstrated that changes in physical activity were likely to happen in patients with better preserved exercise tolerance; however, the correlation between changes in exercise tolerance and changes in exercise capacity per se were not good.[13,14] Furthermore, we showed that increases in physical activity were possible without alterations in lung function or exercise tolerance in patients with rather well-preserved baseline lung function and exercise tolerance.[15] From this, it is clear that changes in physical activity behavior are difficult to achieve in absence of sufficient physical fitness (exercise tolerance, muscle strength) but, once a threshold level of fitness is reached, changes in physical activity dissociate from further improvements in exercise tolerance.

Other factors that are needed to change physical activity behavior are motivation, self-efficacy (the confidence one can do an activity),[16] the belief that physical activity is not harmful, and the willingness to engage in activities despite symptoms. The social environment also plays an important role. Patients with active spouses are themselves more active than patients with a similar impairment and less active loved ones.[17] Along these lines, patients (particularly men) who engage in grandparenting and those who walk a dog have also been reported more active for a given functional capacity.[18] Health insurance companies are currently starting to set up initiatives that include incentives to engage in physical activity.[19,20] Although this has not been studied in COPD specifically, it may provide an additional stimulus for behavior change. A final factor that may be important, particularly in COPD patients, is the season and climate or air pollution.[21] Patients with COPD are less likely to be active in winter conditions[22] or on days with particularly hot weather. In addition, physical activity is not advised for these patients on days with elevated levels of air pollution because this may directly and adversely affect their health.[23] The environment in which patients need to carry out physical activity may also be challenging in itself. A study from the United Kingdom, for example, showed that the time that crossing lights remain green is simply too short for almost all people referred to pulmonary rehabilitation to cross a road safely.[24] This unsafe feeling may prohibit patients to walk outdoors.

> Although a minimal level of fitness is required to enable patients to be physically active in daily life, further increases in fitness are not necessarily translated into more physical activity.

HOW TO ENHANCE PHYSICAL ACTIVITY

Knowledge of the prerequisites for physical activity and exercise can help in designing interventions to enhance physical activity. However, the authors and others[25] advocate that proper patient selection may also be of importance. Broadly speaking, 2 types of patients exist. The first group of patients are those with truly limited exercise tolerance. The second group are patients with sufficient exercise tolerance to engage in physical activity. In the first group, the emphasis on physical activity can be questioned as a feasible goal for treatment. In the second group, increasing physical activity can be achieved through comprehensive strategies.

Patients with Limited Capacity

Three studies from the authors' group, as well as studies reported by others, support the concept that changing physical activity is difficult, if not impossible, in patients with severely impaired exercise capacity. In a post hoc analysis of a study successfully using telecoaching as an intervention to enhance physical activity, subjects with a 6MWD less than 450 m were less likely to respond to the behavioral intervention. Similarly, in a study investigating physical activity in subjects with a 6MWD distance less than 350 m referred to pulmonary rehabilitation, the likelihood of a meaningful increase (600–1000 steps per day[26]) was only 16%. In subjects with a better baseline 6MWD, the likelihood was 3-fold higher.[13] In severely disabled subjects who were discharged from the hospital, a step counter–based program was also not effective to regain physical activity.[27] In a COPD cohort that was rather severe in terms of exercise limitation, Nolan and colleagues[28] also did not find benefits in adding a behavioral intervention to enhance physical activity.

It is currently unclear whether a fixed threshold exists for exercise capacity below which improvements in physical activity are difficult to obtain. In a study on pulmonary rehabilitation, the authors identified 350 m in a 6MWD test as a possible cutpoint; however, this needs to be prospectively confirmed. This threshold coincides with the functional exercise tolerance, in which the variability in physical activity seems to become larger, meaning that it is possible for patients to engage in physical activity once this exercise tolerance is reached.

Also, 350 m is near the cutoff value identified as the threshold value in a 6MWT in which survival becomes compromised.[29]

In patients with low exercise tolerance, the focus of interventions should be to enhance physical fitness. This is achieved through optimal bronchodilator therapy, which enhances the ventilatory capacity by alleviating airflow obstruction and reducing dynamic hyperinflation (further discussion in the topic is provided in The Pathophysiology of Dyspnea and Exercise Intolerance in COPD). In selected patients, exercise capacity can also be enhanced by lung volume reduction. High-intensity exercise training tackles the nonrespiratory consequences of exercise limitation in the cardiovascular and muscular system, and can be associated with these therapies. It is beyond the scope of this article to provide a comprehensive overview of all options to achieve optimal fitness. This is discussed in detail elsewhere.[30] In proper exercise training paradigms, high-intensity exercise training is alternated with periods of rest, allowing the skeletal muscle to recover from the training overload. In that sense, too much stimulation through physical activity outside an intensive training program may actually be deleterious to muscle adaptations in patients in whom regular physical activity may be close to their maximal exercise tolerance.[31] Whether this could jeopardize a healthy balance between recovery and high-intensity exercise should be further studied.

> Improving fitness is important to allow patients with poor exercise tolerance to engage in more physical activity.

Patients with Sufficient Exercise Tolerance

Once patients attain sufficient exercise tolerance, enhancing physical activity can become the main focus of the (nonpharmacological) treatment. In such patients, this goal can be achieved in the short term, even without any efforts to further enhance exercise tolerance.[14,15,32] Adherence to the guidelines for physical activity becomes important. To that end, behavioral strategies need to be embedded in the treatment. A taxonomy for behavior approaches was recently introduced by Susan Michie and colleagues.[33] The techniques most frequently or successfully adopted to enhance physical activity are the self-monitoring of physical activity behavior combined with realistic and collaborative goal-setting and the provision of effective feedback to physical activity behavior. This is easily implemented by using a step counter and dynamic goal-setting.[14,32,34–36]

Static goals (maintained for the duration of the study with little feedback from health care providers) proved to be less successful.[37] Smartphone applications can be used to facilitate the interaction with patients. Although some patients still experience difficulties using a smartphone, the use of a step counter and, particularly, the contact with health care providers were judged by patients as essential components of such an intervention.[38] Although results of studies adopting these techniques with adequate health care provider support were encouraging, the design of applications and using persuasive methodology, such as dialogue support, primary task support, or social support, can be further adapted to the individual patient preference.[39] As can be expected, behavior interventions may not be sufficient or effective in all patients (**Table 1**). Other internal and external barriers may prohibit patients from engaging in regular physical activities. Tackling these barriers in a collaborative relationship with the patient may lead to individual success. As an example, 2 studies identified safe, walkable trails in the community near the subjects where they could walk and exercise.[40,41] These studies suggested significant gains in physical activity in subjects who used the trails. Another study used Nordic walking as a group therapy to enhance physical activity[42] and showed that even at follow-up most of the subjects remained engaged in Nordic walking.

To increase fitness or maintain it after a conventional rehabilitation program it may also be important to ensure physical activity at sufficient intensity in the lifestyle of the patient. Provision of feedback based only on steps per day misses out on that opportunity. In the future, it may be possible and feasible to also provide feedback on the intensity of the physical activity.

To cope comfortably with physical activity, optimal pharmacotherapy seems to be essential. This improves exercise tolerance to some extent but also reduces symptoms during exercise (and physical activity), which improves the experience patients have with physical activity.[15,43] In addition, optimal pharmacotherapy also prevents exacerbations,[44–46] which have a devastating effect on physical activity levels. Patients with frequent exacerbations have more rapid decline in physical activity[47,48] and, therefore, the prevention of exacerbations is an important step to maintain physical activity levels.

> Behavioral interventions associated with a careful removal of barriers and limitations to regular physical activity are the suggested strategies for patients with sufficient exercise tolerance.

Physical Activity in Chronic Respiratory Diseases 401

Table 1
Factors that may contribute to the physical activity in patients with chronic diseases

	Modifiable by Enhancing Capacity or Pharmacotherapy	Modifiable by Enhancing Capacity or Exercise Training in Groups	Modifiable by Behavior Therapy	Modifiable by Social Interventions	Modifiable by Altering Environment	Not Modifiable or Modifiable by Policy Measures
Lung function	✓	✓	—	—	—	—
Exercise tolerance	✓	✓	—	—	—	—
Awareness of behavior	—	—	✓	—	—	—
Self-efficacy	—	✓	✓	—	—	—
Mood status	—	✓	✓	—	—	—
Health beliefs	—	—	✓	—	—	—
Motivation	—	—	✓	—	—	—
Social contacts	—	✓	—	✓	—	—
Activity levels of loved ones	—	—	—	✓	—	—
Group activities	—	—	—	✓	—	—
Walkable neighborhoods	—	—	—	—	✓	—
Safe neighborhoods	—	—	—	—	✓	—
Health insurance incentive	—	—	—	—	✓	—
Climate	—	—	—	—	—	✓
Air pollution	—	—	—	—	—	✓

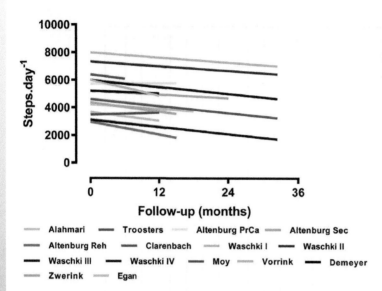

Fig. 2. Decline in physical activity as assessed in steps per day in several studies published in the peer reviewed literature (for references, see text). Waschki I through IV refer to the severity of COPD (mild, I; moderate, II; severe, III; and very severe, IV). Altenburg PrCa refers to the 'primary care cohort', Altenburg Sec refers to the 'secondary care cohort', Altenburg Reh refers to the 'rehabilitation cohort'. All data are the control groups in case of interventional designs.

MAINTAINING PHYSICAL ACTIVITY AS A LONG-TERM GOAL

Physical activity declines with increasing age. The rate of decline of physical activity is not very well studied in patients with COPD. Only a few cohort studies have investigated decline in physical activity and follow-up has been relatively short (**Fig. 2**).[35,47,49–56]

No studies have so far compared longitudinal changes in physical activity between subjects with and without COPD. The decline in physical activity calculated over all the clinical cohorts presented in **Fig. 1** was approximately equal to −450 steps per day per year, with a wide range across studies. Factors known to be associated to decline in physical activity are exacerbations,[47,49] better baseline physical activity,[51] and lung function impairment.[51] Long-term changes in physical activity mirrored decline in health-related quality of life and deterioration in lung function.[52] Surprisingly, interventions have until now mainly focused on improving physical activity. In view of the progressive nature of COPD it might be of equal importance to study how physical activity levels can be maintained for as long as possible. Two studies have looked at the long-term effect of a mobile phone[37] or Internet-based[53] platform to support physical activity but failed to show long-term effects. Probably, interaction with health care providers to adjust the behavior strategy adopted and maintain adherence is needed for long-term behavior change. In addition, when patients suffer from exacerbations, they will acutely lose function,[48] which needs to be restored, in conjunction with reactivation once physical fitness is regained. Further research is needed to discover the best approach in individual stable and exacerbating patients. It is reasonable to speculate that any intervention that reduces the number of exacerbations in the long term will lead to better preservation of physical activity. To that end, a study looking at the effects of more optimal pharmacotherapy with an impact on exacerbation rate, or other therapies that favorably affect exacerbation rate, would benefit from the use of physical activity as a key secondary end point.

SUMMARY

Physical activity is best measured by the assessment of voluntary movements of patients, using accelerometers. Changing physical activity is complex because it requires sufficient exercise tolerance and physical fitness, and requires behavior change. Much progress has been made in identifying candidates for behavioral interventions; however, work needs to be done regarding long-term strategies to maintain improvements or prevent decline in physical activity.

ACKNOWLEDGMENTS

HDM is a postdoctoral fellow of FWO Flanders #12H7517N, FMR is supported by The National Council for Scientific and Technological Development (CNPq), Brazil (249579/2013-8). TT is supported by FWO-Flanders #G.0871.13.

REFERENCES

1. Piercy KL, Troiano RP, Ballard RM, et al. The physical activity guidelines for Americans. JAMA 2018; 320(19):2020–8.
2. Caspersen CJ, Powell KE, Christenson GM. Physical activity, exercise, and physical fitness: definitions

and distinctions for health-related research. Public Health Rep 1985;100(2):126–31.

3. Watz H, Pitta F, Rochester CL, et al. An official European Respiratory Society statement on physical activity in COPD. Eur Respir J 2014;44(6):1521–37.

4. Van Remoortel H, Hornikx M, Langer D, et al. Risk factors and comorbidities in the preclinical stages of chronic obstructive pulmonary disease. Am J Respir Crit Care Med 2014;189(1):30–8.

5. Sergi G, Coin A, Marin S, et al. Body composition and resting energy expenditure in elderly male patients with chronic obstructive pulmonary disease. Respir Med 2006;100(11):1918–24.

6. Layec G, Haseler LJ, Hoff J, et al. Evidence that a higher ATP cost of muscular contraction contributes to the lower mechanical efficiency associated with COPD: preliminary findings. Am J Physiol Regul Integr Comp Physiol 2011;300(5):R1142–7.

7. Rabinovich RA, Louvaris Z, Raste Y, et al. Validity of physical activity monitors during daily life in patients with COPD. Eur Respir J 2013;42(5):1205–15.

8. Van Remoortel H, Raste Y, Louvaris Z, et al. Validity of six activity monitors in chronic obstructive pulmonary disease: a comparison with indirect calorimetry. PLoS One 2012;7(6):e39198.

9. Demeyer H, Burtin C, Van Remoortel H, et al. Standardizing the analysis of physical activity in patients with COPD following a pulmonary rehabilitation program. Chest 2014;146(2):318–27.

10. den Hoed M, Brage S, Zhao JH, et al. Heritability of objectively assessed daily physical activity and sedentary behavior. Am J Clin Nutr 2013;98(5):1317–25.

11. Klimentidis YC, Raichlen DA, Bea J, et al. Genome-wide association study of habitual physical activity in over 377,000 UK Biobank participants identifies multiple variants including CADM2 and APOE. Int J Obes (Lond) 2018;42(6):1161–76.

12. Bauman AE, Reis RS, Sallis JF, et al. Correlates of physical activity: why are some people physically active and others not? Lancet 2012;380(9838):258–71.

13. Osadnik C, Loeckx M, Louvaris Z, et al. The likelihood of improving physical activity after pulmonary rehabilitation is increased in patients with COPD who have better exercise tolerance. Int J Chron Obstruct Pulmon Dis 2018;13:3515–27.

14. Demeyer H, Louvaris Z, Frei A, et al. Physical activity is increased by a 12-week semiautomated telecoaching programme in patients with COPD: a multicentre randomised controlled trial. Thorax 2017; 72(5):415–23.

15. Troosters T, Maltais F, Leidy N, et al. Effect of bronchodilation, exercise training, and behavior modification on symptoms and physical activity in chronic obstructive pulmonary disease. Am J Respir Crit Care Med 2018;198(8):1021–32.

16. Hartman JE, Boezen HM, de Greef MH, et al. Physical and psychosocial factors associated with physical activity in patients with chronic obstructive pulmonary disease. Arch Phys Med Rehabil 2013; 94(12):2396–402.e7.

17. Mesquita R, Nakken N, Janssen DJA, et al. Activity levels and exercise motivation in patients with COPD and their resident loved ones. Chest 2017; 151(5):1028–38.

18. Arbillaga-Etxarri A, Gimeno-Santos E, Barberan-Garcia A, et al. Socio-environmental correlates of physical activity in patients with chronic obstructive pulmonary disease (COPD). Thorax 2017;72(9):796–802.

19. Mitchell MS, Goodman JM, Alter DA, et al. Financial incentives for exercise adherence in adults: systematic review and meta-analysis. Am J Prev Med 2013; 45(5):658–67.

20. Patel MS, Foschini L, Kurtzman GW, et al. Using wearable devices and smartphones to track physical activity: initial activation, sustained use, and step counts across sociodemographic characteristics in a national sample. Ann Intern Med 2017;167(10):755–7.

21. Alahmari AD, Mackay AJ, Patel AR, et al. Influence of weather and atmospheric pollution on physical activity in patients with COPD. Respir Res 2015;16:71.

22. Furlanetto KC, Demeyer H, Sant'anna T, et al. Physical activity of patients with COPD from regions with different climatic variations. COPD 2017;14(3):276–83.

23. Sinharay R, Gong J, Barratt B, et al. Respiratory and cardiovascular responses to walking down a traffic-polluted road compared with walking in a traffic-free area in participants aged 60 years and older with chronic lung or heart disease and age-matched healthy controls: a randomised, crossover study. Lancet 2018;391(10118):339–49.

24. Nolan CM, Kon SSC, Patel S, et al. Gait speed and pedestrian crossings in COPD. Thorax 2018;73(2): 191–2.

25. Singh S. Physical activity and pulmonary rehabilitation - a competing agenda? Chron Respir Dis 2014;11(4):187–9.

26. Demeyer H, Burtin C, Hornikx M, et al. The minimal important difference in physical activity in patients with COPD. PLoS One 2016;11(4):e0154587.

27. Hornikx M, Demeyer H, Camillo CA, et al. The effects of a physical activity counseling program after an exacerbation in patients with Chronic Obstructive Pulmonary Disease: a randomized controlled pilot study. BMC Pulm Med 2015;15:136.

28. Nolan CM, Maddocks M, Canavan JL, et al. Pedometer step count targets during pulmonary rehabilitation in chronic obstructive pulmonary disease. A randomized controlled trial. Am J Respir Crit Care Med 2017;195(10):1344–52.

29. Singh SJ, Puhan MA, Andrianopoulos V, et al. An official systematic review of the European Respiratory Society/American Thoracic Society: measurement properties of field walking tests in chronic respiratory disease. Eur Respir J 2014;44(6):1447–78.

30. Camillo CA, Osadnik CR, van Remoortel H, et al. Effect of "add-on" interventions on exercise training in individuals with COPD: a systematic review. ERJ Open Res 2016;2(1) [pii:00078-2015].

31. Lahaije AJ, van Helvoort HA, Dekhuijzen PN, et al. Physiologic limitations during daily life activities in COPD patients. Respir Med 2010;104(8):1152–9.

32. Mendoza L, Horta P, Espinoza J, et al. Pedometers to enhance physical activity in COPD: a randomised controlled trial. Eur Respir J 2015;45(2):347–54.

33. Michie S, Wood CE, Johnston M, et al. Behaviour change techniques: the development and evaluation of a taxonomic method for reporting and describing behaviour change interventions (a suite of five studies involving consensus methods, randomised controlled trials and analysis of qualitative data). Health Technol Assess 2015;19(99):1–188.

34. Moy ML, Collins RJ, Martinez CH, et al. An internet-mediated pedometer-based program improves health-related quality-of-life domains and daily step counts in COPD: a randomized controlled trial. Chest 2015;148(1):128–37.

35. Altenburg WA, ten Hacken NH, Bossenbroek L, et al. Short- and long-term effects of a physical activity counselling programme in COPD: a randomized controlled trial. Respir Med 2015;109(1):112–21.

36. Wan ES, Kantorowski A, Homsy D, et al. Promoting physical activity in COPD: insights from a randomized trial of a web-based intervention and pedometer use. Respir Med 2017;130:102–10.

37. Vorrink SN, Kort HS, Troosters T, et al. A mobile phone app to stimulate daily physical activity in patients with chronic obstructive pulmonary disease: development, feasibility, and pilot studies. JMIR Mhealth Uhealth 2016;4(1):e11.

38. Loeckx M, Rabinovich RA, Demeyer H, et al. Smartphone-based physical activity telecoaching in chronic obstructive pulmonary disease: mixed-methods study on patient experiences and lessons for implementation. JMIR 2018;6(12):e200.

39. Bartlett YK, Webb TL, Hawley MS. Using persuasive technology to increase physical activity in people with chronic obstructive pulmonary disease by encouraging regular walking: a mixed-methods study exploring opinions and preferences. J Med Internet Res 2017;19(4):e124.

40. Pleguezuelos E, Pérez ME, Guirao L, et al. Improving physical activity in patients with COPD with urban walking circuits. Respir Med 2013; 107(12):1948–56.

41. Arbillaga-Etxarri A, Gimeno-Santos E, Barberan-Garcia A, et al. Long-term efficacy and effectiveness of a behavioural and community-based exercise intervention (Urban Training) to increase physical activity in patients with COPD: a randomised controlled trial. Eur Respir J 2018;52(4) [pii:1800063].

42. Breyer MK, Breyer-Kohansal R, Funk GC, et al. Nordic walking improves daily physical activities in COPD: a randomised controlled trial. Respir Res 2010;11:112.

43. Watz H, Troosters T, Beeh KM, et al. ACTIVATE: the effect of aclidinium/formoterol on hyperinflation, exercise capacity, and physical activity in patients with COPD. Int J Chron Obstruct Pulmon Dis 2017;12:2545–58.

44. Vogelmeier CF, Criner GJ, Martinez FJ, et al. Global strategy for the diagnosis, management, and prevention of chronic obstructive lung disease 2017 report: GOLD executive summary. Eur Respir J 2017;49(3) [pii:1700214].

45. Vestbo J, Papi A, Corradi M, et al. Single inhaler extrafine triple therapy versus long-acting muscarinic antagonist therapy for chronic obstructive pulmonary disease (TRINITY): a double-blind, parallel group, randomised controlled trial. Lancet 2017;389(10082):1919–29.

46. Wedzicha JA, Banerji D, Chapman KR, et al. Indacaterol-glycopyrronium versus salmeterol-fluticasone for COPD. N Engl J Med 2016;374(23):2222–34.

47. Demeyer H, Costilla-Frias M, Louvaris Z, et al. Both moderate and severe exacerbations accelerate physical activity decline in COPD patients. Eur Respir J 2018;51(1) [pii:1702110].

48. Alahmari AD, Kowlessar BS, Patel AR, et al. Physical activity and exercise capacity in patients with moderate COPD exacerbations. Eur Respir J 2016;48(2):340–9.

49. Alahmari AD, Patel AR, Kowlessar BS, et al. Daily activity during stability and exacerbation of chronic obstructive pulmonary disease. BMC Pulm Med 2014;14:98.

50. Troosters T, Sciurba FC, Decramer M, et al. Tiotropium in patients with moderate COPD naive to maintenance therapy: a randomised placebo-controlled trial. NPJ Prim Care Respir Med 2014;24:14003.

51. Clarenbach CF, Sievi NA, Haile SR, et al. Determinants of annual change in physical activity in COPD. Respirology 2017;22(6):1133–9.

52. Waschki B, Kirsten AM, Holz O, et al. Disease progression and changes in physical activity in patients with chronic obstructive pulmonary disease. Am J Respir Crit Care Med 2015;192(3):295–306.

53. Moy ML, Martinez CH, Kadri R, et al. Long-term effects of an internet-mediated pedometer-based walking program for chronic obstructive pulmonary disease: randomized controlled trial. J Med Internet Res 2016;18(8):e215.

54. Vorrink SN, Kort HS, Troosters T, et al. Efficacy of an mHealth intervention to stimulate physical activity in COPD patients after pulmonary rehabilitation. Eur Respir J 2016;48(4):1019–29.

55. Egan C, Deering BM, Blake C, et al. Short term and long term effects of pulmonary rehabilitation on physical activity in COPD. Respir Med 2012;106(12):1671–9.

56. Zwerink M, van der Palen J, Kerstjens HA, et al. A community-based exercise programme in COPD self-management: two years follow-up of the COPE-II study. Respir Med 2014;108(10):1481–90.

Exercise Pathophysiology in Interstitial Lung Disease

Yannick Molgat-Seon, PhD[a,b], Michele R. Schaeffer, PhD[a,b], Christopher J. Ryerson, MD[a,c], Jordan A. Guenette, PhD[a,b,c],*

KEYWORDS

- Dyspnea - Exercise intolerance - Hypoxemia - Idiopathic pulmonary fibrosis
- Pulmonary gas exchange - Restrictive ventilatory impairment

KEY POINTS

- Patients with interstitial lung disease (ILD) have reduced lung volumes, poor pulmonary gas exchange efficiency, and impaired cardiovascular function. In addition, patients with ILD may have skeletal muscle dysfunction.
- Although ILD primarily affects the lungs, the mechanisms of exercise limitation in ILD are related to a combination of factors that include impaired pulmonary gas exchange and abnormalities in pulmonary mechanics as well as cardiovascular function.
- Overall, the pathophysiologic features of ILD have a significant detrimental impact on the integrative response to exercise, which results in exercise intolerance and exertional dyspnea.

INTRODUCTION

Interstitial lung disease (ILD) refers to a diverse group of disorders characterized by inflammation and/or fibrosis of the lung parenchyma.[1] The various forms of ILD can be classified into major categories (**Fig. 1**), including: ILDs resulting from connective tissue disease, environmental exposure-related ILDs, granulomatous ILDs, idiopathic interstitial pneumonias, as well as other relatively rare forms of ILD that do not fit within the aforementioned categories. Given that all ILD subtypes involve some degree of inflammation and/or fibrosis of the lung parenchyma, they share a common pattern of physiologic abnormalities.[2] Patients with ILD typically have reduced pulmonary function, as evidenced by a restrictive ventilatory defect and impaired pulmonary gas exchange, they commonly experience dyspnea, and they usually have poor exercise tolerance.[3–5]

The overarching premise for this review, as outlined in **Fig. 2**, is that the pathophysiology of ILD increases the perceived intensity of exertional dyspnea and contributes to exercise intolerance. Together, exertional dyspnea and exercise intolerance may lead to physical activity avoidance and progressive deconditioning, which further exacerbates the functional consequences of ILD. Within this review, the authors summarize the primary pathophysiologic features of patients with ILD and their effects on the integrative response to exercise.

PATHOPHYSIOLOGY

The pathogenesis of ILD is complex and diverse but generally involves diffuse remodeling of the lungs resulting from systemic or direct injury.[2] Briefly, when the lungs are injured, inflammatory cells are recruited to the site of injury to initiate the wound

Disclosure Statement: The authors have no relevant disclosures.
a Centre for Heart Lung Innovation, St. Paul's Hospital, 166-1081 Burrard Street, Vancouver, British Columbia V6T 1Y6, Canada; b Department of Physical Therapy, Faculty of Medicine, University of British Columbia, 212 Friedman Building, 2177 Wesbrook Mall, Vancouver, British Columbia V6T 1Z3, Canada; c Division of Respiratory Medicine, Faculty of Medicine, University of British Columbia, Gordon and Leslie Diamond Health Care Centre, 7th Floor, 2775 Laurel Street, Vancouver, British Columbia V5Z 1M9, Canada
* Corresponding author. Centre for Heart Lung Innovation, St. Paul's Hospital, 166-1081 Burrard Street, Vancouver, British Columbia V6T 1Y6, Canada.
E-mail address: jordan.guenette@hli.ubc.ca

Clin Chest Med 40 (2019) 405–420
https://doi.org/10.1016/j.ccm.2019.02.011
0272-5231/19/© 2019 Elsevier Inc. All rights reserved.

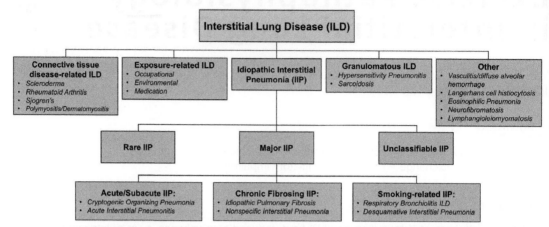

Fig. 1. Classification of ILD. (*Data from* Ryerson CJ, Collard HR. Update on the diagnosis and classification of ILD. Curr Opin Pulm Med 2013;19(5):453–9; and Travis WD, Costabel U, Hansell DM, et al. An official American Thoracic Society/European Respiratory Society statement: update of the international multidisciplinary classification of the idiopathic interstitial pneumonias. Am J Respir Crit Care Med 2013;188(6):733–48.)

healing process.[6] The inflammatory cells then release reactive oxygen species, cytokines, chemokines, and growth factors that either resolve the inflammation and repair the injury or promote further expansion of inflammatory cell infiltration, thereby causing more damage. In the latter case, the persistence of inflammatory cells damages the tissues of the extracellular matrix, which can promote fibrosis. However, it is noteworthy that persistent inflammation in the lungs can occur in the

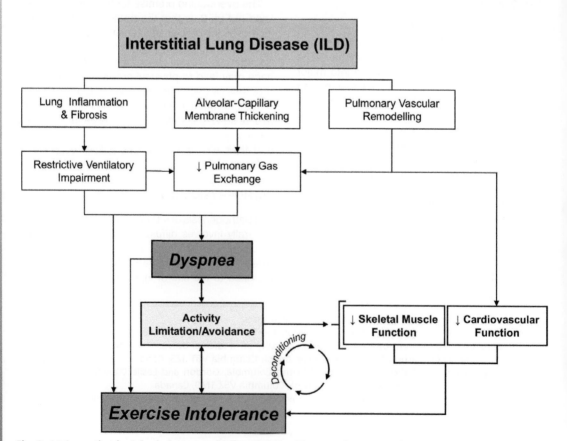

Fig. 2. Major pathophysiologic features of ILD and their effects on dyspnea and exercise tolerance.

absence of fibrosis, as is often the case in cryptogenic organizing pneumonia and desquamative interstitial pneumonia. Conversely, other ILD subtypes are characterized by extensive fibrosis with minimal amounts of chronic inflammation (eg, idiopathic pulmonary fibrosis [IPF]). Moreover, although the term "interstitial" is used as a qualifier to describe the site of pathology, in many cases other structures of the respiratory system are affected, including the airways and the pleura.[7] In addition, the pulmonary circulation is often affected, as shown in patients with IPF.[8] Overall, persistent inflammation and/or the formation of fibrotic tissue within the lungs significantly alters their structural and mechanical properties, and the pathophysiologic effects of ILD can be readily observed in the context of pulmonary function testing[9] (**Table 1**). Moreover, a pathologic reduction in cardiovascular function is a relatively common feature in ILD, particularly when significant lung fibrosis is present.[10]

Lung Compliance

Lung remodeling in ILD decreases compliance and increases the static recoil pressure[11] (see **Table 1**). Low lung compliance can be attributed to reductions in alveolar size and distensibility, an increase in alveolar surface tension, a decrease in lung volumes, or a combination thereof[11–14]; many of these factors are present in ILD. Given that lung compliance and volume are linearly related, it is unsurprising that the pathologic reduction in lung compliance noted in ILD can be ascribed, in large part, to a reduced lung volume.[13] However, Gibson and Pride[11] noted that in patients with fibrosing alveolitis, the reduction in lung volume does not entirely account for the decrease in lung compliance, suggesting that other mechanisms are also involved. Although direct evidence linking changes in alveolar size, distensibility, and surface tension with measures of compliance are lacking, some studies provide important insights. For example, constant k, which describes the shape of the pressure-volume curve of the lungs and provides a volume-corrected index of compliance,[15] is linearly related to the extent of lung fibrosis in patients with IPF and hypersensitivity pneumonitis.[16] This suggests that the formation of fibrotic tissue in the lungs alters its elastic properties independently from changes in lung volume. In addition, abnormalities in the bronchoalveolar lavage content of surfactant that may increase alveolar surface tension have been documented in patients with ILD.[17] Overall, the loss of lung compliance in ILD seems to be primarily related to a reduction

Table 1
Effect of interstitial lung disease (ILD) on measures of resting pulmonary function

Pulmonary Function Measures	ILD vs Health
Lung Compliance	
C_{dyn}, cmH$_2$O·l^{-1}	↓
C_{stat}, cmH$_2$O·l^{-1}	↓
Static Recoil Pressure	
$P_{st(100\%TLC)}$, cmH$_2$O	↑
$P_{st(50\%VC)}$, cmH$_2$O	↔
Lung Volumes	
TLC, l	↓
VC, l	↓
IC, l	↓
FRC, l	↓
ERV, l	↓
RV, l	↓
RV/TLC, %	↔ ↑
Spirometry	
FVC, l	↓
FEV$_1$, l	↓
FEV$_1$/FVC, %	↔ ↑
FEF$_{25\%-75\%}$, l·s^{-1}	↔ ↑
PEF, l·s^{-1}	↔ ↓
Diffusing Capacity	
DLCO, ml·mm Hg^{-1}·min^{-1}	↓
V$_A$, l	↓
DLCO/V$_A$, ml·mm Hg^{-1}·min^{-1}·l^{-1}	↓
Arterial Blood Gases	
Pao$_2$, mm Hg	↓
Paco$_2$, mm Hg	variable

Abbreviations: C_{dyn}, dynamic compliance; C_{stat}, static compliance; DLCO, diffusion capacity of the lungs for carbon monoxide; ERV, expiratory reserve volume; FEF$_{25\%-75\%}$, forced expired flow between 25% and 75% of forced vital capacity; FEV$_1$, forced expired volume in 1 s; FRC, functional residual capacity; FVC, forced vital capacity; IC, inspiratory capacity; ILD, interstitial lung disease; Paco$_2$, arterial partial pressure of carbon dioxide; Pao$_2$, arterial partial pressure of oxygen; PEF, peak expired flow; $P_{st(100\%TLC)}$, static recoil pressure of the lungs at 100% of total lung capacity; $P_{st(50\%VC)}$, static recoil pressure of the lungs at 50% of vital capacity; RV, residual volume; TLC, total lung capacity; V$_A$, alveolar volume; VC, vital capacity.

in lung volume with a secondary contribution from a stiffening of the lungs resulting from the formation of fibrotic tissue within the parenchyma.

A decrease in lung volume does not fully explain the low compliance (ie, high elastance) typically seen in patients with ILD: fibrosis, abnormalities in the elastic properties of the lung interstitium, and high alveolar surface tension may contribute to increased elastic recoil of the lungs.

Lung Volumes and Spirometry

ILD causes a progressive reduction in static lung volumes and capacities.[3] Specifically, patients with ILD have a reduced total lung capacity, vital capacity, functional residual capacity, and residual volume compared with healthy individuals (**Fig. 3**; see **Table 1**). The loss in lung volume is thought to be due to a combination of factors, including a loss of alveolar units, the filling of the alveoli with inflammatory materials and edema, as well as fibroproliferation.[18] However, lung volume subdivisions do not decline uniformly. The decrease in total lung capacity is driven by a reduction in vital capacity.[19] Conversely, the declines in functional residual capacity and residual volume are small in relation to the reduction in vital capacity.[20] It follows that the ratio of residual volume to total lung capacity is frequently elevated in ILD, particularly in those with severe

ILD who have experienced a significant decline in vital capacity.[20] As ILD progresses, so too does the reduction in lung volumes. Thus, it is logical that the reduction in lung volumes is associated with increased mortality.[19] Yet, lung volumes may be preserved in patients with ILD who have comorbid emphysema,[21] which affects the prediction of mortality based on reductions in lung volume alone.[22]

The ability to generate expired flow increases as a function of lung volume. Thus, it would be reasonable to speculate that patients with ILD, with their reduced lung volumes, would also have a corresponding decrease in their ability to generate expired flow. However, patients with ILD have preserved, and in some cases even increased, mid-expiratory flows (ie, forced expiratory flows from 25% to 75% of vital capacity).[23,24] As the compliance of the lungs decreases, static recoil pressure increases reciprocally, thereby increasing the force driving expired flow at a given lung volume.[25] Although maximal expiratory flows are often lower in patients with ILD than height- and sex-matched healthy individuals when comparisons are made in absolute terms (ie, in $l \cdot s^{-1}$), expiratory flows are similar or even higher than in healthy individuals when corrected for lung volume[24,26] (see **Fig. 3**).

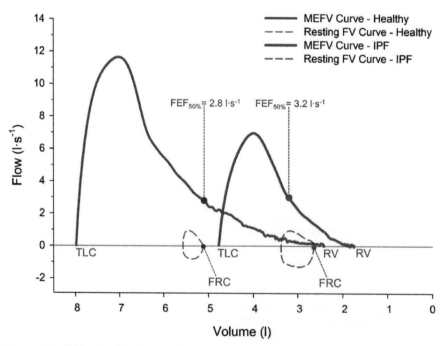

Fig. 3. MEFV curves (*solid lines*) and resting tidal flow-volume curves (dashed lines) in a man with IPF (*red lines*) and an age-, height-, and sex-matched healthy individual (*blue lines*). FEF$_{50\%}$, forced expired flow at 50% of forced vital capacity; FRC, functional residual capacity; IPF, idiopathic pulmonary fibrosis; MEFV, maximum expiratory flow-volume; RV, residual volume; TLC, total lung capacity.

Since total lung capacity (TLC) is generally reduced to a greater extent than residual volume (RV), the RV/TLC ratio may increase in patients with ILD: this should not be misinterpreted as evidence of gas trapping.

Pulmonary Gas Exchange

Gas exchange abnormalities are a hallmark feature of ILD.[27] The diffusion capacity of the lungs for carbon monoxide, an indicator of pulmonary gas exchange efficiency, is reduced in patients with ILD[28,29] (see **Table 1**). In addition, most patients with ILD are hypoxemic at rest, as indicated by a low arterial oxygen saturation (SaO_2) and arterial partial pressure of oxygen (Pao_2)[30,31] (see **Table 1**). Given the detrimental effect of ILD on pulmonary gas exchange efficiency, one might expect arterial partial pressure of carbon dioxide ($Paco_2$) to be elevated; however, most patients with ILD are able to increase minute ventilation ($\dot{V}_E$) in order to prevent hypercapnia.[32] Thus, these patients usually have a normal or mildly reduced $Paco_2$ (due to slight alveolar hyperventilation), and only in the terminal stages of the disease do they retain carbon dioxide[20] (see **Table 1**). The aforementioned increase in resting $\dot{V}_E$ also increases the alveolar partial pressure of oxygen, and because increasing $\dot{V}_E$ has a greater beneficial effect on the maintenance of $Paco_2$ than Pao_2, the alveolar-to-arterial partial pressure of oxygen gradient ($PA-aO_2$) widens.[33] The putative mechanisms of gas exchange impairment in ILD include diffusion limitation, ventilation-perfusion mismatching, and intrapulmonary shunt.[7]

Impaired diffusion of gas between the alveoli and the pulmonary capillaries results from a thickening of the alveolar-capillary membrane and a reduction in pulmonary capillary blood volume.[34] Morphometric analyses of the lungs of patients with ILD indicate that the thickness of the alveolar-capillary membrane is approximately two-fold larger than in healthy individuals,[35] which is likely the product of the combined effects of destruction, thickening, and infiltration of the membrane.[28] Pulmonary capillary blood volume is also reduced in ILD, presumably due to the destruction, obstruction, and/or compression of the pulmonary capillaries, particularly in cases where significant fibrosis is present.[36,37] Accordingly, previous studies have shown that membrane diffusion capacity is impaired and pulmonary capillary blood volume is reduced in patients with ILD and that both of these factors seem to contribute equally to reduced diffusion capacity of the lungs for carbon monoxide (further discussion in this topic is provided in Incorporating Lung Diffusing Capacity for Carbon Monoxide to Clinical Decision Making in Chest Medicine).[28]

The pathogenesis of most ILDs does not affect the lungs homogenously, rather the pattern of lung inflammation and fibrosis is often described as "patchy,"[38] which can be observed using high-resolution computed tomography imaging (**Fig. 4**). It follows that the distribution of ventilation within the lungs is correspondingly nonuniform.[39] Similarly, the abovementioned destruction, obstruction, or compression of the pulmonary capillaries in ILD[8] also supports the notion that the distribution of blood flow within the lungs is likely impaired. The pathologic disruption in the distribution of ventilation and perfusion within

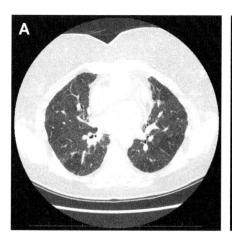
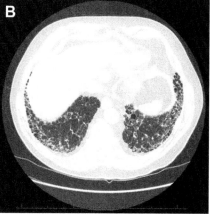

Fig. 4. High-resolution computed tomography of a 51-year-old woman with hypersensitivity pneumonitis that shows mild peripheral reticulation, ground glass, and mosaic attenuation (panel A) and a 79-year-old man with IPF that shows a usual interstitial pneumonia pattern of peripheral and lower-lung predominant reticulation, traction bronchiectasis, and honeycombing, without significant ground glass, mosaic attenuation, or nodularity (panel B).

lungs of patients with ILD do not always coincide spatially. The resulting scenario is a mismatch between the distribution of ventilation and perfusion within the lungs. Based on studies using the multiple inert gas elimination technique, resting hypoxemia in ILD can mostly be explained by ventilation-perfusion mismatch.[31,40]

It has also been suggested that intrapulmonary shunts may contribute to hypoxemia in ILD, whereby poorly oxygenated blood bypasses the ventilated regions of the lungs. Morphologic assessments of the lungs of patients with ILD and pulmonary hypertension suggest that the pathogenesis of ILD may lead to the enlargement of existing precapillary pulmonary anastomoses.[41] Indeed, studies in patients with ILD have reported shunt fractions ranging from 2% to 5% of cardiac output at rest.[31,40] However, given their magnitude, the current consensus is that in most patients, intrapulmonary shunts contribute minimally to resting hypoxemia.

Contrary to common belief, thickening of the alveolar-capillary membrane is not the main mechanism leading to impaired pulmonary gas exchange in ILD. In fact, ventilation-perfusion mismatch assumes a prominent role in most patients at rest.

Cardiovascular Function

The pathogenesis of ILD often involves obliteration of the pulmonary capillary bed and remodeling of the pulmonary vasculature.[42,43] In addition, many patients with ILD are hypoxemic at rest, thereby resulting in hypoxic pulmonary vasoconstriction.[44] The aforementioned factors contribute to increased pulmonary vascular resistance and an associated increase in pulmonary artery pressure.[42] Defining the degree of cardiovascular involvement in ILD is complicated by the variability in ILD cause and pathophysiology. The ILD subtypes most commonly associated with elevated pulmonary arterial pressure are idiopathic pulmonary fibrosis (IPF), sarcoidosis, connective tissue disease-related ILD, and histiocytosis.[45] In some cases, mean pulmonary arterial pressure can exceed 25 mm Hg, at which point overt pulmonary hypertension is said to be present.[46] Across ILDs, the estimated prevalence of pulmonary hypertension is ~15%[47]; however, the prevalence is higher in specific forms of ILD that have significant pulmonary vascular involvement, such as IPF, where the prevalence can be as high as 55% in patients with advanced disease.[48] Given that the pulmonary vasculature as well as the right and left ventricles of the heart represent a pathophysiologic

continuum, it is unsurprising that right and left ventricular function can also be impaired in ILD.[10] Retrograde transmission of the elevated pulmonary arterial pressure increases pressure within the right ventricle. Thus, to maintain cardiac output, the right ventricle must perform more work to overcome the elevated pulmonary vascular resistance, which places a significant amount of stress on the right ventricular wall.[49] Over time, patients with ILD can develop right ventricular hypertrophy and ultimately right ventricular failure.[50] Indeed, *cor pulmonale* often characterizes the terminal stages of ILD.[51] As the function of the right ventricle declines, its stroke volume decreases and contraction time increases.[52] The prolonged right ventricular contraction time and decreased stroke volume can lead to contractile asynchrony between the left and right ventricles as well as a leftward shift of the interventricular septum, which impairs left ventricular filling.[52] Collectively, in patients with ILD who have a significant degree of pulmonary vascular involvement, cardiovascular function is often reduced, as evidenced by elevated pulmonary arterial pressures, right ventricular dysfunction, and in some cases left ventricular dysfunction.

The key central hemodynamic abnormalities in patients with advanced ILD relate to impaired right ventricular function, which, depending on the severity of associated pulmonary hypertension and leftward shift of the interventricular septum, may dynamically interfere with left ventricular structure and function.

PATHOPHYSIOLOGIC RESPONSES TO EXERCISE

The pathophysiologic features of ILD have a detrimental influence on the physiologic and sensory responses to exercise. Although ILD primarily affects the lungs, decrements in cardiovascular and skeletal muscle function have also been documented.[10,53] Based on our current understanding of exercise pathophysiology in ILD, it seems that the pathologic reductions in pulmonary, cardiovascular, and skeletal muscle function collectively contribute to worsening exertional dyspnea and reduced exercise tolerance. As a result, patients with ILD tend to avoid exercise, as indicated by their low physical activity levels in comparison to healthy individuals,[54] which then leads to progressive deconditioning and a worsening of the pathophysiologic and sensory consequences of ILD (see **Fig. 2**). Herein, a detailed description of the main pathophysiologic consequences of ILD and their associated impacts on the integrative response to exercise is provided. An illustrative case (#2) is provided in Unraveling the Causes of Unexplained Dyspnea: The Value of Exercise Testing).

Ventilatory Responses

The most obvious effect of ILD on the physiologic response to exercise relates to the respiratory system. The pathologic effects of ILD on the mechanical and functional properties of the lungs result in (1) ventilatory inefficiency; (2) alterations to breathing patterns and the regulation of operating lung volumes; (3) a propensity toward expiratory flow limitation; and (4) an increase in the energetic cost of breathing.

During exercise, $\dot{V}_E$ increases to meet the demands associated with increased oxygen uptake ($\dot{V}O_2$) and carbon dioxide production ($\dot{V}CO_2$). However, the restrictive ventilatory impairment in ILD decreases the respiratory system's capacity to increase $\dot{V}_E$, as indicated by a low maximal voluntary ventilation.[55] Moreover, ILD results in ventilatory inefficiency, whereby $\dot{V}_E$ at a given exercise intensity is higher compared with healthy individuals[55] (**Fig. 5**A). The increased ventilatory response to exercise in ILD is due to ventilation-perfusion mismatch, which is present at rest and often persists during exercise, as well as the stimulatory effects of arterial hypoxemia and metabolic acidosis on ventilatory drive.[56] Thus, many patients with ILD use a relatively large fraction of their available ventilatory capacity during exercise (ie, the quotient of $\dot{V}_E$ and either maximal voluntary ventilation or maximal ventilatory capacity), with reported values ranging from 43% to 88% at peak exercise.[55,57–59]

The ventilatory response to exercise in ILD is further complicated by the effect of a restrictive ventilatory impairment on breathing patterns and operational lung volumes. Because vital capacity is reduced in ILD, tidal volume reaches a plateau (typically at ~50%–60% of vital capacity) at a lower $\dot{V}_E$ and exercise intensity than in healthy individuals[55] (**Fig. 5**B). Because tidal volume expansion is limited in ILD, patients must rely on increasing breathing frequency in order to achieve further increases in $\dot{V}_E$ (**Fig. 5**C). This rapid and shallow breathing pattern, which is often present

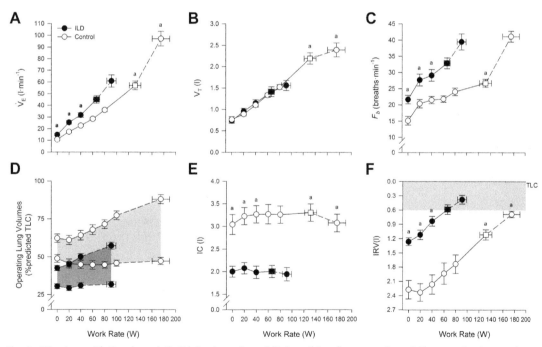

Fig. 5. Minute ventilation (panel A), tidal volume (panel B), breathing frequency (panel C), operating lung volumes (panel D), inspiratory capacity (panel E), and inspiratory reserve volume (panel F) during incremental cycle exercise in patients with ILD and age-matched healthy controls. Circles represent data points at discrete work rates or at peak exercise, and squares represent the tidal volume–minute ventilation inflection points. The shaded area in panel F represents the minimal IRV reached by both groups at the end of exercise. [a] P<.05 ILD versus control subjects. F_b, breathing frequency; IC, inspiratory capacity; IRV, inspiratory reserve volume; TLC, total lung capacity; $\dot{V}_E$, minute ventilation; V_T, tidal volume. (*Reprinted* with permission of the American Thoracic Society. Copyright © 2018 American Thoracic Society. Faisal A, Alghamdi BJ, Ciavaglia CE, et al. Common mechanisms of dyspnea in chronic interstitial and obstructive lung disorders. Am J Respir Crit Care Med. 2016;193(3):299–309. The American Journal of Respiratory and Critical Care Medicine is an official journal of the American Thoracic Society.)

at rest,[20] is a characteristic response to exercise in patients with ILD[55] and has important consequences on the mechanical cost of breathing as well as on pulmonary gas exchange efficiency.

In addition, the restrictive ventilatory pattern in ILD influences the regulation of operating lung volumes, whereby end-inspiratory lung volume and end-expiratory lung volume are shifted downward relative to healthy individuals when expressed as a percentage of predicted total lung capacity[55] (**Fig. 5**D). The pathologic reduction in total lung capacity implies that when compared with healthy individuals, patients with ILD have a lower inspiratory capacity and inspiratory reserve at rest and throughout exercise (**Fig. 5**E, F). In fact, patients with ILD reach a critically low inspiratory reserve volume at a lower exercise intensity than healthy individuals (see **Fig. 5**F), which contributes to an increase in the perceived intensity of dyspnea.[55,59]

The combination of ventilatory inefficiency and a tachypneic breathing pattern during exercise suggests that patients with ILD are likely to reach their maximum capacity to generate expired flow, a concept known as expiratory flow limitation. In this scenario, further increases in expiratory pressure generation do not result in a corresponding increase in flow, which can result in alveolar

hypoventilation as well as an increased mechanical and metabolic cost of breathing.[60] Although patients with ILD are predisposed to developing expiratory flow limitation during exercise, it is not a universal phenomenon.[58] For patients with ILD who are capable of exercising at relatively high intensities or who have marked ventilatory inefficiency, expiratory flow limitation might occur during exercise (**Fig. 6**A). In contrast, patients who terminate exercise early, presumably due to factors unrelated to ventilatory constraints, may not exhibit expiratory flow limitation (**Fig. 6**B).

The mechanical work of breathing is substantially increased in ILD, both at rest and during exercise, due to the pathologic changes to the mechanical properties of the lungs, ventilatory inefficiency, expiratory flow limitation (if present), and restrictive ventilatory impairment. The compliance of the lungs is reduced in ILD, whereby a given change in volume requires a greater change in transpulmonary pressure compared with healthy individuals.[55] Moreover, there is a curvilinear relationship between the work of breathing and $\dot{V}_E$, and since $\dot{V}_E$ is higher for a given metabolic rate in patients with ILD relative to their healthy counterparts, so too is the work of breathing.[55] However, as previously mentioned, patients with ILD initially increase $\dot{V}_E$

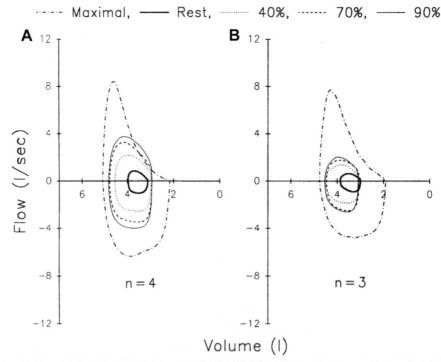

Fig. 6. Composite averaged maximum expiratory flow-volume curves as well as composite averaged tidal flow-volume loops at rest, 40%, 70%, and 90% of peak exercise intensity in patients with ILD who reported terminating incremental testing due to intolerable dyspnea (panel A) or leg fatigue (panel B). (*From* Marciniuk DD, Sridhar G, Clemens RE, et al. Lung volumes and expiratory flow limitation during exercise in interstitial lung disease. J Appl Physiol 1994;77(2):970; with permission.)

by expanding tidal volume and quickly reach the less compliant portion of the respiratory system's pressure volume curve where further tidal volume expansion occurs at the expense of a substantial degree of viscoelastic work. Thus, patients with ILD avoid excessive elastic loading by increasing breathing frequency in order to increase $\dot{V}_E$. This approach is effective because the resistive work of breathing is normal in ILD.[18] However, although the adoption of a rapid and shallow breathing pattern may minimize the viscoelastic work of breathing, it also prevents the reduction in the dead space to tidal volume ratio typically observed during exercise and increases the likelihood of experiencing expiratory flow limitation. The absence of a reduction in the dead space to tidal volume ratio during exercise reduces ventilatory efficiency and negatively affects pulmonary gas exchange.[33]

> An abnormally high ventilatory response to exercise, which can only be met by a fast and shallow breathing pattern (as an attempt to minimize the elastic work of breathing), increases the overall metabolic cost of breathing in patients with ILD.

Pulmonary Gas Exchange

During exercise, whole-body $\dot{V}O_2$ increases above resting levels, thereby requiring a greater rate of oxygen diffusion into the blood via the lungs to sustain aerobic metabolism. For patients with ILD, the decrements in resting pulmonary gas exchange efficiency are worsened during exercise.[27] Because the ability to increase diffusion capacity during exercise is limited, arterial oxygen content tends to decrease. The resulting consequence is the development of exercise-induced arterial hypoxemia (ie, a reduction in SaO_2 to <94% or $\geq$4% from rest, and/or Pao_2 $\geq$10 mm Hg from rest[61]). Although some patients with ILD are not hypoxemic at rest, virtually all patients with ILD experience some level of arterial hypoxemia during exercise.[62] Moreover, they exhibit a greater degree of arterial desaturation during a 6-minute walk test than patients with chronic obstructive pulmonary disease[63]; however, the degree of exercise-induced arterial hypoxemia varies substantially between ILD subtypes.[27,62] Although resting hypoxemia in ILD is primarily related to ventilation-perfusion mismatch, exercise-induced arterial hypoxemia can be largely ascribed to diffusion limitation and reduced mixed-venous partial pressure of oxygen (PvO_2).[27]

Diffusion limitation in ILD is due to a reduction in both pulmonary capillary blood volume and membrane diffusion capacity.[28] During exercise, the

destruction of the pulmonary capillary bed means that fewer pulmonary capillaries can be recruited in the setting of increased cardiac output. Accordingly, the time during which erythrocytes are in contact with the alveolar capillary membrane is reduced to ~0.1- to 0.6 seconds.[64] When erythrocyte transit time becomes less than 0.2 seconds, oxygen equilibrium becomes compromised, which contributes to a widening $PA\text{-}aO_2$.[18] In contrast to other forms of chronic lung disease where significant diffusion limitation is not evident during exercise,[27] diffusion limitation increases $PA\text{-}aO_2$ during exercise in patients with ILD,[31,65] thereby contributing to exercise-induced arterial hypoxemia.

According to the Fick equation, $\dot{V}O_2$ is the product of cardiac output and oxygen extraction at the level of the skeletal muscle. It follows that an increase in $\dot{V}O_2$ can be the result of an increase in cardiac output, oxygen extraction, or both. Assuming that $\dot{V}O_2$, cardiac output, and oxygen extraction are fixed during a bout of steady-state exercise, a patient with ILD is likely to have a lower arterial oxygen content than a healthy individual due to the effect of ILD on pulmonary gas exchange efficiency. In this scenario, it is logical that venous oxygen content (and PvO_2) would also be lower during exercise in ILD than in healthy individuals. Indeed, patients with ILD have a low mixed venous PvO_2 during exercise,[31,66] which worsens the widening of $PA\text{-}aO_2$ and further contributes to exercise-induced arterial hypoxemia. It is also noteworthy that in patients with attendant cardiovascular dysfunction, PvO_2 may be further diminished due to the limited capacity to increase cardiac output.[18] In order to achieve a given $\dot{V}O_2$, ILD patients with cardiovascular dysfunction likely rely on increasing oxygen extraction to a greater extent than increases in cardiac output.

> Increased flow of poorly oxygenated mixed venous blood through lung regions with low ventilation-perfusion ratios largely explains the exertional hypoxemia experienced by most patients with moderate to severe ILD.

Cardiovascular Function

The effect of ILD pathophysiology on cardiovascular function during exercise is variable and largely depends on the underlying disease process as well as the degree of pulmonary vascular involvement. In general, patients with ILD have a similar cardiac output than healthy individuals at rest, despite having higher pulmonary artery pressures[67] (**Fig. 7**). During a low absolute exercise intensity (eg, $\dot{V}O_2$ of 0.75 l·min^{-1}), patients

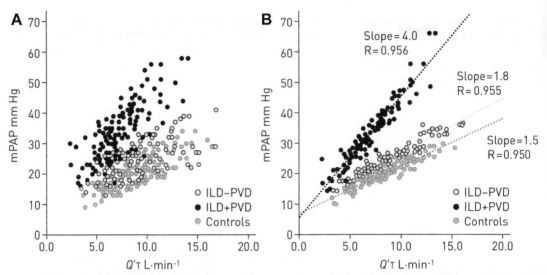

Fig. 7. Pulmonary arterial pressure-flow relationships in patients with ILD with (+) or without (−) PVD and in healthy controls. Minute-by-minute measures of mPAP indexed to cardiac output (Q'_T) are presented as raw values (panel *A*) and Poon fit data (panel *B*) in all subjects. mPAP, mean pulmonary arterial pressure; PVD, pulmonary vascular dysfunction; Q'_T, cardiac output. (*Reproduced* with permission of the © ERS 2019. From Degani-Costa LH, Levarge B, Digumarthy SR, Eisman AS, Harris RS, Lewis GD. Pulmonary vascular response patterns during exercise in interstitial lung disease. European Respiratory Journal 46(3):738–749; DOI: 10.1183/09031936.00191014 Published 31 August 2015.)

with ILD are still capable of increasing cardiac output to an equivalent degree as seen in healthy individuals.[67,68] However, at higher exercise intensities, cardiac output is diminished in patients with ILD,[67,68] which likely results in inadequate oxygen delivery to the exercising skeletal muscle, leading to exercise termination at relatively low absolute intensities.[18] The blunted cardiac output response to exercise in ILD is due to the increased pulmonary vascular resistance, which is brought on by the destruction of pulmonary capillaries and hypoxic pulmonary vasoconstriction.[31] In healthy humans, pulmonary vascular resistance decreases dramatically during exercise in order to accommodate the marked increase in cardiac output and mitigate the increase in pulmonary artery pressure. However, the loss of pulmonary capillaries in ILD interferes with vascular recruitment and distention in the lungs, thereby preventing the normally observed decrease in pulmonary vascular resistance during exercise. In addition, arterial hypoxemia results in a further increase in pulmonary vascular tone via hypoxemic pulmonary vasoconstriction.[31,69] The resulting effect is an exaggerated pulmonary artery pressure response to exercise in ILD, whereby a given increase in cardiac output causes a greater increase in mean pulmonary artery pressure than observed in healthy individuals[67] (see **Fig. 7**). The elevated pulmonary artery pressure during exercise increases right ventricular afterload, which can reduce stroke

volume and ultimately cardiac output.[70] Left ventricular afterload may also be elevated in ILD due to the effect of large intrathoracic pressure swings resulting from the high work of breathing, which can further reduce stroke volume.[18] The effect of a high pulmonary artery pressure response during exercise on functional capacity is highlighted by the fact that in patients with IPF and right ventricular dysfunction, sildenafil (a pulmonary vasodilator) improves exercise capacity.[71] The magnitude of increase in pulmonary artery pressure during exercise is variable between the various ILD subtypes.[72] For example, even with adjustment for ILD severity, patients with IPF are more likely to have elevated pulmonary artery pressure at rest and during exercise than those with most other forms of ILD.[10]

Given the abovementioned impairment in cardiovascular function coupled with potential deconditioning, the heart rate response to submaximal exercise is usually higher in patients with ILD than in healthy individuals for a given absolute exercise intensity.[73] However, patients with ILD commonly have low heart rates at peak exercise due to cessation of exercise before a physiologic maximum is reached.[74] Yet, patients with ILD with significant degrees of cardiovascular involvement, such as scleroderma[75] or sarcoidosis,[73] often have a low cardiac reserve at peak exercise, indicating that exercise limitation is likely the result of cardiovascular factors in these patients.[74]

Exercise usually worsens the central hemodynamic abnormalities observed at rest in patients with ILD: for instance, the right ventricular afterload increases out of proportion to cardiac output, leading to higher pulmonary arterial pressures.

Skeletal Muscle Function

Skeletal muscle dysfunction is emerging as an important systemic consequence of ILD that likely contributes to exercise intolerance.[53,76] The term "skeletal muscle dysfunction" is used to reflect the morphologic changes to the skeletal muscle that result in a degradation in function (ie, muscle strength, endurance, and/or resistance to fatigue) of the limb muscles (further discussion in the topic is provided in The Relevance of Limb Muscle Dysfunction In COPD: A Review for Clinicians).[77,78] Although considered a separate entity from the limb muscles, the structure and function of the respiratory muscles are also thought to be adversely affected in ILD, albeit to a lesser extent (further discussion in the topic is provided in Respiratory Muscle assessment in Clinical Practice).[53] Current studies have not identified the exact mechanisms of skeletal muscle dysfunction in ILD; however, a host of factors that are known to decrease skeletal muscle function are commonly observed in patients with ILD, including physical deconditioning, malnutrition, arterial hypoxemia, oxidative stress, pulmonary and systemic inflammation, and corticosteroid use.[53] When present, skeletal muscle dysfunction hastens metabolic acidosis during exercise as well as the onset of exercise-induced skeletal muscle fatigue. It follows that skeletal muscle dysfunction likely influences the physiologic response to exercise in ILD.

Studies in a variety of ILD subtypes indicate that quadriceps muscle strength is reduced relative to normative values in healthy individuals.[79–82] Moreover, after adjusting for body mass, quadriceps strength seems to be lower in patients with IPF than in those with chronic obstructive pulmonary disease.[83] Although limited evidence is available, it stands to reason that the loss in quadriceps muscle strength in ILD is related to changes in morphology. Indeed, a recent study in patients with advanced IPF indicates that rectus femoris cross-sectional area was 19% lower compared with healthy age-matched controls. The clinical relevance of skeletal muscle dysfunction is underscored by the fact that the loss in quadriceps muscle strength in ILD is associated with the degree of impairment in functional capacity[79,82] and that functional capacity is a significant predictor of both quality of life[84] and mortality.[85]

The data relating to the effect of ILD on respiratory muscle function are equivocal. It seems intuitive that skeletal muscle function is likely to be globally affected, whereby the respiratory muscle function would be reduced to a similar degree compared with other skeletal muscles. However, the increased work of breathing and the decreased ventilatory efficiency in ILD likely result in chronic "loading" of the respiratory muscles that preserves their function. Indeed, respiratory muscle strength, as indicated by maximal respiratory pressures, seem to be relatively preserved in ILD.[58,86] Conversely, another report suggests that patients with ILD have impaired diaphragmatic force-generating capacity relative to healthy controls.[87]

Impaired appendicular muscle function is a common feature in patients with advanced ILD, likely contributing to increase the neural afferent inputs that stimulate ventilation.

Sensory Responses

The negative consequences of ILD on pulmonary, cardiovascular, and skeletal muscle function increase the perceived intensity of dyspnea and/or leg discomfort during exercise. Patients with ILD report higher dyspnea intensity ratings for a given $\dot{V}_E$ and work rate compared with healthy individuals[55,59,88] (**Fig. 8**). Although the mechanisms of dyspnea are complex and multifactorial, there is evidence that exertional dyspnea intensity is a reflection of increased neural respiratory drive in healthy individuals as well as those with chronic respiratory disease (further discussion in the topic is provided in The Pathophysiology of Dyspnea and Exercise Intolerance in COPD).[55,89,90] Thus, the increased dyspnea intensity ratings in patients with ILD can be partly attributed to factors that increase neural respiratory drive, such as ventilatory inefficiency, constraints on tidal volume expansion, and pulmonary gas exchange impairment.[90] Indeed, dyspnea intensity ratings during cardiopulmonary exercise testing in patients with ILD are significantly associated with (1) $\dot{V}_E$ relative to maximum, (2) electromyography of the diaphragm relative to maximum (a surrogate measure of neural respiratory drive), (3) tidal volume relative to vital capacity, (4) neuromechanical uncoupling (ie, the ratio between electromyography of the diaphragm relative to maximum and tidal volume relative to vital capacity), and (5) increasing esophageal pressure relative to maximum (an index of increased contractile respiratory muscle effort).[55,59,89]

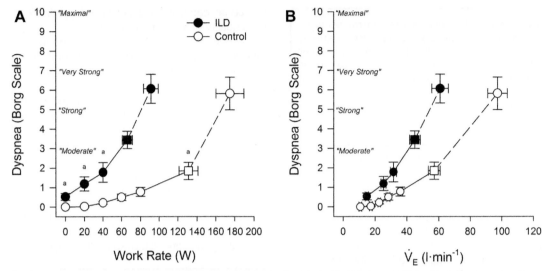

Fig. 8. Dyspnea as a function of work rate (panel *A*) and minute ventilation (panel *B*) during incremental cycle exercise in patients with ILD and age-matched healthy controls. Circles represent data points at discrete work rates and at peak exercise, and squares represent the tidal volume–minute ventilation inflection points. [a] $P<.05$ for ILD versus control subjects. $\dot{V}_E$, minute ventilation. (*Reprinted* with permission of the American Thoracic Society. Copyright © 2018 American Thoracic Society. Faisal A, Alghamdi BJ, Ciavaglia CE, et al. Common mechanisms of dyspnea in chronic interstitial and obstructive lung disorders. Am J Respir Crit Care Med. 2016;193(3):299–309. The American Journal of Respiratory and Critical Care Medicine is an official journal of the American Thoracic Society.)

Perceived dyspnea quality during exercise also differs between patients with ILD and healthy individuals.[59] Although both populations report an increased sensation of "work and effort to breathe" during exercise, patients with ILD report a sensation of "unsatisfied inspiration" at peak exercise.[55,59,90] Although the precise physiologic mechanisms have not been identified, it has been suggested that the perception of "unsatisfied inspiration" during exercise in ILD is likely the result of an awareness of a greater neural respiratory drive needed to support a given level of ventilation in the setting of constraints on tidal volume expansion.[55,89,91]

Patients with ILD who experience ventilatory constraints during exercise are more likely to discontinue exercise because of intolerable dyspnea than those who do not, whereas the latter are more likely to terminate exercise due to leg discomfort[58] (see **Fig. 6**). Exercise-induced arterial hypoxemia may also contribute to increased perceived leg discomfort and consequent exercise cessation, because reduced oxygen delivery to the peripheral locomotor muscles can result in increased muscle fatigue and metabolic acidosis.[92] In addition, skeletal muscle dysfunction may contribute to increased sensations of both dyspnea and/or leg discomfort due to reductions in respiratory and locomotor muscle oxidative capacity, thereby resulting in premature peripheral muscle fatigue.[53] However, direct experimental data supporting this idea are lacking.

> Regardless of the specific mechanism (ventilatory inefficiency, inspiratory volume constraints, hypoxemia, ergo-receptor stimulation, sympathetic overexcitation), a high respiratory neural drive at a given work rate largely explains exertional breathlessness in patients with ILD.

MECHANISMS OF EXERCISE LIMITATION

Given the numerous pathologic consequences of ILD on the physiologic and sensory responses to exercise, defining the precise mechanisms of exercise limitation is challenging. Because ILD primarily affects the lungs, it is reasonable to assume that the associated derangements in the ventilatory response to exercise would primarily contribute to exercise limitation. Indeed, imposing an additional ventilatory stimulus by adding external dead space to the breathing circuit during incremental cycling reduces exercise capacity and increases dyspnea compared with incremental exercise without additional dead space in patients with ILD.[93] The logical conclusion from this finding is that the inability to further increase $\dot{V}_E$ during incremental exercise with additional dead space indicates that exercise intolerance is brought on by ventilatory limitation. Conversely, providing high amounts of supplemental oxygen (ie, 60%) in combination with additional dead space (to prevent the decrease in $\dot{V}_E$ associated with breathing supplemental oxygen) during incremental exercise results in improved exercise capacity compared with breathing ambient air with no additional dead space.[94] Thus, it would seem that pulmonary gas exchange impairment is even more important than ventilatory limitation when considering the causes of exercise limitation in ILD. Others have argued that circulatory dysfunction is the primary predictor of exercise capacity based on retrospective correlative analyses of data from cardiopulmonary exercise tests in a relatively large sample of patients with ILD.[95] Moreover, it is entirely possible that skeletal muscle dysfunction may also contribute to exercise limitation in ILD[53]; however, direct evidence supporting this hypothesis is currently lacking. Despite the fact that exercise limitation in ILD has been separately ascribed to ventilatory limitation,[93] impairments in pulmonary gas exchange,[94] and cardiovascular function,[95] a far more plausible scenario is that these factors collectively lead to exercise limitation in this population.[5] The relative contribution of each pathophysiologic feature of ILD is likely to vary based on the ILD subtype, disease severity, presence of comorbidities, and the degree of functional decline.

> The relative contribution of ventilation, lung mechanics, pulmonary gas exchange, and cardiovascular function to exercise intolerance varies in patients with ILD: cardiopulmonary exercise testing might prove valuable to untangle the most prominent physiologic abnormalities in individual patients.

SUMMARY

ILD is a devastating category of diseases that affects primarily the lungs but also the pulmonary vasculature and the heart. At rest, patients with ILD have restrictive ventilatory impairment, poor pulmonary gas exchange, and in many cases, decreased cardiovascular function. In addition, a growing body of evidence indicates that some patients with ILD have skeletal muscle dysfunction. The pathologic features of ILD are worsened during exercise, resulting in increased dyspnea and poor exercise tolerance. Our current understanding of the pathophysiology of exercise in ILD suggests that exercise limitation is related to the combined influences of mechanical ventilatory constraints, impaired pulmonary gas exchange, and reduced cardiovascular function.

ACKNOWLEDGMENTS

YMS was supported by fellowships from the Michael Smith Foundation for Health Research (MSFHR) and the British Columbia Lung Association (BCLA). MRS was supported by a fellowship from the BCLA. CJR was supported by a Scholar Award from the MSFHR. JAG was supported by a Clinical Rehabilitation New Investigator Award from the Canadian Institutes of Health Research and a Scholar Award from the MSFHR.

REFERENCES

1. King TE Jr. Clinical advances in the diagnosis and therapy of the interstitial lung diseases. Am J Respir Crit Care Med 2005;172(3):268–79.
2. Tinghe RM, Noble PW. Inflammation in the pathogenesis of interstitial lung disease. In: Schwarz MI, King TE, editors. Interstitial lung disease. 5th edition. Shelton (CT): People's Medical Publishing House; 2011. p. 281–314.
3. Chetta A, Marangio E, Olivieri D. Pulmonary function testing in interstitial lung diseases. Respiration 2004; 71(3):209–13.
4. Collard HR, Pantilat SZ. Dyspnea in interstitial lung disease. Curr Opin Support Palliat Care 2008;2(2): 100–4.
5. Holland AE. Exercise limitation in interstitial lung disease - mechanisms, significance and therapeutic options. Chron Respir Dis 2010;7(2):101–11.
6. Bagnato G, Harari S. Cellular interactions in the pathogenesis of interstitial lung diseases. Eur Respir Rev 2015;24(135):102–14.
7. Cosgrove GP, Schwarz MI. Approach to the evaluation and diagnosis of intersititial lung disease. In: Schwarz MI, King TE, editors. Interstitial lung disease. 5th edition. Shelton (CT): People's Medical Publishing House; 2011. p. 3–33.
8. Farkas L, Gauldie J, Voelkel NF, et al. Pulmonary hypertension and idiopathic pulmonary fibrosis: a tale of angiogenesis, apoptosis, and growth factors. Am J Respir Cell Mol Biol 2011;45(1):1–15.
9. Baydur A. Pulmonary physiology in interstitial lung disease: recent developments in diagnostic and prognostic implications. Curr Opin Pulm Med 1996; 2(5):370–5.
10. Panagiotou M, Church AC, Johnson MK, et al. Pulmonary vascular and cardiac impairment in interstitial lung disease. Eur Respir Rev 2017; 26(143).
11. Gibson GJ, Pride NB. Pulmonary mechanics in fibrosing alveolitis: the effects of lung shrinkage. Am Rev Respir Dis 1977;116(4):637–47.
12. McCormack FX, King TE Jr, Voelker DR, et al. Idiopathic pulmonary fibrosis. Abnormalities in the bronchoalveolar lavage content of surfactant protein A. Am Rev Respir Dis 1991;144(1):160–6.
13. Thompson MJ, Colebatch HJ. Decreased pulmonary distensibility in fibrosing alveolitis and its relation to decreased lung volume. Thorax 1989;44(9):725–31.

14. Knudson RJ, Kaltenborn WT. Evaluation of lung elastic recoil by exponential curve analysis. Respir Physiol 1981;46(1):29–42.

15. Gibson GJ. Lung volumes and elasticity. Clin Chest Med 2001;22(4):623–35, vii.

16. Sansores RH, Ramirez-Venegas A, Perez-Padilla R, et al. Correlation between pulmonary fibrosis and the lung pressure-volume curve. Lung 1996;174(5):315–23.

17. Gunther A, Schmidt R, Nix F, et al. Surfactant abnormalities in idiopathic pulmonary fibrosis, hypersensitivity pneumonitis and sarcoidosis. Eur Respir J 1999;14(3):565–73.

18. Parker CM, Fitzpatrick MF, O'Donnell DE. Physiology of interstitial lung disease. In: Schwarz MI, King TE, editors. Interstitial lung disease. 5th edition. Shelton (CT): People's Medical Publishing House; 2011. p. 61–84.

19. Martinez FJ, Flaherty K. Pulmonary function testing in idiopathic interstitial pneumonias. Proc Am Thorac Soc 2006;3(4):315–21.

20. Javaheri S, Sicilian L. Lung function, breathing pattern, and gas exchange in interstitial lung disease. Thorax 1992;47(2):93–7.

21. Mura M, Zompatori M, Pacilli AM, et al. The presence of emphysema further impairs physiologic function in patients with idiopathic pulmonary fibrosis. Respir Care 2006;51(3):257–65.

22. Schmidt SL, Nambiar AM, Tayob N, et al. Pulmonary function measures predict mortality differently in IPF versus combined pulmonary fibrosis and emphysema. Eur Respir J 2011;38(1):176–83.

23. Berend N. Respiratory disease and respiratory physiology: putting lung function into perspective interstitial lung disease. Respirology 2014;19(7):952–9.

24. Jayamanne DS, Epstein H, Goldring RM. The influence of lung volume on expiratory flow rates in diffuse interstitial lung disease. Am J Med Sci 1978;275(3):329–36.

25. Lambert RK, Wilson TA, Hyatt RE, et al. A computational model for expiratory flow. J Appl Physiol Respir Environ Exerc Physiol 1982;52(1):44–56.

26. Boros PW, Franczuk M, Wesolowski S. Value of spirometry in detecting volume restriction in interstitial lung disease patients. Spirometry in interstitial lung diseases. Respiration 2004;71(4):374–9.

27. Young IH, Bye PT. Gas exchange in disease: asthma, chronic obstructive pulmonary disease, cystic fibrosis, and interstitial lung disease. Compr Physiol 2011;1(2):663–97.

28. Wemeau-Stervinou L, Perez T, Murphy C, et al. Lung capillary blood volume and membrane diffusion in idiopathic interstitial pneumonia. Respir Med 2012;106(4):564–70.

29. Levinson RS, Metzger LF, Stanley NN, et al. Airway function in sarcoidosis. Am J Med 1977;62(1):51–9.

30. Oliveira RK, Pereira CA, Ramos RP, et al. A haemodynamic study of pulmonary hypertension in chronic hypersensitivity pneumonitis. Eur Respir J 2014;44(2):415–24.

31. Agusti AG, Roca J, Gea J, et al. Mechanisms of gas-exchange impairment in idiopathic pulmonary fibrosis. Am Rev Respir Dis 1991;143(2):219–25.

32. West JB. Causes of carbon dioxide retention in lung disease. N Engl J Med 1971;284(22):1232–6.

33. Risk C, Epler GR, Gaensler EA. Exercise alveolar-arterial oxygen pressure difference in interstitial lung disease. Chest 1984;85(1):69–74.

34. Roughton FJ, Forster RE. Relative importance of diffusion and chemical reaction rates in determining rate of exchange of gases in the human lung, with special reference to true diffusing capacity of pulmonary membrane and volume of blood in the lung capillaries. J Appl Physiol 1957;11(2):290–302.

35. Cassan SM, Divertie MB, Brown AL Jr. Fine structural morphometry on biopsy specimens of human lung. 2. Diffuse idiopathic pulmonary fibrosis. Chest 1974;65(3):275–8.

36. Renzoni EA, Walsh DA, Salmon M, et al. Interstitial vascularity in fibrosing alveolitis. Am J Respir Crit Care Med 2003;167(3):438–43.

37. Kubo H, Nakayama K, Yanai M, et al. Anticoagulant therapy for idiopathic pulmonary fibrosis. Chest 2005;128(3):1475–82.

38. Martin MD, Chung JH, Kanne JP. Idiopathic pulmonary fibrosis. J Thorac Imaging 2016;31(3):127–39.

39. Read J, Williams RS. Pulmonary ventilation; blood flow relationships in intersititial disease of the lungs. Am J Med 1959;27:545–50.

40. Wagner PD, Dantzker DR, Dueck R, et al. Distribution of ventilation-perfusion ratios in patients with interstitial lung disease. Chest 1976;69(2 Suppl):256–7.

41. Turner-Warwick M. Precapillary systemic-pulmonary anastomoses. Thorax 1963;18:225–37.

42. Seeger W, Adir Y, Barbera JA, et al. Pulmonary hypertension in chronic lung diseases. J Am Coll Cardiol 2013;62(25 Suppl):D109–16.

43. Nathan SD, Noble PW, Tuder RM. Idiopathic pulmonary fibrosis and pulmonary hypertension: connecting the dots. Am J Respir Crit Care Med 2007;175(9):875–80.

44. Zangiabadi A, De Pasquale CG, Sajkov D. Pulmonary hypertension and right heart dysfunction in chronic lung disease. Biomed Res Int 2014;2014:739674.

45. Shino MY, Lynch JP 3rd, Saggar R, et al. Pulmonary hypertension complicating interstitial lung disease and COPD. Semin Respir Crit Care Med 2013;34(5):600–19.

46. Simonneau G, Gatzoulis MA, Adatia I, et al. Updated clinical classification of pulmonary hypertension. J Am Coll Cardiol 2013;62(25 Suppl):D34–41.

47. Andersen CU, Mellemkjaer S, Hilberg O, et al. Pulmonary hypertension in interstitial lung disease: prevalence, prognosis and 6 min walk test. Respir Med 2012;106(6):875–82.

48. Papakosta D, Pitsiou G, Daniil Z, et al. Prevalence of pulmonary hypertension in patients with idiopathic pulmonary fibrosis: correlation with physiological parameters. Lung 2011;189(5):391–9.

49. Bogaard HJ, Abe K, Vonk Noordegraaf A, et al. The right ventricle under pressure: cellular and molecular mechanisms of right-heart failure in pulmonary hypertension. Chest 2009;135(3):794–804.

50. Kolb TM, Hassoun PM. Right ventricular dysfunction in chronic lung disease. Cardiol Clin 2012;30(2):243–56.

51. Weitzenblum E, Ehrhart M, Rasaholinjanahary J, et al. Pulmonary hemodynamics in idiopathic pulmonary fibrosis and other interstitial pulmonary diseases. Respiration 1983;44(2):118–27.

52. Vonk Noordegraaf A, Galie N. The role of the right ventricle in pulmonary arterial hypertension. Eur Respir Rev 2011;20(122):243–53.

53. Panagiotou M, Polychronopoulos V, Strange C. Respiratory and lower limb muscle function in interstitial lung disease. Chron Respir Dis 2016;13(2):162–72.

54. Nishiyama O, Yamazaki R, Sano H, et al. Physical activity in daily life in patients with idiopathic pulmonary fibrosis. Respir Investig 2018;56(1):57–63.

55. Faisal A, Alghamdi BJ, Ciavaglia CE, et al. Common mechanisms of dyspnea in chronic interstitial and obstructive lung disorders. Am J Respir Crit Care Med 2016;193(3):299–309.

56. Van Meerhaeghe A, Scano G, Sergysels R, et al. Respiratory drive and ventilatory pattern during exercise in interstitial lung disease. Bull Eur Physiopathol Respir 1981;17(1):15–26.

57. Dias OM, Baldi BG, Ferreira JG, et al. Mechanisms of exercise limitation in patients with chronic hypersensitivity pneumonitis. ERJ Open Res 2018;4(3).

58. Marciniuk DD, Sridhar G, Clemens RE, et al. Lung volumes and expiratory flow limitation during exercise in interstitial lung disease. J Appl Physiol 1994;77(2):963–73.

59. O'Donnell DE, Chau LK, Webb KA. Qualitative aspects of exertional dyspnea in patients with interstitial lung disease. J Appl Physiol 1998;84(6):2000–9.

60. Dominelli PB, Render JN, Molgat-Seon Y, et al. Precise mimicking of exercise hyperpnea to investigate the oxygen cost of breathing. Respir Physiol Neurobiol 2014;201:15–23.

61. Dempsey JA, Wagner PD. Exercise-induced arterial hypoxemia. J Appl Physiol 1999;87(6):1997–2006.

62. Agusti AG, Roca J, Rodriguez-Roisin R, et al. Different patterns of gas exchange response to exercise in asbestosis and idiopathic pulmonary fibrosis. Eur Respir J 1988;1(6):510–6.

63. Du Plessis JP, Fernandes S, Jamal R, et al. Exertional hypoxemia is more severe in fibrotic interstitial lung disease than in COPD. Respirology 2018;23(4):392–8.

64. Hamer J. Cause of low arterial oxygen saturation in pulmonary fibrosis. Thorax 1964;19:507–14.

65. Jernudd-Wilhelmsson Y, Hornblad Y, Hedenstierna G. Ventilation-perfusion relationships in interstitial lung disease. Eur J Respir Dis 1986;68(1):39–49.

66. Eklund A, Broman L, Broman M, et al. V/Q and alveolar gas exchange in pulmonary sarcoidosis. Eur Respir J 1989;2(2):135–44.

67. Degani-Costa LH, Levarge B, Digumarthy SR, et al. Pulmonary vascular response patterns during exercise in interstitial lung disease. Eur Respir J 2015;46(3):738–49.

68. Bush A, Busst CM. Cardiovascular function at rest and on exercise in patients with cryptogenic fibrosing alveolitis. Thorax 1988;43(4):276–83.

69. Hawrylkiewicz I, Izdebska-Makosa Z, Grebska E, et al. Pulmonary haemodynamics at rest and on exercise in patients with idiopathic pulmonary fibrosis. Bull Eur Physiopathol Respir 1982;18(3):403–10.

70. Troy LK, Young IH, Lau EM, et al. Exercise pathophysiology and the role of oxygen therapy in idiopathic interstitial pneumonia. Respirology 2016;21(6):1005–14.

71. Collard HR, Anstrom KJ, Schwarz MI, et al. Sildenafil improves walk distance in idiopathic pulmonary fibrosis. Chest 2007;131(3):897–9.

72. Caminati A, Cassandro R, Harari S. Pulmonary hypertension in chronic interstitial lung diseases. Eur Respir Rev 2013;22(129):292–301.

73. Baughman RP, Gerson M, Bosken CH. Right and left ventricular function at rest and with exercise in patients with sarcoidosis. Chest 1984;85(3):301–6.

74. Marciniuk DD, Gallagher CG. Clinical exercise testing in interstitial lung disease. Clin Chest Med 1994;15(2):287–303.

75. Schwaiblmair M, Behr J, Fruhmann G. Cardiorespiratory responses to incremental exercise in patients with systemic sclerosis. Chest 1996;110(6):1520–5.

76. Holland AE. Functional capacity in idiopathic pulmonary fibrosis: looking beyond the lungs. Respirology 2015;20(6):857–8.

77. Mador MJ, Bozkanat E. Skeletal muscle dysfunction in chronic obstructive pulmonary disease. Respir Res 2001;2(4):216–24.

78. Maltais F, Decramer M, Casaburi R, et al. An official American Thoracic Society/European Respiratory Society statement: update on limb muscle

dysfunction in chronic obstructive pulmonary disease. Am J Respir Crit Care Med 2014;189(9): e15–62.

79. Nishiyama O, Taniguchi H, Kondoh Y, et al. Quadriceps weakness is related to exercise capacity in idiopathic pulmonary fibrosis. Chest 2005;127(6): 2028–33.

80. Spruit MA, Thomeer MJ, Gosselink R, et al. Skeletal muscle weakness in patients with sarcoidosis and its relationship with exercise intolerance and reduced health status. Thorax 2005;60(1):32–8.

81. Mendoza L, Gogali A, Shrikrishna D, et al. Quadriceps strength and endurance in fibrotic idiopathic interstitial pneumonia. Respirology 2014;19(1): 138–43.

82. Watanabe F, Taniguchi H, Sakamoto K, et al. Quadriceps weakness contributes to exercise capacity in nonspecific interstitial pneumonia. Respir Med 2013; 107(4):622–8.

83. Kozu R, Senjyu H, Jenkins SC, et al. Differences in response to pulmonary rehabilitation in idiopathic pulmonary fibrosis and chronic obstructive pulmonary disease. Respiration 2011;81(3):196–205.

84. Chang JA, Curtis JR, Patrick DL, et al. Assessment of health-related quality of life in patients with interstitial lung disease. Chest 1999;116(5):1175–82.

85. Wallaert B, Monge E, Le Rouzic O, et al. Physical activity in daily life of patients with fibrotic idiopathic interstitial pneumonia. Chest 2013;144(5):1652–8.

86. Garcia-Rio F, Pino JM, Ruiz A, et al. Accuracy of noninvasive estimates of respiratory muscle effort during spontaneous breathing in restrictive diseases. J Appl Physiol 2003;95(4):1542–9.

87. Walterspacher S, Schlager D, Walker DJ, et al. Respiratory muscle function in interstitial lung disease. Eur Respir J 2013;42(1):211–9.

88. O'Donnell DE, Ora J, Webb KA, et al. Mechanisms of activity-related dyspnea in pulmonary diseases. Respir Physiol Neurobiol 2009;167(1):116–32.

89. Schaeffer MR, Ryerson CJ, Ramsook AH, et al. Neurophysiological mechanisms of exertional dyspnoea in fibrotic interstitial lung disease. Eur Respir J 2018;51(1):1701726.

90. O'Donnell DE, Elbehairy AF, Berton DC, et al. Advances in the evaluation of respiratory pathophysiology during exercise in chronic lung diseases. Front Physiol 2017;8:82.

91. Schaeffer MR, Ryerson CJ, Ramsook AH, et al. Effects of hyperoxia on dyspnoea and exercise endurance in fibrotic interstitial lung disease. Eur Respir J 2017;49(5).

92. Amann M, Regan MS, Kobitary M, et al. Impact of pulmonary system limitations on locomotor muscle fatigue in patients with COPD. Am J Physiol Regul Integr Comp Physiol 2010;299(1):R314–24.

93. Marciniuk DD, Watts RE, Gallagher CG. Dead space loading and exercise limitation in patients with interstitial lung disease. Chest 1994;105(1):183–9.

94. Harris-Eze AO, Sridhar G, Clemens RE, et al. Role of hypoxemia and pulmonary mechanics in exercise limitation in interstitial lung disease. Am J Respir Crit Care Med 1996;154(4 Pt 1):994–1001.

95. Hansen JE, Wasserman K. Pathophysiology of activity limitation in patients with interstitial lung disease. Chest 1996;109(6):1566–76.

Clinical and Physiologic Implications of Negative Cardiopulmonary Interactions in Coexisting Chronic Obstructive Pulmonary Disease-Heart Failure

J. Alberto Neder, MD, PhD, FRCPC, FERS[a],*,
Alcides Rocha, MD, PhD[b], Danilo C. Berton, MD, PhD[c],
Denis E. O'Donnell, MD, FRCPI, FRCPC, FERS[d]

KEYWORDS

- Lung function • Cardiopulmonary interactions • Cardiopulmonary exercise testing • Dyspnea
- Chronic obstructive pulmonary disease

KEY POINTS

- Chronic obstructive pulmonary disease (COPD) and heart failure (HF) frequently coexist in practice, being important causes of disability and poor quality of life in the elderly.
- Complex interactions between the cardiocirculatory consequences of COPD and the respiratory effects of HF influence the physiologic abnormalities typically seen in each disease either at rest or on exertion.
- Understanding those interactions is clinically relevant for the correct interpretation of pulmonary function and cardiopulmonary exercise testing results.
- Pharmacologic treatment approaches based on (patho)physiologic concepts may have important beneficial effects on clinical outcomes, including symptom control and exercise tolerance.

INTRODUCTION

Heart failure with reduced ejection fraction (HF) is a common and disabling comorbidity of chronic obstructive pulmonary disease (COPD).[1] The prevalence of comorbid COPD-HF is higher than expected by their individual occurrence, particularly in the elderly.[2,3] Although increased proinflammatory and hyperoxidative stresses may partially justify this frequent association,[4] it seems mainly explained by a key risk factor common to COPD and ischemic heart disease: cigarette smoking. Owing to the continuous increase in age expectance,[5] rise in

Disclosure Statement: No author has any relationship with a commercial company that has a direct financial interest in subject matter or materials discussed in article or with a company making a competing product.
[a] Laboratory of Clinical Exercise Physiology, Division of Respirology and Sleep Medicine, Department of Medicine, Kingston Health Science Center, Queen's University, Richardson House, 102 Stuart Street, Kingston, Ontario K7L 2V6, Canada; [b] Heart Failure-COPD Outpatients Service and Pulmonary Function and Clinical Exercise Physiology Unit (SEFICE), Division of Respirology, Federal University of Sao Paulo, Sao Paulo, Brazil; [c] Division of Respirology, Federal University of Rio Grande do Sul, Porto Alegre, Brazil; [d] Respiratory Investigation Unit, Division of Respirology and Sleep Medicine, Kingston Health Science Center, Queen's University, Kingston, Ontario, Canada
* Corresponding author.
E-mail address: alberto.neder@queensu.ca

Clin Chest Med 40 (2019) 421–438
https://doi.org/10.1016/j.ccm.2019.02.006
0272-5231/19/© 2019 Elsevier Inc. All rights reserved.

COPD incidence[6] and the stable prevalence of HF,[7] comorbid COPD-HF will constitute an even more relevant public health issue in the next few decades.[8]

There is a wide variability in the prevalence of HF in patients with COPD and vice versa (ranging from ~10% to 25%). Higher prevalence rates are found in elderly patients with more severe COPD who are admitted in tertiary centers, in which full PFTs, transthoracic echocardiogram, and brain natriuretic peptide (BNP) measurements are readily available.

Dyspnea that is characteristically worsened, or precipitated, by exertion is the chief complaint in either COPD or HF.[8] Clinical, laboratorial, and imaging findings are dubious with regard to the presence and severity of the comorbid condition.[3] In practice, therefore, these patients are frequently referred to a pulmonary function test (PFT) laboratory in one of the following scenarios:

- A query for potential COPD in a smoker or ex-smoker with HF who remains dyspneic despite maximization of cardiovascular therapy;
- A patient with HF without the diagnosis of a respiratory disease who has been hospitalized due to a lower respiratory tract infection deemed to represent a "COPD exacerbation";
- A patient with known COPD and coronary artery disease with out-of-proportion dyspnea (to functional impairment indicated by previous PFTs); or
- Longitudinal assessment of a patient with COPD-HF with progressing dyspnea and exercise intolerance.

In any of these circumstances, the PFT laboratory might prove valuable information to assist on clinical decision making. There is, however, a noticeable paucity of information to guide the chest physician on how best to incorporate the information provided by the PFT laboratory in the clinical management of patients with COPD-HF.

In the present article, therefore, we firstly present the key respiratory functional consequences of HF and the main cardiocirculatory effects of COPD. We then outline the practical implications of those negative cardiopulmonary interactions on the interpretation of resting PFTs and cardiopulmonary exercise tests (CPETs). We finalize by presenting the potential impact of physiologic abnormalities in the currently available alternatives for the pharmacologic treatment of HF and COPD. Because of space constraints, we 'do not discuss the potential consequences of overlapping COPD-HF with preserved ejection fraction.[9]

RESPIRATORY CONSEQUENCES OF HEART FAILURE

Lower changes in lung volume relative to variations in transpulmonary pressure (ie, poor lung compliance) is the key abnormality observed in patients with chronic, moderate to severe HF. The mechanisms behind lung "stiffening"[10] in stable HF are multiple and inter-related:

- Accumulation of extravascular lung water;[11,12]
- Increased intrathoracic blood volume and chronic pulmonary congestion;[13]
- Septal thickening;[14]
- The space-occupying effects of an enlarged heart[15]; and, in some patients,
- Inspiratory muscle weakness.[16]

Moreover, low radial distending forces exerted on the bronchial wall because of low lung volumes, peribronchial edema, vascular engorgement of bronchovascular sheaths, and increased airway smooth muscle contractility may lead to varied degrees of (usually mild) airflow limitation.[17,18] Impaired pulmonary perfusion (low capillary blood volume) in areas of relatively preserved ventilation may increase the dead space (V_D), which, in association with a low tidal volume (V_T), increases the (V_D)/V_T ratio, that is, the "wasted" fraction of the breath. Hydrostatic injury due to recurrent edema, subendothelial fibrosis, and altered alveolar fluid clearance may impair the alveolar-capillary membrane conductance thereby worsening the efficiency of the lung as a gas exchanger.[19]

Routine PFTs in a patient with moderate to severe, but stable, HF usually shows a mild restrictive ventilatory defect with a trend to low lung diffusing factor for carbon monoxide (D_{LCO}) and diffusing coefficient for carbon monoxide (K_{CO}) (unless a sizable pleural effusion or massive cardiomegaly lead to a high K_{CO}, ie, a pattern of "extraparenchymal" restriction). Arterial blood gases measurements reveal normal-low Pa_{O_2} and Pa_{CO_2}. Low maximal "static" inspiratory pressures might be seen in a subset of patients.

The above-mentioned derangements are associated with many abnormalities on standard PFTs:[20,21]

- A "restrictive ventilatory defect" (**Fig. 1**) of highly variable severity, which is characterized by low total lung capacity (TLC) and forced vital capacity (FVC) with normal or, occasionally, increased forced expiratory volume in 1 second (FEV_1)/FVC ratio;

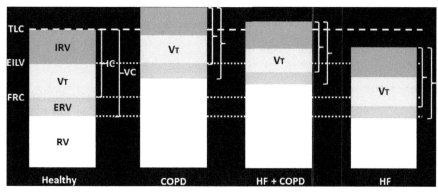

Fig. 1. Effects of chronic HF (CHF), COPD, and their overlap on resting lung volumes and capacities in nonseverely obese subjects.[17,20,21,38,86] Note that patients with combined diseases present with a variable combination of obstructive (COPD) and restrictive abnormalities (CHF). See text for further elaboration. EILV, end-inspiratory lung volume; ERV, expiratory reserve volume; FRC, functional residual capacity; IC, inspiratory capacity; IRV, inspiratory reserve volume; RV, residual volume; TLC, total lung capacity; VC, vital capacity; VT, tidal volume. (*From* Neder JA, Rocha A, Alencar MCN, et al. Current challenges in managing comorbid heart failure and COPD. Expert Rev Cardiovasc Ther 2018;16(9):655; with permission.)

- Low mid-expiratory flows (forced expiratory flow at 25%–75% of FVC (FEF$_{25\%-75\%}$) either because of impaired small airway function or the direct effects of a low FVC;
- A relatively preserved residual volume (RV) (unless the patient is morbidly obese or there is mild gas trapping owing to early closure of the small airways)[22];
- A low inspiratory capacity (IC) due to greater decrements in TLC than functional residual capacity (FRC); and, depending on disease severity,
- Low D$_{LCO}$ usually associated with normal or slightly reduced D$_{LCO}$/alveolar volume (V$_A$) ratio (K$_{CO}$) and largely preserved V$_A$/TLC ratio (further discussion in this topic is provided in Incorporating Lung Diffusing Capacity for Carbon Monoxide to Clinical Decision Making in Chest Medicine).[23]

CARDIOCIRCULATORY EFFECTS OF CHRONIC OBSTRUCTIVE PULMONARY DISEASE

The potential negative effects of COPD on central hemodynamics have long been recognized.[24] Although their clinical relevance is likely greater in situations associated with worsening lung mechanics (such as disease exacerbation or invasive positive pressure ventilation with high tidal volume), some of those abnormalities might be present in response to acute-on-chronic hyperinflation (eg, exercise).[25] It is rather axiomatic that their negative consequences tend to be worse in patients with an already compromised cardiac function (ie, HF) (**Fig. 2**):[8,26]

- High mean intrathoracic pressure compressing the inferior vena cava and right atrium, thereby decreasing venous return and right ventricle preload;
- High intrinsic positive end-expiratory pressure and hypoxia-induced pulmonary vasoconstriction increasing right ventricular afterload;
- The latter, in particular, may lead to a leftward shift of the interventricular septum, thereby precluding the left ventricle to reach the optimal geometry to maximize stroke volume for a given preload; and
- Larger swings in intrapleural pressure with consequent increase in left ventricular transmural pressure and afterload.

The importance of a low cardiac output secondary to negative cardiopulmonary interactions, particularly on exertion, should not be overlooked in COPD-HF: as shown in **Fig. 3**, patients with HF with similar resting hemodynamics present with lower leg blood flow, which parallels the impairment in central hemodynamics.[27] It is also conceivable that part of the cardiac output may be redirected from the peripheral muscles to the overloaded respiratory muscles, particularly at higher levels of ventilation in severely hyperinflated patients.[28,29] Abnormalities in peripheral vascular control and sympathetic overexcitation may also contribute to impair O$_2$ delivery to the contracting peripheral muscles (further discussion in the topic is provided in Respiratory Determinants of Exercise Limitation: Focus on Phrenic Afferents and The Lung Vasculature).[27]

> Increased left ventricular filling is important to minimize decrements in stroke volume in HF with reduced ejection fraction. Hyperinflation and gas trapping due to COPD are known to impair left ventricular filling, which may further hamper cardiac output on exertion in COPD-HF.

INTERPRETATION OF COMMON PULMONARY FUNCTION TESTS IN CHRONIC OBSTRUCTIVE PULMONARY DISEASE-HEART FAILURE
Ventilation

Low FVC in a patient with COPD with airflow limitation (reduced FEV_1/FVC) more commonly reflects a larger increase in RV (gas trapping) than TLC (thoracic hyperinflation) (**Table 1**).[25] In the appropriate clinical scenario, however, this can be ascribed to the restrictive effects of coexistent HF, that is, low TLC. In fact, the negative effects of HF on FVC may lead to a false-negative for airflow limitation if FVC decreases more than FEV_1 thereby "normalizing" FEV_1/FVC.[30] This is more likely to occur if the patient is obese, because high body mass characteristically reduces FVC[31]; of note, obesity is highly prevalent in COPD-HF.[2] Regardless of the severity of airflow limitation, part of the FEV_1 impairment might be a result of the restrictive effects of HF per se. It follows that there is a risk of overestimating COPD severity by FEV_1 alone in COPD-HF[32]; moreover, a "fast" decline in FEV_1 over time might in fact reflect a progressive decrease in FVC due to worsening HF. As in most circumstances, spirometry should be repeated after an inhaled short-acting bronchodilator even if FEV_1/FVC is preserved: a volume response to inhaled bronchodilator (significant and proportional increases in FVC and FEV_1)[33] might uncover an obstruction that had been obscured by a low FVC at baseline.

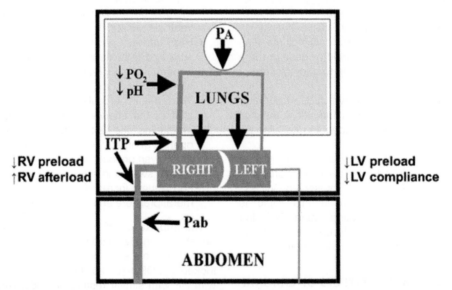

Fig. 2. Schematic illustration of the potential hemodynamic effects of gas trapping and lung hyperinflation secondary to expiratory flow limitation in patients with COPD. Right heart preload might be negatively influenced by hypercapnia-induced venous blood pooling, intraabdominal compression of splanchnic vessels (particularly inferior vena cava), and high mean intrathoracic pressure (ITP). Lung hyperinflation and a high intrinsic positive end-expiratory pressure (PEEPi) may compress the large and small pulmonary arterial vessels and the heart chambers: this effect, in association with high pulmonary capillary pressures due to left ventricular failure and alveolar (alv) hypoxia, increases the afterload of the right ventricle. Left ventricular stroke volume can be compromised by lower filling pressures, hypoxia-induced myocardial stiffness, and decreased compliance due to a leftward shift of the interventricular septum by the overdistended right ventricle. The latter, in particular, may interfere with the "ideal" left ventricular length-tension relationship for the prevailing filling pressure (Frank-Starling mechanism). Low dynamic lung compliance and high PEEPi require a more negative intrapleural pressure, particularly at the start of inspiration; consequently, left ventricular transmural pressure and left ventricular afterload increase. The latter may also increase secondary to high systemic vascular resistance induced by sympathetic overexcitation. Those abnormalities jointly lead to low right and left stroke volume, particularly under the stress of exercise. (*From* O'Donnell DE, Laveneziana P, Webb K, et al. Chronic obstructive pulmonary disease: clinical integrative physiology. Clin Chest Med 2014;35(1):60; with permission.)

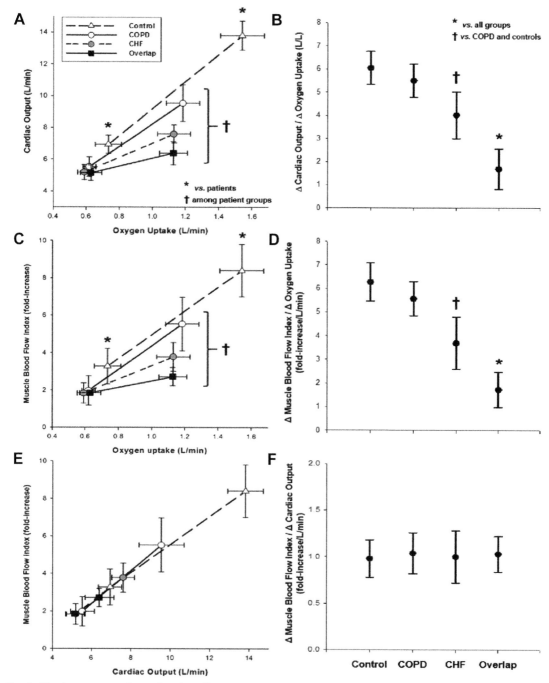

Fig. 3. The importance of exertional cardiac output in impairing muscle blood flow in patients with coexisting COPD-HF ("overlap"). Note that despite similar resting hemodynamics, overlap patients presented with lower increases in cardiac output than their counterparts with HF (*upper panels*). Those negative cardiopulmonary interaction led to proportional decreases in muscle blood flow (*middle* and *lower panels*). "Δ" is the difference between 20% and 80% peak work rate. (*From* Oliveira MF F Arbex F, Alencar MC, et al. Heart failure impairs muscle blood flow and endurance exercise tolerance in COPD. COPD 2016;13(4):5; with permission.)

Spirometry alone can also increase the risk of a false-positive result for COPD in patients with HF. For instance, β-blockers may disproportionately reduce FEV_1 compared with FVC, leading to a low FEV_1/FVC.[17] As FEV_1/FVC decreases with age in both genders, the 0.7 threshold to indicate airflow limitation may overcall COPD in an elderly smoker with HF (see **Table 1**). Using the lower

Table 1
Common findings on routine PFTs in patients with comorbid COPD-HF (the abnormalities are influenced by the relative severity of each disease, clinical (in)stability, and obesity, among others)

	Potential interpretative challenges and their clinical consequences
Spirometry	
⇓ FVC	• Decrement in FVC might be larger than expected from COPD-induced gas trapping • If greater than FEV_1 decrease, preserved FEV_1/FVC may lead to a false-negative for airflow limitation • When low FVC is mainly determined by HF, alleviation of lung congestion is associated with rapid improvement in FVC
⇓ FEV_1	• Overestimation of the functional impairment caused by COPD • Decrease in FEV_1 in serial measurements might be related to HF rather than COPD worsening
⇓ $FEF_{25\%-75\%}$	• Influenced by a low FVC due to HF-related restriction: mid-expiratory flows may relate variably to the severity of small airway dysfunction
Lung volumes	
⇓ or ⇔ TLC	• Combined (obstructive and restrictive) ventilatory defect; potential "normalization" of TLC, that is, no evidence of thoracic hyperinflation in some patients
⇑ RV	• Pronounced decrement in FVC when associated with low TLC • If high, useful to confirm the presence of COPD-related gas trapping
⇑ or ⇔ FRC	• Useful to confirm the presence of COPD-related lung hyperinflation
⇓ IC	• Marked decrement in the volume available for tidal volume expansion, a key correlate of dyspnea
Respiratory Muscles	
⇓ MIP	• May reflect the compound effects of functional weakness due to COPD-related gas trapping with HF-induced weakness
Gas exchange	
⇓ to ⇓⇓ D_{LCO}	• May overestimate the impact of COPD on gas exchange efficiency (ie, disproportional to emphysema burden) • May lead to out-of-proportion decrease in D_{LCO} relative to the severity of FEV_1 impairment • Increase the likelihood of resting or exertional hypoxemia • Strong correlate of dyspnea and exercise intolerance in COPD-HF
⇑ V_D/V_T	• Marked increment contributing to increase exertional ventilation and dyspnea
⇔ or ⇓ Pa_{O_2}	• Hypoxemia depends on COPD severity and, secondarily, to HF control (congestion)
Variable Pa_{CO_2}	• Hypercapnia depends mainly on COPD severity • If low, important source of excessive exertional ventilation and dyspnea

Abbreviations: ⇑, increase; ⇓, decrease; ⇔, unaltered; D_{LCO}, lung diffusing capacity for carbon monoxide; $FEF_{25\%-75\%}$, forced expiratory flow between 25% and 75% of FVC; FEV_1, forced expiratory volume in one second; FRC, functional residual capacity; FVC, forced vital capacity; IC, inspiratory capacity; MIP, maximal inspiratory pressure; Pa, arterial partial pressure; RV, residual volume; TLC, total lung capacity; V_D, dead space; V_T, tidal volume.

limit of normal of FEV_1/FVC as the defining cutoff for airflow limitation may help to decrease the false-positives for COPD.[34] To avoid the erroneous interpretation that an (usually mild-to-moderate) obstructive defect following an acute decompensation of HF is due to COPD,[18] spirometry should be performed 3 to 4 weeks after clinical stabilization.[35] A positive methacholine challenge test may also be found during or immediately after an episode of HF decompensation,[36] and it should not be misinterpreted as indicating an intrinsic airway disease in this specific scenario.

A combined obstructive and restrictive ventilatory defect is characteristically seen in patients with COPD-HF. In a patient with known COPD who had been longitudinally followed with PFTs, the constrictive effects of HF may disproportionally lessen thoracic hyperinflation (high TLC) compared with gas trapping (high FRC and/or RV). The resulting decrements in FVC are variably related to a lower FEV_1: in some circumstance (eg, a patient with mild airflow limitation and reduced FVC due to gas trapping and/or obesity), a larger decrement in FVC than FEV_1 may "normalize" the FEV_1/FVC ratio.

Measurements of "static" lung volumes are helpful in clarifying potentially equivocal results from spirometry, particularly the meaning of a low FVC. In this context, gas trapping due to COPD may be readily identified by a high RV (eg, >120% predicted) and RV/TLC.[32] However, morbid obesity can decrease RV[31]; thus, a normal RV in a severely obese patient with HF should not be seen as evidence against COPD in a patient at risk. It should also be remembered that TLC within normal range may result from the opposing effects of COPD-induced hyperinflation and HF-related restriction (see **Fig. 1**).[32] If the latter prevails, airflow limitation and gas trapping may coexist with restriction (mixed disorder) with an ample list of differential diagnoses, including HF. Patients with COPD-HF may present with particularly low IC due to the combination of a high FRC (COPD) with a low TLC (HF) (see **Fig. 1**). Thus, the mechanical inspiratory limits for V_T expansion can be easily reached at lower levels of ventilation, leading to exertional dyspnea.[17] Of note, decreases in the so-called inspiratory fraction (IC/TLC ratio) may fail to reflect the severity of gas trapping as seen in COPD alone if TLC decreases more than IC in individual patients with COPD-HF.

Gas Exchange

Patients with coexisting COPD-HF commonly present with "out-of-proportion" (to emphysema burden) decrements in D_{LCO} (see **Table 1**). K_{CO} is also variably reduced but an apparently normal value may reflect a low V_A (and a low V_A/TLC ratio) as a result of impaired gas distribution.[37] In practice, longitudinal decrements in D_{LCO}, particularly over a short period of time, might reflect HF worsening rather than emphysema progression. The physiologic dead space (V_D/V_T ratio) is invariably increased, as is the alveolar-arterial O_2 gradient.[38] Whether this proves severe enough to decrease Pa_{O2} depends largely on the severity of COPD and, to a lesser extent, to lung congestion secondary to HF. Because of the increased respiratory neural drive associated with HF, some patients with COPD-HF may present with a trend to hypocapnia, a finding with important implications for ventilatory control and exertional dyspnea in comorbid HF-COPD (**Fig. 4**).[39] It is also possible that chronic cerebral vasoconstriction due to hypocapnia (**Fig. 5**)[40] may impair cerebrovascular reactivity to CO_2[41] leading to increased [H^+] close to the central chemoreceptors with thereby contributing to hyperventilation in selected patients with HF-COPD.

Clinical interpretation of a low D_{LCO} in a patient with comorbid COPD-HF should consider the potential cumulative effects of: emphysema, low "alveolar volume" secondary to ventilation distribution inhomogeneity and low lung volumes, ventilation-perfusion inequality, poor pulmonary blood flow due to low cardiac output, impaired alveolar-capillary membrane conductance, and anemia.

PATTERNS OF RESPONSE TO INCREMENTAL CARDIOPULMONARY EXERCISE TESTS IN CHRONIC OBSTRUCTIVE PULMONARY DISEASE-HEART FAILURE

Understanding the complex interaction among the mechanisms leading to exertional symptoms in COPD-HF might provide useful insights into the potential targets for disease management (**Fig. 6**).[42] Thus, CPETs can be valuable to determine if symptomatic patients are primarily limited by critical mechanical-ventilatory constraints and/or hypoxemia (suggesting a greater role for COPD)[43] or, alternatively, exercise is interrupted because of complaints of severe leg discomfort and preserved mechanical reserves (suggesting a dominant contribution of HF) (see also Unraveling the Causes of Unexplained Dyspnea: The Value of Exercise Testing). CPETs usually show a highly variable combination of findings typical of each disease as follows:

- Impaired muscle blood flow (in association with low Ca_{O2} in some patients) and bioenergetics leading to poor muscle O_2 delivery coupled with increasing contribution of anaerobic metabolism to adenosine triphosphate regeneration. As depicted in **Fig. 7**, this is shown by:[44]
  a. A shallow O_2 uptake ($\dot{V}O_2$)-work rate (WR) relationship (or even a downward inflection on at abnormally low WR);
  b. An early lactate ("anaerobic") threshold; and,
  c. An increased sense of leg effort at a given WR.
- Impaired stroke volume suggested (in a patient not treated with a β-blocker) by:
  a. An earlier and more rapid rise in heart rate as a function of $\dot{V}O_2$; and
  b. A low submaximal and maximal ($\dot{V}O_2$/heart rate ratio (O_2 pulse), particularly if there is a discernible plateau in O_2 pulse (provided an increased muscle O_2 extraction is

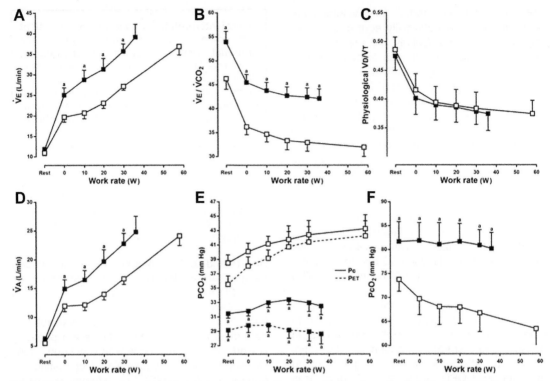

Fig. 4. The relevance of hypocapnia in increasing exertional ventilation in patients with COPD-HF. Hypocapnic patients (*closed circles*) presented with high minute (*A*) and alveolar (*D*) ventilation and poorer ventilatory efficiency (*B*) despite similar physiologic dead space (*C*) than their counterparts with normal-high capillary P_{CO_2} (*open symbols*) (*E*). Despite better preserved arterial oxygenation (*F*), higher ventilation in hypocapnic led to earlier attainment of critical mechanical constraints and intolerable dyspnea (not shown). [a]$P<.05$ for between-group comparisons at rest, standardized work rates and the highest work rate attained by all subjects in a given group. $\dot{V}A$, alveolar ventilation; Pc, capillary (arterialized) partial pressure; PET, end-tidal partial pressure; VD/VT, dead space/tidal volume ratio. (Reprinted with permission of the American Thoracic Society. Copyright © 2019 American Thoracic Society. Rocha A, Arbex FF, Sperandio PA, Souza A, Biazzim L, Mancuso F, et al. Excess Ventilation in COPD-heart Failure Overlap: Implications for Dyspnea and Exercise Intolerance. Am J Respir Crit Care Med. 2017 Nov 15;196:1264–1274. The American Journal of Respiratory and Critical Care Medicine is an official journal of the American Thoracic Society.)

unable to compensate for the low stroke volume).

- Increased ventilation ($\dot{V}E$) relative to metabolic demands secondary to heightened central and peripheral chemoreflexes (see also Update on Chemoreception: Influence on Cardiorespiratory Regulation and Patho-Physiology) and sympathetic activation (all contributing to a $Paco_2$, which is lower than otherwise expected by the severity of COPD)[39] plus a high VD/VT (see also Pulmonary Limitations in Heart Failure)[45]:
  a. A high submaximal $\dot{V}E/\dot{V}CO_2$ ratio, commonly as a consequence of a steep $\dot{V}E - \dot{V}CO_2$ slope and a normal-low $\dot{V}E - \dot{V}CO_2$ intercept;[39,46]
  b. A low end-tidal CO_2 (P_{ETCO_2}) that frequently fails to increase with disease progression;

and, if exercise is not precociously interrupted by a heightened sense of leg effort and/or dyspnea;
  c. Low ventilatory reserves as suggested by a high $\dot{V}E$/maximal voluntary ventilation ratio either at submaximal or peak exercise (>0.7–0.8);

- An early attainment of critical inspiratory constraints as a consequence of a normal or low "ceiling" (TLC), worsening expiratory flow limitation, and variable degrees of dynamic hyperinflation[47] (**Fig. 7**) (further discussion in the topic is provided in The Pathophysiology of Dyspnea and Exercise Intolerance in COPD):
  a. Low resting IC that remains stable or further decreases with exercise progression;

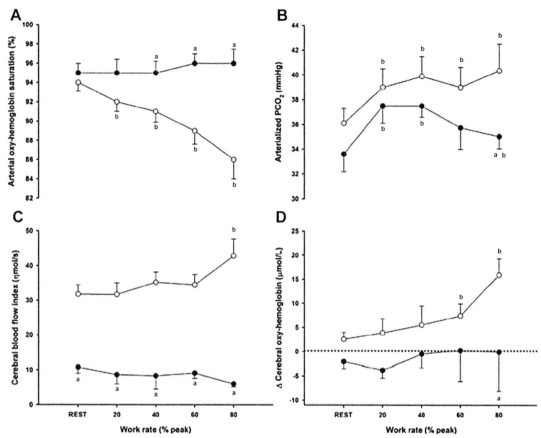

Fig. 5. Prefrontal cerebral blood flow (*C*) and oxygenation (*D*) as a function of exercise intensity in COPD (*open symbols*) and COPD-HF (*closed symbols*). Note that the latter group presented with impaired cerebral hemodynamics despite better preserved arterial oxygen saturation (*A*), a finding associated with lower arterialized partial pressure of carbon dioxide (*B*). [a] Between-group differences at a given time point; [b] Intragroup differences versus rest. (*From* Oliveira MF, Alencar MC, Arbex F, et al. Effects of heart failure on cerebral blood flow in COPD: Rest and exercise. Respir Physiol Neurobiol 2016;221:44; with permission.)

b. High V_T/IC and end-inspiratory lung volume/TLC ratios reflecting a critically low inspiratory reserve volume leading to a V_T plateau;

c. A large fraction of the tidal flow-volume loop overlapping the maximal tidal flow-volume loop with a change to a trapezoid shape, and

d. Increased dyspnea scores for a given WR and $\dot{V}E$.

Those mechanical abnormalities might be hastened if excessive ventilatory stimuli adds to a prolonged circulatory time to promote cycles of waxing and waning ventilation (exercise oscillatory ventilation) (**Fig. 8**) (further discussion in the topic is provided in Exertional Periodic Breathing in Heart Failure: Mechanisms and Clinical Implications).[48,49]

There are some specific clinical scenarios in which CPET can be particularly valuable in patients with suspected COPD-HF:

- In a smoker or ex-smoker with HF, the attainment of early critical inspiratory constraints (with or without a low breathing reserve) associated with a simultaneous increase in dyspnea as a function of WR and ventilation, occasionally accompanied by an unexpectedly high $\dot{V}E - \dot{V}CO_2$ intercept (as HF usually leads to a low intercept), indicate that COPD is contributing to patient's exercise intolerance.

- Conversely, preserved lung-mechanical reserves associated with dyspnea scores that increase in tandem with a heightened ventilatory response is not consistent with a mechanistic role for COPD to explain patient's exertional symptoms.

- An exaggerated ventilatory response to exertion in a patient with COPD (eg, a high $\dot{V}E - \dot{V}CO_2$ slope, a low $\dot{V}E - \dot{V}CO_2$ intercept, a low P_{ETCO_2} that fails to increase with exercise progression), which is deemed out-of-proportion to emphysema burden or pulmonary hypertension may, in the right clinical context, raise the suspicion of underlying HF.

- Identification of exertional oscillatory ventilation in a patient with COPD should prompt a more detailed cardiovascular investigation to rule out HF or another cause of exertional oscillatory ventilation (eg, atrial fibrillation, severe left atrial dilatation, central sleep apnea) (see also Exertional periodic breathing in heart failure: mechanisms and clinical implications).

CHRONIC OBSTRUCTIVE PULMONARY DISEASE PATHOPHYSIOLOGY: IMPLICATIONS FOR HEART FAILURE TREATMENT
β-Blockers

β-Blockers are associated with positive clinical outcomes in patients with COPD with or without coexistent HF.[50] Owing to the fear of worsening bronchoconstriction and gas trapping due to β_2-blockade, the diagnosis of COPD frequently inhibits the prescription of β-blockers in COPD-HF.[51] Thus, drugs with higher selectivity to β_1-receptors are generally preferred over nonselective β-blockers.[51] Although the undesirable effects of nonselective β-blockade on lung mechanics are commonly mild and transitory, patients with COPD-HF with lower FEV_1 and/or more severe gas trapping are at greater risk to report worsening dyspnea with nonselective medications. Although there is a lack of evidence based in large studies, patients with a pronounced "flow" response to inhaled bronchodilator (ie, large increase in FEV_1 but not in FVC) seem to be at higher risk of significant bronchoconstriction after β-blockade. Excessive chronotropic control after β-blockade might hamper the cardiac output response to exertion thereby contributing to poor exercise tolerance in some patients with COPD-HF.[52]

Selective β_1-blockers with slow uptitration of dosing should be preferred in patients with COPD-HF. This is particularly relevant in patients with poorer lung function (eg, FEV_1 < 1 L and/or RV > 200% predicted). In case of worsening bronchoconstriction, antimuscarinics may be used to temporarily control bronchoconstriction.

Diuretics

Diuretics are expected to decrease left ventricular filling pressures and the stimulation of juxtacapillary receptors, an important source of high neural respiratory drive and dyspnea in HF with or without COPD.[53] Lower pulmonary artery occlusion pressure may also help in decreasing right ventricular afterload and the leftward shift of the interventricular septum.[54] Less lung congestion is known to improve lung compliance and airway function, thereby reducing the work of breathing.[20,53] Thus, lower lung congestion secondary to diuretics may lessen the respiratory neural drive and improve neuromechanical coupling in COPD-HF.[55] Conversely, cardiac output in patients with COPD-HF might be particularly sensitive to changes in preload because of the negative effects of hyperinflation and abnormal lung mechanics.[25] Thus, relative hypovolemia caused by excessive diuresis may decrease cardiac output in the case of critical decrements in the filling pressures of the right and left atria.[8] It should also be emphasized that leg edema in COPD-HF may be caused by right ventricle failure and/or hypercapnia; moreover, peripheral edema is inconsistently related to lung congestion in these patients.[56] In this context, excessive diuresis may promote a hemodynamic status of relative hypovolemia leading to critical decrements in venous return and stroke volume.[8] Diuretic-induced metabolic alkalosis may lead to compensatory alveolar hypoventilation and further deterioration of arterial blood gases.[57] In fact, there is recent evidence that incident use of diuretics is independently associated with mortality in COPD.[58]

The "ideal" dose of diuretics in COPD-HF (which frequently changes dynamically over time) should be the lowest effective in relieving lung congestion and dyspnea while preserving cardiac output at rest and on exertion.

Renin-Angiotensin-Aldosterone Blockers

Renin-angiotensin-aldosterone blockers have been associated with slower emphysema progression in smokers[59] and FEV_1 decline in COPD,[60] as well as reductions in COPD-related hospitalizations and mortality.[51,61] Some physiologic investigations suggest that, if well tolerated, angiotensin-converting enzyme inhibitors (ACEIs) are particularly advantageous in patients with COPD-HF vis-à-vis the improvement in ventilatory and pulmonary gas exchange efficiency[62,63] and D_{LCO}[64] found in HF. Of note, controversy remains regarding to

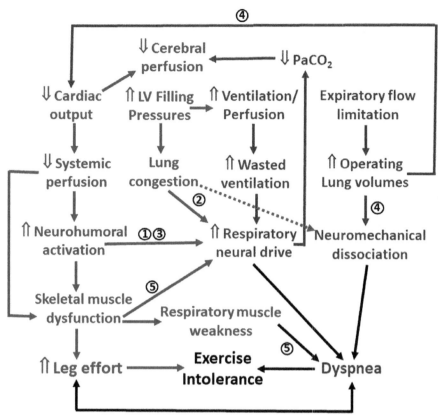

Fig. 6. A schematic representation of the pathophysiological linkages between HF (*red*) and COPD (*green*), which leads to poor exercise tolerance as a result of a sense of excessive leg effort and dyspnea. Low cardiac output associated with heightened sympathetic excitation impairs muscle blood flow and O_2 delivery increasing leg effort (*left*). The resulting overexcitation of muscle ergorreceptors and early lactacidosis, in addition to neurohumoral activation and lung congestion, are powerful stimulants of the drive to breathe (respiratory neural drive). The respiratory neural drive is further increased due to coexistent COPD as a large fraction of the breath is wasted in the dead space (VD) (*center*). Some patients ventilate in excess to the amount needed to overcome the increased VD: the consequent alveolar hyperventilation lead to hypocapnia, which, in association with a low cardiac output, impairs cerebral blood flow. Low cerebral blood flow, in turn, may decrease motor output to muscles and disturb cerebral vascular reactivity to changes in P_{CO_2} leading to sustained ventilatory stimuli. Higher operating lung volumes (lung hyperinflation) secondary to COPD (*right*) increase mean intrathoracic pressure and intrabreath swings in pleural pressure, which may impair venous return and increase left ventricle afterload, respectively. High respiratory neural drive and abnormal lung mechanics (partially related to low lung compliance due to congestion [*dashed line*]) jointly increase dyspnea for a given work rate and ventilation. High ventilation and abnormal lung mechanics increase the work of weaker inspiratory muscles, further worsening dyspnea in selected patients. Some patients may over-rate an uncomfortable sensation in the presence of another distressing symptom; thus, leg effort and dyspnea may potentiate each other (*bottom*). The main sites of action of the foundations of HF-COPD treatment, pertaining to symptom control, are shown (β-blockers [1], diuretics [2], renin-angiotensin blockers [3], bronchodilators [4], and exercise training [5]). See text for a detailed discussion. (*From* Neder JA, Rocha A, Alencar MCN, et al. Current challenges in managing comorbid heart failure and COPD. Expert Rev Cardiovasc Ther 2018;16(9):657; with permission.)

whether ACEIs or angiotensin receptor blockers are associated with lower risk of COPD exacerbation or pneumonia. Although COPD does not seem to increase the risk of ACEI-induced angioedema or cough,[65] the latter is particularly undesirable as it may incorrectly suggest poor control of COPD. Thus, worsening of cough on ACEI administration should prompt immediate switch to an angiotensin receptor blocker. There is no evidence so far that patients with COPD-HF should be denied the positive effects of the dual-acting angiotensin receptor neprilisyn inhibitors seen in patients with New York Heart Association class II or III HF.[66,67] Nevertheless, decreased expression of neprilisyn under hypoxia led to pulmonary arterial remodeling and a higher risk of pulmonary

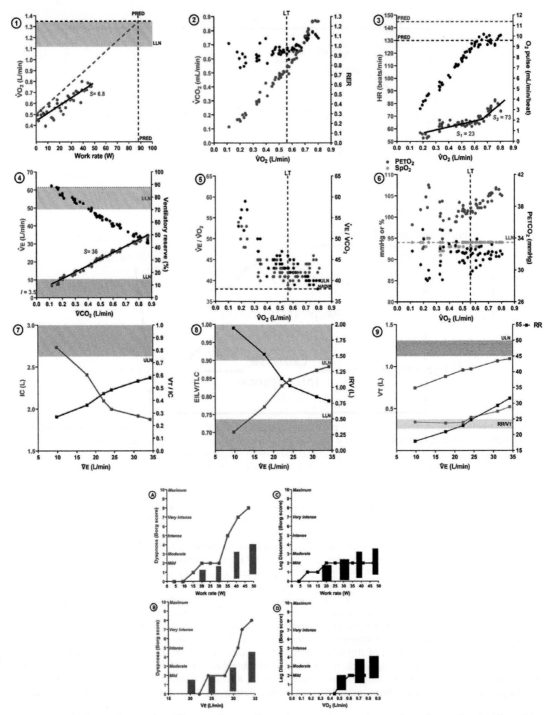

Fig. 7. Metabolic/cardiovascular (*first row*), ventilatory/gas exchange (*second row*), mechanical/breathing pattern (*third row*), and sensory (*bottom graphs*) responses to incremental cycle ergometer exercise in a 74-year-old man with HF (LVEF = 34%)-COPD (FEV$_1$ = 58% predicted). Key abnormalities in which HF likely had a dominant role: a blunted increase in O$_2$ uptake (V̇O$_2$) as a function of work rate (WR) indicating poor O$_2$ delivery to the contracting peripheral muscles (*panel 1*), an early lactate threshold (LT) (*panel 2*), and a plateau in O$_2$ pulse at a low WR, suggesting impaired stroke volume and/or poor muscle O$_2$ extraction (*panel 3*). Key abnormalities primarily linked to COPD: a progressive decline in inspiratory capacity (IC) indicating dynamic hyperinflation (*panel 7*), the attainment of critical mechanical inspiratory constraints at a minute ventilation (V̇E) of ~ 30 L/min (*panel 8*) leading to a blunted increase in tidal volume (V$_T$) (*panel 9*), and a sharp

hypertension in animal models[68]; of note, neprilisyn levels may be reduced in the lungs of patients with COPD.[69] These potential negative effects should be tempered with the vasodilatory and antiproliferative activity of natriuretic peptides, which characteristically increase after the use of angiotensin receptor neprilisyn inhibitors.[70]

- Hydralazine/nitrates may worsen gas exchange and pulmonary hypertension in COPD-HF, thereby requiring close monitoring of these undesirable side effects.
- Little is currently known about the effects of ivabradine on exertional cardiac output in COPD-HF: if used, it should be considered only as an add-on therapy after careful optimization of β-blocker therapy.
- Owing to increased risk (eg, right ventricle inotropism may worsen pulmonary hypertension leading to right ventricular failure, toxicity, worsening of COPD-related multifocal atrial tachycardia), digitalis should be useful only as an adjunct to control atrial fibrillation on top of β-blockers in patients with COPD-HF.
- Although nonshockable rhythm is more frequent in COPD, particularly if associated with atrial fibrillation, an implantable cardioverter defibrillator should not be denied to patients with COPD-HF.

HEART FAILURE PATHOPHYSIOLOGY: IMPLICATIONS FOR CHRONIC OBSTRUCTIVE PULMONARY DISEASE TREATMENT
Bronchodilators

There is a long-standing controversy on the cardiovascular risks involved in the administration of bronchodilators in HF, including tachycardia (β2 stimulation, muscarinic M_2 receptor blockade, reflex tachycardia due to peripheral vasodilation), tachyarrhythmias, and increased myocardial O_2 demands.[71] Although retrospective studies and real-life data did not find a clear link between bronchodilators and morbimortality in COPD-HF, no large randomized control trial has included a sizable fraction of patients with

HF to specifically test their safety in this specific subpopulation.

It should also be emphasized that bronchodilators may also have some important beneficial consequences in COPD-HF (see **Fig. 2**)[72-75]:

- Less pronounced swings in intrapleural pressures and lower mean intrathoracic pressure due to less gas trapping may improve venous return, reduce compression of the pulmonary vasculature and the cardiac fossae, and decrease left ventricle transmural pressure;
- Lower work of breathing on exertion may decrease the requirements for blood perfusion of the respiratory muscles, thereby improving peripheral muscle blood flow;[76,77]
- Enhanced clearance of lung extravascular water leading to higher lung compliance and D_{LCO};[78,79]
- β_2 stimulation, particularly when administered in association with a β_1-blocker, may have an antiapoptotic effect[80] and stimulate cardiac progenitor cells to differentiation.[81]

The use of rescuing short-acting bronchodilators should be minimized by providing a more stable and sustained control of dyspnea over the 24-hour period. At this point in time, it remains unclear whether monotherapy with a long-acting β_2-adrenergic or antimuscarinic is safer than their combination in symptomatic patients with COPD-HF.[82] Despite their weak bronchodilatory effects and low therapeutic index, slow-release methylxanthines might prove useful in selected patients with COPD-HF because of their (usually mild) antiinflammatory, inotropic, diuretic, and ergogenic effects.[83]

- There is a theoretic rationale to avoid frequent use of short-acting bronchodilators in COPD-HF due to their summative cardiovascular effects throughout the day.
- Owing to the synergy between β_2-adrenoceptor stimulation and β_1 blockade in myocardial repair, a full or near full β_2-agonist might confer advantages on a long-term basis in COPD-HF.

---

increase in dyspnea (*bottom panels, left*). The following abnormalities were likely influenced by both HF and COPD: an excessive V̇E relative to metabolic demand (CO2 output, V̇CO2) either expressed as a slope (*panel 4*) or as a ratio (*panel 5*), and a low end-tidal P_{CO_2} (P_{ETCO_2}) associated with a borderline decrease in O_2 saturation by pulse oximetry (Sp_{O_2}) (*panel 6*). EILV, end-inspiratory lung volume; HR, heart rate; *I*, intercept; IRV, inspiratory reserve volume; LLN, lower limit of normal; LT, estimated lactate threshold; pred, predicted; $_{RER}$, respiratory exchange ratio; RR, respiratory rate; *S*, slope; TLC, total lung capacity; ULN, upper limit of normal. (*From* Neder JA, Rocha A, Alencar MCN, et al. Current challenges in managing comorbid heart failure and COPD. Expert Rev Cardiovasc Ther 2018;16(9):659; with permission.)

- Long-acting antimuscarinics with a shorter onset of action, shorter circulating time, and a higher affinity to M_3 receptors (compared with M_2) are preferable to minimize the risk of undesirable side effects in COPD-HF.

Corticosteroids

Low-to-moderate doses of an inhaled corticosteroid may lessen the COPD exacerbation burden in patients with a clear history of "frequent" (at least 2 per year in the preceding 2 years) or "life-threatening" (at least 1 prompting hospitalization) exacerbations.[6] A more liberal approach might be applicable to patients with associated asthma and/or high blood eosinophils.[84] The use of oral

corticosteroids should be restricted to the treatment of exacerbations (frequently in association with antibiotics), avoiding prolonged courses (ie, 7–10 days) because of the risk of fluid retention and worsening lung congestion.

Oxygen

The rationale for O_2 supplementation to lessen the hypoxic drive and improve tissue O_2 delivery[27] is rather straightforward in patients with COPD-HF who are overtly hypoxemic. It should be noted that the severity of hypoxemia might not be as pronounced as expected from resting lung function impairment in the subset of patients with chronic hypocapnia and alveolar hyperventilation (see **Fig. 4**).[39]

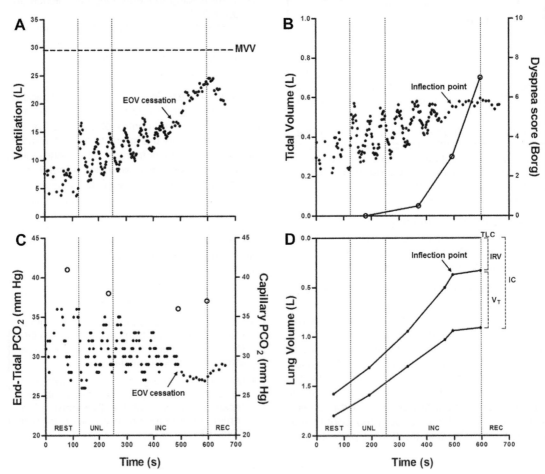

Fig. 8. Physiologic and perceptual responses to incremental exercise in a patient with COPD-HF (woman: age, 63 years; height, 146 cm) presenting with exercise oscillatory ventilation (EOV). Cycles of waxing and vanning of tidal volume (V_T) (B) and end-tidal partial pressure for carbon dioxide (Pco_2) (C) associated with progressive gas trapping led to earlier attainment of critical inspiratory constraints (inflection point) (D) and abrupt cessation of the oscillations (A). Under those circumstances (high neural drive and mechanical impediment), dyspnea ratings sharply increased (B). IC, inspiratory capacity; IRV, inspiratory reserve volume; MVV, maximal voluntary ventilation; TLC, total lung capacity. (*From* Rocha A, Arbex FF, Alencar MC, et al. Physiological and sensory consequences of exercise oscillatory ventilation in heart failure-COPD. Int J Cardiol 2016;224:448; with permission.)

SUMMARY

The coexistence of a failing heart with defective lungs offers a unique opportunity to translate classical concepts of cardiorespiratory pathophysiology to the clinical care of patients. For instance, interpretation of PFTs and CPETs in a patient with COPD needs to take into consideration the respiratory and systemic effects of HF and vice versa. Although comorbid COPD-HF does not change the foundations of the treatment of each disease, HF treatment might need to be modified to address its potential effects on COPD-related symptoms, particularly breathlessness. The treatment of COPD should aim to achieve the most feasible compromise between dyspnea control and cardiovascular toxicity. In any circumstance, it is out of debate that patients with COPD-HF are best managed by multidisciplinary (co-led by respirologists and cardiologists) and multiprofessional (including specialist nurses and physiotherapists) health care teams devoted to the management of elderly patients with multiple comorbidities.[8,85]

REFERENCES

1. Rutten FH, Cramer M-JM, Lammers J-WJ, et al. Heart failure and chronic obstructive pulmonary disease: an ignored combination? Eur J Heart Fail 2006;8(7):706–11.
2. Pirina P, Martinetti M, Spada C, et al. Prevalence and management of COPD and heart failure comorbidity in the general practitioner setting. Respir Med 2017; 131:1–5.
3. Pellicori P, Salekin D, Pan D, et al. This patient is not breathing properly: is this COPD, heart failure, or neither? Expert Rev Cardiovasc Ther 2017;15(5): 389–96.
4. van Mourik Y, Bertens LCM, Cramer MJM, et al. Unrecognized heart failure and chronic obstructive pulmonary disease (COPD) in frail elderly detected through a near-home targeted screening strategy. J Am Board Fam Med 2014;27(6): 811–21.
5. Vetrano DL, Palmer K, Marengoni A, et al. Frailty and multimorbidity: a systematic review and meta-analysis. J Gerontol A Biol Sci Med Sci 2018. https://doi.org/10.1093/gerona/gly110.
6. Vestbo J, Hurd SS, Agustí AG, et al. Global strategy for the diagnosis, management, and prevention of chronic obstructive pulmonary disease: GOLD executive summary. Am J Respir Crit Care Med 2013;187(4):347–65.
7. Savarese G, Lund LH. Global public health burden of heart failure. Card Fail Rev 2017;3(1):7–11.

8. Neder JA, Rocha A, Alencar MCN, et al. Current challenges in managing comorbid heart failure and COPD. Expert Rev Cardiovasc Ther 2018;16(9):653–73.
9. Borlaug BA. The pathophysiology of heart failure with preserved ejection fraction. Nat Rev Cardiol 2014;11(9):507–15.
10. Agostoni P, Pellegrino R, Conca C, et al. Exercise hyperpnea in chronic heart failure: relationships to lung stiffness and expiratory flow limitation. J Appl Physiol (1985) 2002;92(4):1409–16.
11. Chase SC, Taylor BJ, Cross TJ, et al. Influence of thoracic fluid compartments on pulmonary congestion in chronic heart failure. J Card Fail 2017;23(9): 690–6.
12. Chase SC, Fermoyle CC, Wheatley CM, et al. The effect of diuresis on extravascular lung water and pulmonary function in acute decompensated heart failure. ESC Heart Fail 2018;5(2):364–71.
13. Ries AL, Gregoratos G, Friedman PJ, et al. Pulmonary function tests in the detection of left heart failure: correlation with pulmonary artery wedge pressure. Respiration 1986;49(4):241–50.
14. Hosenpud JD, Stibolt TA, Atwal K, et al. Abnormal pulmonary function specifically related to congestive heart failure: comparison of patients before and after cardiac transplantation. Am J Med 1990; 88(5):493–6.
15. Olson TP, Beck KC, Johnson BD. Pulmonary function changes associated with cardiomegaly in chronic heart failure. J Card Fail 2007;13(2):100–7.
16. Kelley RC, Ferreira LF. Diaphragm abnormalities in heart failure and aging: mechanisms and integration of cardiovascular and respiratory pathophysiology. Heart Fail Rev 2017;22(2):191–207.
17. Magnussen H, Canepa M, Zambito PE, et al. What can we learn from pulmonary function testing in heart failure? Eur J Heart Fail 2017;19(10):1222–9.
18. Brenner S, Güder G, Berliner D, et al. Airway obstruction in systolic heart failure–COPD or congestion? Int J Cardiol 2013;168(3):1910–6.
19. Agostoni PG, Bussotti M, Palermo P, et al. Does lung diffusion impairment affect exercise capacity in patients with heart failure? Heart 2002;88(5):453–9.
20. Apostolo A, Giusti G, Gargiulo P, et al. Lungs in heart failure. Pulm Med 2012;2012:952741.
21. Olson TP, Denzer DL, Sinnett WL, et al. Prognostic value of resting pulmonary function in heart failure. Clin Med Insights Circ Respir Pulm Med 2013;7:35–43.
22. Torchio R, Gulotta C, Greco-Lucchina P, et al. Closing capacity and gas exchange in chronic heart failure. Chest 2006;129(5):1330–6.
23. Mettauer B, Lampert E, Charloux A, et al. Lung membrane diffusing capacity, heart failure, and heart transplantation. Am J Cardiol 1999;83(1):62–7.
24. Bishop JM. Cardiovascular complications of chronic bronchitis and emphysema. Med Clin North Am 1973;57(3):771–80.

25. O'Donnell DE, Laveneziana P, Webb K, et al. Chronic obstructive pulmonary disease: clinical integrative physiology. Clin Chest Med 2014;35(1): 51–69.

26. Oliveira MF, Zelt JTJ, Jones JH, et al. Does impaired O2 delivery during exercise accentuate central and peripheral fatigue in patients with coexistent COPD-CHF? Front Physiol 2014;5:514.

27. Oliveira MF, F Arbex F, Alencar MC, et al. Heart failure impairs muscle blood flow and endurance exercise tolerance in COPD. COPD 2016;13(4):407–15.

28. Chiappa GR, Queiroga F, Meda E, et al. Heliox improves oxygen delivery and utilization during dynamic exercise in patients with chronic obstructive pulmonary disease. Am J Respir Crit Care Med 2009;179(11):1004–10.

29. Amann M, Regan MS, Kobitary M, et al. Impact of pulmonary system limitations on locomotor muscle fatigue in patients with COPD. Am J Physiol Regul Integr Comp Physiol 2010;299(1):R314–24.

30. Güder G, Brenner S, Störk S, et al. Chronic obstructive pulmonary disease in heart failure: accurate diagnosis and treatment. Eur J Heart Fail 2014; 16(12):1273–82.

31. O'Donnell DE, Ciavaglia CE, Neder JA. When obesity and chronic obstructive pulmonary disease collide. Physiological and clinical consequences. Ann Am Thorac Soc 2014;11(4):635–44.

32. Güder G, Rutten FH, Brenner S, et al. The impact of heart failure on the classification of COPD severity. J Card Fail 2012;18(8):637–44.

33. Deesomchok A, Webb KA, Forkert L, et al. Lung hyperinflation and its reversibility in patients with airway obstruction of varying severity. COPD 2010; 7(6):428–37.

34. Cooper BG, Stocks J, Hall GL, et al. The Global Lung Function Initiative (GLI) Network: bringing the world's respiratory reference values together. Breathe (Sheff) 2017;13(3):e56–64.

35. Minasian AG, van den Elshout FJ, Dekhuijzen PR, et al. Serial pulmonary function tests to diagnose COPD in chronic heart failure. Transl Respir Med 2014;2(1):12.

36. Evans SA, Kinnear WJ, Watson L, et al. Breathlessness and exercise capacity in heart failure: the role of bronchial obstruction and responsiveness. Int J Cardiol 1996;57(3):233–40.

37. Davis C, Sheikh K, Pike D, et al. Ventilation heterogeneity in never-smokers and COPD: comparison of pulmonary functional magnetic resonance imaging with the poorly communicating fraction derived from plethysmography. Acad Radiol 2016;23(4):398–405.

38. Wasserman K, Zhang YY, Gitt A, et al. Lung function and exercise gas exchange in chronic heart failure. Circulation 1997;96(7):2221–7.

39. Rocha A, Arbex FF, Sperandio PA, et al. Excess ventilation in COPD-heart failure overlap: implications for dyspnea and exercise intolerance. Am J Respir Crit Care Med 2017;196(10):1264–74.

40. Oliveira MF, Arbex F, Alencar MCN, et al. Heart failure impairs cerebral oxygenation during exercise in patients with COPD. Eur Respir J 2013; 42(5):1423.

41. Treptow E, Oliveira MF, Soares A, et al. Cerebral microvascular blood flow and CO2 reactivity in pulmonary arterial hypertension. Respir Physiol Neurobiol 2016;233:60–5.

42. Neder JA, Laveneziana P, Ward SA, et al. CPET in clinical practice. Recent advances, current challenges and future directions. In: Palange P, Laveneziana P, Neder JA, et al., editors. Clinical exercise testing. vol. 80. European Respiratory Monograph. Lausanne: European Respiratory Society; 2018. p. x-xxv.

43. O'Donnell DE, Elbehairy AF, Faisal A, et al. Exertional dyspnoea in COPD: the clinical utility of cardiopulmonary exercise testing. Eur Respir Rev 2016;25(141):333–47.

44. Neder JA, Berton DC, Rocha A, et al. Abnormal patterns of response to Incremental CPET. In: Palange P, Laveneziana P, Neder JA, et al, editors. Clinical exercise testing. European Respiratory Monograph, vol. 80. Lausanne: European Respiratory Society; 2018. p. 34–58.

45. Agostoni P, Cattadori G, Bussotti M, et al. Cardiopulmonary interaction in heart failure. Pulm Pharmacol Ther 2007;20(2):130–4.

46. Smith JR, Van Iterson EH, Johnson BD, et al. Exercise ventilatory inefficiency in heart failure and chronic obstructive pulmonary disease. Int J Cardiol 2018. https://doi.org/10.1016/j.ijcard.2018.09.007.

47. O'Donnell DE, Elbehairy AF, Berton DC, et al. Advances in the evaluation of respiratory pathophysiology during exercise in chronic lung diseases. Front Physiol 2017;8:82.

48. Corrà U. Exercise oscillatory ventilation in heart failure. Int J Cardiol 2016. https://doi.org/10.1016/j.ijcard.2016.02.122.

49. Rocha A, Arbex FF, Alencar MCN, et al. Physiological and sensory consequences of exercise oscillatory ventilation in heart failure-COPD. Int J Cardiol 2016;224:447–53.

50. Leitao Filho FS, Alotaibi NM, Yamasaki K, et al. The role of beta-blockers in the management of chronic obstructive pulmonary disease. Expert Rev Respir Med 2018;12(2):125–35.

51. Roversi S, Fabbri LM, Sin DD, et al. Chronic obstructive pulmonary disease and cardiac diseases. An urgent need for integrated care. Am J Respir Crit Care Med 2016;194(11):1319–36.

52. Magrì D, Palermo P, Cauti FM, et al. Chronotropic incompetence and functional capacity in chronic heart failure: no role of β-blockers and β-blocker dose. Cardiovasc Ther 2012;30(2):100–8.

53. Ellison DH, Felker GM. Diuretic treatment in heart failure. N Engl J Med 2018;378(7):684–5.

54. Barr RG, Bluemke DA, Ahmed FS, et al. Percent emphysema, airflow obstruction, and impaired left ventricular filling. N Engl J Med 2010;362(3):217–27.

55. Mahler DA, O'Donnell DE. Recent advances in dyspnea. Chest 2015;147(1):232–41.

56. Clark AL, Cleland JGF. Causes and treatment of oedema in patients with heart failure. Nat Rev Cardiol 2013;10(3):156–70.

57. Prieto de Paula JM, Franco Hidalgo S, Borge Gallardo L, et al. The importance of identifying the association between metabolic alkalosis and respiratory acidosis. Arch Bronconeumol 2012;48(2):65–6.

58. Vozoris NT, Wang X, Austin PC, et al. Incident diuretic drug use and adverse respiratory events among older adults with chronic obstructive pulmonary disease. Br J Clin Pharmacol 2018;84(3): 579–89.

59. Parikh MA, Aaron CP, Hoffman EA, et al. Angiotensin-converting inhibitors and angiotensin II receptor blockers and longitudinal change in percent emphysema on computed tomography. The multiethnic study of atherosclerosis lung study. Ann Am Thorac Soc 2017;14(5):649–58.

60. Petersen H, Sood A, Meek PM, et al. Rapid lung function decline in smokers is a risk factor for COPD and is attenuated by angiotensin-converting enzyme inhibitor use. Chest 2014;145(4):695–703.

61. Mancini GBJ, Etminan M, Zhang B, et al. Reduction of morbidity and mortality by statins, angiotensin-converting enzyme inhibitors, and angiotensin receptor blockers in patients with chronic obstructive pulmonary disease. J Am Coll Cardiol 2006;47(12): 2554–60.

62. Guazzi M, Melzi G, Marenzi GC, et al. Angiotensin-converting enzyme inhibition facilitates alveolar-capillary gas transfer and improves ventilation-perfusion coupling in patients with left ventricular dysfunction. Clin Pharmacol Ther 1999;65(3):319–27.

63. Guazzi M, Palermo P, Pontone G, et al. Synergistic efficacy of enalapril and losartan on exercise performance and oxygen consumption at peak exercise in congestive heart failure. Am J Cardiol 1999;84(9): 1038–43.

64. Guazzi M, Agostoni P, Guazzi MD. Modulation of alveolar-capillary sodium handling as a mechanism of protection of gas transfer by enalapril, and not by losartan, in chronic heart failure. J Am Coll Cardiol 2001;37(2):398–406.

65. Sebastian JL, McKinney WP, Kaufman J, et al. Angiotensin-converting enzyme inhibitors and cough. Prevalence in an outpatient medical clinic population. Chest 1991;99(1):36–9.

66. McMurray JJV, Packer M, Desai AS, et al. Angiotensin-neprilysin inhibition versus enalapril in heart failure. N Engl J Med 2014;371(11):993–1004.

67. Yancy CW, Jessup M, Bozkurt B, et al. 2017 ACC/AHA/HFSA Focused Update of the 2013 ACCF/AHA Guideline for the Management of Heart Failure: a report of the American College of Cardiology/American Heart Association Task Force on Clinical Practice Guidelines and the Heart Failure Society of America. Circulation 2017;136(6):e137–61.

68. Dempsey EC, Wick MJ, Karoor V, et al. Neprilysin null mice develop exaggerated pulmonary vascular remodeling in response to chronic hypoxia. Am J Pathol 2009;174(3):782–96.

69. Wick MJ, Buesing EJ, Wehling CA, et al. Decreased neprilysin and pulmonary vascular remodeling in chronic obstructive pulmonary disease. Am J Respir Crit Care Med 2011;183(3):330–40.

70. Liczek M, Panek I, Damiański P, et al. Neprilysin inhibitors as a new approach in the treatment of right heart failure in the course of chronic obstructive pulmonary disease. Adv Respir Med 2018. https://doi.org/10.5603/ARM.a2018.0028.

71. Singh S, Loke YK, Enright P, et al. Pro-arrhythmic and pro-ischaemic effects of inhaled anticholinergic medications. Thorax 2013;68(1):114–6.

72. Hohlfeld JM, Vogel-Claussen J, Biller H, et al. Effect of lung deflation with indacaterol plus glycopyrronium on ventricular filling in patients with hyperinflation and COPD (CLAIM): a double-blind, randomised, crossover, placebo-controlled, single-centre trial. Lancet Respir Med 2018;6(5):368–78.

73. Stone IS, Barnes NC, James W-Y, et al. Lung deflation and cardiovascular structure and function in chronic obstructive pulmonary disease. a randomized controlled trial. Am J Respir Crit Care Med 2016; 193(7):717–26.

74. Segreti A, Fiori E, Calzetta L, et al. The effect of indacaterol during an acute exacerbation of COPD. Pulm Pharmacol Ther 2013;26(6):630–4.

75. Cosentino ER, Degli Esposti D, Miceli R, et al. Coexisting heart failure and chronic obstructive pulmonary disease: report of two cases treated with indacaterol/glycopyrronium. Respiration 2018; 95(Suppl 1):3–5.

76. Dempsey JA, Romer L, Rodman J, et al. Consequences of exercise-induced respiratory muscle work. Respir Physiol Neurobiol 2006;151(2–3):242–50.

77. Borghi-Silva A, Carrascosa C, Oliveira CC, et al. Effects of respiratory muscle unloading on leg muscle oxygenation and blood volume during high-intensity exercise in chronic heart failure. Am J Physiol Heart Circ Physiol 2008;294(6):H2465–72.

78. Agostoni P, Palermo P, Contini M. Respiratory effects of beta-blocker therapy in heart failure. Cardiovasc Drugs Ther 2009;23(5):377–84.

79. Chase SC, Wheatley CM, Olson LJ, et al. Impact of chronic systolic heart failure on lung structure-function relationships in large airways. Physiol Rep 2016;4(13) [pii:e12867].

80. Matera MG, Martuscelli E, Cazzola M. Pharmacological modulation of beta-adrenoceptor function in patients with coexisting chronic obstructive pulmonary disease and chronic heart failure. Pulm Pharmacol Ther 2010;23(1):1–8.

81. Rinaldi B, Donniacuo M, Sodano L, et al. Effects of chronic treatment with the new ultra-long-acting β2-adrenoceptor agonist indacaterol alone or in combination with the β1-adrenoceptor blocker metoprolol on cardiac remodelling. Br J Pharmacol 2015; 172(14):3627–37.

82. Calzetta L, Rogliani P, Matera MG, et al. A systematic review with meta-analysis of dual bronchodilation with LAMA/LABA for the treatment of stable chronic obstructive pulmonary disease. Chest 2016. https://doi.org/10.1016/j.chest.2016.02.646.

83. Dini FL, Pasini G, Cortellini G, et al. Methylxanthine drug therapy in chronic heart failure associated with hypoxaemia: double-blind placebo-controlled clinical trial of doxofylline versus theophylline and bamifylline. Int J Clin Pharmacol Res 1993;13(6): 305–16.

84. Leung JM, Sin DD. Asthma-COPD overlap syndrome: pathogenesis, clinical features, and therapeutic targets. BMJ 2017;358:j3772.

85. Kastner M, Cardoso R, Lai Y, et al. Effectiveness of interventions for managing multiple high-burden chronic diseases in older adults: a systematic review and meta-analysis. CMAJ 2018;190(34):E1004–12.

86. Souza AS, Sperandio PA, Mazzuco A, et al. Influence of heart failure on resting lung volumes in patients with COPD. J Bras Pneumol 2016;42(4):273–8.

Pulmonary Limitations in Heart Failure

Ivan Cundrle Jr, MD, PhD[a,b,c], Lyle J. Olson, MD[d], Bruce D. Johnson, PhD[d],*

KEYWORDS

- Heart failure • Cardiopulmonary exercise testing • Ventilatory efficiency

KEY POINTS

- Heart failure is associated with airway obstruction, reduced lung volume, impaired gas exchange, and abnormal ventilatory control.
- Abnormal ventilatory control in patients with heart failure manifests as hyperventilation at rest, during exercise, and even with sleep.
- Cardiopulmonary exercise testing detects abnormalities of gas exchange and ventilatory control.
- Selected cardiopulmonary exercise testing parameters including minute ventilation per unit of carbon dioxide production slope and oscillatory breathing have been strongly associated with prognosis of patients with heart failure.

INTRODUCTION

The heart and lungs are intimately related anatomically and physiologically because they share the enclosed thoracic cavity, are exposed to similar intrathoracic pressures, have a common surface area, and are hemodynamically linked because the lungs accept nearly the entire cardiac output.[1] Hence, changes in cardiac function may directly influence lung function because of alterations in cardiac preload and afterload, including venous return and cardiac transmural pressure. Heart failure directly affects (1) lung mechanics because of congestion and increased heart size, which promote airway obstruction and lung restriction[1,2]; (2) high pulmonary pressures as well as pulmonary congestion contribute to remodeling of the pulmonary capillaries, increased ventilation-perfusion mismatch, and decreased alveolar-capillary diffusion[3,4]; and (3) disordered ventilatory control, including

hyperventilation at rest, during exercise, and with sleep.[5–7] These pulmonary system changes cause decreased breathing reserve combined with enhanced ventilation for a given metabolic demand (minute ventilation [V_E]/pulmonary carbon dioxide output [V_{CO_2}] ratio) at rest and during exercise (further discussion in the topic is provided in Clinical and Physiological Implications of Negative Cardiopulmonary Interactions in Coexisting COPD-Heart Failure).[7,8] This article discusses heart failure (HF)–related changes in lung mechanics, gas exchange, and ventilatory control as well as their impact on the limitation of exercise capacity, sleep disordered breathing, and prognosis of patients with HF.

LUNG VOLUME AND FLOW IN HEART FAILURE

Pulmonary function is abnormal in patients with HF, including decreased bronchial conductance

Conflicts of interest: None.

Funding: Dr I. Cundrle is supported by Czech Republic Ministry of Health (grant NV18-06-00216); National Program of Sustainability II (MEYS CR) (project no. LQ1605), and by the project FNUSA-ICRC [CZ.1.05/1.1.00/02. 0123 (OP VaVpl)]. Most of the funding for Dr B.D. Johnson's laboratory relative to this article was from NIH grant HL71478.

[a] Department of Anesthesiology and Intensive Care, St. Anne's University Hospital, Pekarska 53, Brno 65691, Czech Republic; [b] Faculty of Medicine, Masaryk University, Brno, Czech Republic; [c] International Clinical Research Center, St. Anne's University Hospital, Brno, Czech Republic; [d] Department of Cardiovascular Diseases, Mayo Clinic, 200 First Street SW, Rochester, MN 55905, USA
* Corresponding author.
E-mail address: johnson.bruce@mayo.edu

Clin Chest Med 40 (2019) 439–448
https://doi.org/10.1016/j.ccm.2019.02.010
0272-5231/19/© 2019 Elsevier Inc. All rights reserved.

chestmed.theclinics.com

and restrictive lung volumes. Moreover, the observed flow limitation and lung restriction may increase the work of breathing, which, in combination with weak respiratory muscles, may increase the sensation of dyspnea in patients with HF.[8] Bronchial flow limitation has been attributed to airway compression (by pulmonary edema) and/or mucosal edema caused by bronchial congestion (**Fig. 1**),[1,8–10] which may develop from either an increase in blood flow or an increase in blood volume without a change of flow caused by increased cardiac filling pressure or pulmonary artery hypertension.[1] Several factors may influence bronchial blood flow in patients with HF, including increased left atrial pressure causing greater pulmonary vascular pressure and bronchial vessel stasis[11]; stretching of the left heart chambers, which may lead to increased bronchial conductance[12]; increase in levels of inflammatory and vasoactive mediators, which may influence vasomotor tone and lead to vasodilatation and congestion of bronchial vessels[13,14]; and chronic hypocapnia, which is a common manifestation of increased left ventricular filling pressures in patients with HF[15] and may also lead to vasodilatation.[16]

Experimental studies have shown fluid overload leads to decrease of the diameter of both small[17] and large airways.[18] Furthermore, pulmonary function test parameters have been shown to improve with diuresis in patients with HF.[19] Agostoni and colleagues[11] observed significantly higher bronchial shunt blood flow in patients with chronic HF than in patients without HF during surgery on cardiopulmonary bypass, suggesting the presence of either dilated or more numerous intrapulmonary bronchial blood vessels in patients with chronic HF. Pulmonary artery hypertension (PAH), a frequent comorbidity in either HF with reduced ejection fraction (HFrEF) or HF with preserved ejection fraction (HFpEF),[20] has been shown to contribute to bronchial airway obstruction by Meyer and colleagues,[21] and others.[22–24]

Physiologic factors that may counteract hydrostatic forces that promote edema formation in the airways include sympathetic nervous system activation with α-adrenergic receptor–mediated vasoconstriction in peribronchiolar vessels, which may reduce congestion.[1] Furthermore, functional capillary remodeling with fibrosis and thickening of the alveolar-capillary membranes caused by

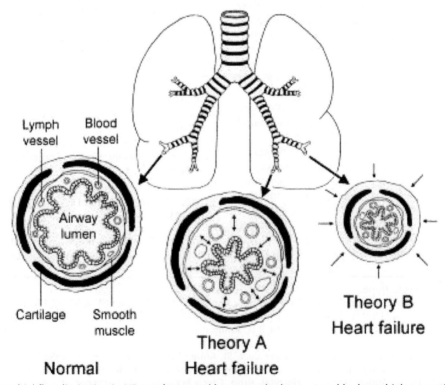

Fig. 1. Bronchial flow limitation in HF may be caused by mucosal edema caused by bronchial congestion, which may develop from either an increase in blood flow or an increase in blood volume (theory A), or by bronchial compression, which may be caused by reduction of intrathoracic space by either increase in heart size or by pulmonary edema (theory B). (*Reprinted from* Ceridon M, Wanner A, Johnson BD. Does the bronchial circulation contribute to congestion in heart failure? Med Hypotheses 2009;73(3):417. Figure 2; with permission.)

chronically increased pulmonary capillary pressure may occur,[25] causing increased resistance to high vascular pressures and interstitial edema development. Lymphatic drainage also progressively increases with the severity of HF,[26] which may serve as another adaptive mechanism to reduce pulmonary congestion.

Olson and colleagues[2] showed a significant relationship between HF severity, heart size, intrathoracic volume, and lung restriction. Cardiac enlargement in HF has been shown by Agostoni and colleagues[27] to promote restrictive lung function. A close relation between pulmonary function and decrease in cardiac volume with heart transplant was shown by McCormack and colleagues.[28]

> Airflow limitation (caused by airway compression by pulmonary edema and/or mucosal edema secondary to bronchial congestion) and lung restriction (linked to cardiomegaly and increased lung elastic recoil) are common consequences of chronic HF.

GAS EXCHANGE CHANGE IN HEART FAILURE

Gas exchange is often abnormal in patients with HF and correlates with disease severity.[29] Several studies have shown decreased lung diffusion factor for carbon monoxide ($D_{L}CO$) in patients with HF.[3,4] The cause is probably multifactorial and involves interstitial edema as well as alveolar-capillary membrane remodeling.[3,4] Furthermore, bronchial obstruction caused by peribronchial edema may reduce ventilation to some pulmonary units, increasing the ventilation-perfusion mismatch and further impairing gas exchange (further discussion in this topic is provided in Incorporating DLCO to Clinical Decision Making in Chest Medicine).

Pulmonary edema increases the distance between alveolar gas and red blood cells and may therefore also impair $D_{L}CO$. However, in healthy people, infusion of normal saline has been associated with worsening of lung mechanics, although not $D_{L}CO$,[30] suggesting alveolar-capillary remodeling may have a greater impact on the $D_{L}CO$ changes observed in patients with HF. Alveolar-capillary remodeling involves fibrosis, thickening of the alveolar-capillary membranes,[25] and β-adrenergic receptor insufficiency of the alveolar epithelium,[31] which may result in inability to effectively clear alveolar fluid.

Impaired $D_{L}CO$ has been associated with poor prognosis[32] as well as low exercise performance.[33] However, adverse remodeling of the alveolar-capillary membrane may not be fully reversible with HF treatment.[34] Only partial improvement of $D_{L}CO$ with heart transplant was shown by Mettauer and colleagues[35] and no change to $D_{L}CO$ with cardiac resynchronization therapy was shown by our group.[36]

Surfactant protein B seems to be a promising marker of alveolar-capillary membrane damage because its levels are not increased in edema with no alveolar damage[37] and have been shown to correlate with HF severity.[38] Moreover, surfactant protein B has been shown to be associated with HF rehospitalization[39] and to be related to $D_{L}CO$,[40] peak oxygen consumption ($\dot{V}O_2$), and $V_E/\dot{V}CO_2$ slope.[38] Surfactant protein B may be a stronger prognostic marker than $D_{L}CO$[41] and, unlike $D_{L}CO$, may decrease with HF clinical improvement.[39]

> The efficiency of intrapulmonary gas exchange can be decreased in HF because of a highly variable combination of interstitial edema, alveolar-capillary membrane remodeling, and ventilation-perfusion mismatch. These abnormalities can be appreciated by the degree of impairment in hemoglobin-corrected $D_{L}CO$.

VENTILATORY CONTROL IN HEART FAILURE

Ventilatory control is frequently abnormal in patients with advanced HF and manifests as hyperventilation at rest,[5] during exercise,[6] and with sleep.[7] The presence of hyperventilation has been associated with decreased functional capacity,[6] more severe symptoms,[42] and increased mortality[43] in patients with HF.

The cause of hyperventilation in patients with HF has not been fully elucidated, and may include activation of pulmonary C-fiber receptors caused by congestion, activation of atrial stretch receptors, ventilation-perfusion mismatch, and low systemic oxygen transfer capacity, as well as increased activation of central and peripheral chemoreflexes and the ergoreflex (further discussion in the topic is provided in Update on Chemoreception: Influence on Cardiorespiratory Regulation and Patho-Physiology).[6,42,44–49] Lactate acidosis was formerly thought to be a major cause of hyperventilation in patients with HF,[50,51] although this concept has now been refuted.[52]

Cardiopulmonary exercise testing (CPET) allows evaluation of the ventilatory response to exercise, which is abnormal in patients with HF despite normal breathing reserve.[8] Normal ventilatory response includes an increase of V_E caused by both increase in tidal volume (V_T) at the beginning

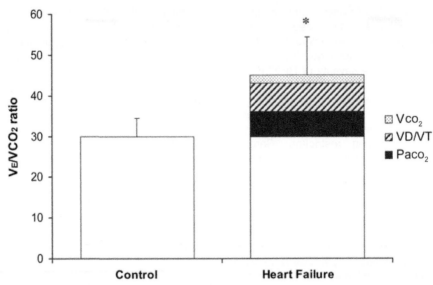

Fig. 2. In HF, both the increased ventilatory drive (low partial pressure of carbon dioxide [$Paco_2$]) and ventilation/perfusion mismatch (high dead space volume to tidal volume ratio [V_D/V_T]) contribute nearly equally to the increase in ventilatory inefficiency (higher V_E/Vco_2). * Significant difference between control and HF groups (p<0.01). (*Reprinted from* Woods PR, Olson TP, Frantz RP, et al. Causes of breathing inefficiency during exercise in heart failure. J Card Fail 2010;16(10):839. Figure 3C; with permission.)

of exercise followed by an increase of breathing frequency (f_b) toward peak exercise.[13] In HF, V_E is significantly increased because of the increase in f_b with little or no increase in V_T.[53] Ventilatory parameters routinely measured during CPET also include ventilatory efficiency (V_E/Vco_2) and partial pressure of end-tidal carbon dioxide ($P_{ET}co_2$).

The V_E/Vco_2 slope identifies and quantifies the magnitude of hyperventilation and has been found to be increased[54,55] and inversely correlated with cardiac output in patients with HF.[55] Importantly, many studies in patients with HF have shown V_E/Vco_2 to be a better predictor of clinical outcome than peak Vo_2.[56–60] Ventilatory efficiency is inversely related to the partial pressure of arterial CO_2 ($Paco_2$) and positively to the dead space/tidal volume ratio (V_D/V_T) by the alveolar gas equation $V_E/Vco_2 = 863/(Paco_2 \times (1 - V_D/V_T))$. From this relationship, it is clear the V_E/Vco_2 may be increased by lowering the $Paco_2$ or increasing the V_D/V_T ratio. Increased stimulation or increased sensitivity of pulmonary receptors, increased sympathetic nerve activity, peripheral and central chemoreceptors, and ergoreceptors may cause hyperventilation and reduction of $Paco_2$. In contrast, the V_D/V_T ratio may be affected by ventilation-perfusion mismatch, including a rapid and shallow breathing pattern.[6] Woods and colleagues[6] quantified the contribution of $Paco_2$ and V_D/V_T to the increased V_E/Vco_2 in patients with HF and found a nearly similar contribution of $Paco_2$ and V_D/V_T (**Fig. 2**).

Low $P_{ET}co_2$ during exercise was also shown to reflect functional, ventilatory, and cardiac performance in patients with HF by Myers and colleagues.[61] Furthermore, rest $P_{ET}co_2$ has also been shown to be useful in HF prognostication[62] and to add incremental prognostic value to V_E/Vco_2 slope.[5] Rest $P_{ET}co_2$ has also been shown to be an independent predictor of left ventricular assist device implantation.[63] $P_{ET}co_2$ has been integrated into 2 CPET scoring systems for adverse event prediction in HF.[64,65] $P_{ET}co_2$ may be decreased by hyperventilation and by increased dead space ventilation; that is, by the same factors that determine V_E/Vco_2,[6] suggesting the parameters are closely related.[61] In our previous studies, we have shown that patients with HF with low $P_{ET}co_2$ and increased V_E/Vco_2 at peak exercise also show low $P_{ET}co_2$ and increased V_E/Vco_2 at rest,[7,66] suggesting factors that promote high V_E/Vco_2 and low $P_{ET}co_2$ may not be limited to exercise.

A high V_E/Vco_2 in HF reflects an excessive ventilation for the prevailing metabolic demand caused by alveolar hyperventilation secondary to increased stimulation or sensitivity of pulmonary receptors, increased sympathetic nerve activity, and chemoreceptor overactivation and/or high wasted ventilation as a consequence of ventilation-perfusion mismatch and a rapid and shallow breathing pattern.

PERIODIC BREATHING, EXERCISE OSCILLATORY VENTILATION, AND CENTRAL SLEEP APNEA

Periodic breathing (PB) is a consequence of respiratory control system instability characterized by waxing and waning of tidal volume with or without interposed apnea[49] caused by oscillations of central respiratory drive.[67] PB may develop at rest,[68] during exercise,[69] or with sleep.[70] It has been shown that PB occurs mostly in the situations in which ventilation is mainly under metabolic control. During sleep it occurs with non–rapid eye movement sleep,[70] and during exercise it is the time when the increased metabolic demand for O_2 consumption and CO_2 production cause respiratory control to decrease, mainly under the influence of the metabolic respiratory control system (further discussion in the topic is provided in Exertional Periodic Breathing in Heart Failure: Mechanisms and Clinical Implications).[71]

Oxygen delivery and CO_2 excretion are physiologically maintained by the respiratory and circulatory systems. Stability of these systems is maintained by several feedback loops involving a central controller comprising peripheral and central chemoreceptors stimulating the brainstem respiratory motor neurons and a peripheral working unit comprising lungs, rib cage, and respiratory muscles.[67] Several factors may destabilize the respiratory control system and produce the PB pattern observed in patients with HF. Prolonged circulatory time may cause delay in the information transfer between lungs and chemoreceptors[72]; increased CO_2 chemosensitivity with increased chemoreceptor gain may lead to overcorrection of $Paco_2$ deviations from the arterial CO_2 set point[69]; and the CO_2 set point may be lowered closer to the apnea threshold by hyperventilation caused by activation of pulmonary C-fibers because of congestion, activation of left atrial stretch receptors by volume overload, ventilation-perfusion mismatch, increased sympathetic nerve activity, or modulation of the ergoreflex.[6,44–49,73] Taken together, PB is a manifestation of control system failure caused by signal underdamping with periodic overshooting and undershooting of ventilation.[67] During sleep, the development of apnea depends mainly on the frequency of oscillations; the lower the frequency, the higher the amplitude and the higher the chance of crossing the CO_2 apnea threshold.[70] Inhalation of 3% CO_2 eliminates Cheyne-Stokes respiration in patients with HFrEF.[74]

In contrast, no association between $Paco_2$ at rest and during exercise and exercise oscillatory ventilation (EOV) (presence, duration, amplitude) was found in the study by Murphy and colleagues.[75] In the same study, EOV was shown to be associated with increased cardiac filling pressure,[75] supporting the concept of activation of pulmonary C-fibers and hyperventilation. However, this observation has been questioned by others who found EOV to disappear during late exercise despite an increase in pulmonary capillary wedge pressure.[76] These observations suggest that EOV pathophysiology is complex and likely involves multiple factors.

The American Heart Association has defined EOV as an oscillatory ventilatory pattern that persists for at least 60% of exercise at an amplitude of 15% or more of the average resting value[77,78] (**Fig. 3**). By CPET, EOV has been detected in 19% to 51% of patients with HFrEF[75] and a similar prevalence has been observed in patients with HFpEF.[79] EOV has been associated with increased risk of death.[73,80] Moreover, the risk of death is further increased in patients with HF with EOV and increased V_E/Vco_2 slope.[81] Guazzi and colleagues[79] found EOV to be the strongest predictor of cardiac events in patients with HFpEF and in patients without clinical manifestations of HF.[82] The risk of death is further increased if EOV is combined with abnormal breathing during sleep.[83] The prevalence of EOV is similar to the prevalence of central sleep apnea (CSA) and the presence of EOV is highly predictive of the presence of CSA,[84] suggesting shared pathophysiology.

In patients with HF, CSA is characterized as a crescendo-decrescendo breathing pattern with hyperventilation alternating with compensatory apnea.[85,86] CSA is considered a consequence of HF,[86–90] is linked to the hemodynamic severity of HF,[91,92] and associated with increased hospital readmission rates[93] and mortality.[94] A previous study by our group showed that patients with HF with CSA have higher central CO_2 chemosensitivity; increased V_E and lower $P_{ET}CO_2$ at rest; higher V_E, V_T, and V_E/Vco_2 ratio and lower $P_{ET}CO_2$ during exercise; and higher V_E/Vco_2 ratio and lower $P_{ET}CO_2$ at peak exercise.[7] Moreover, central CO_2 chemosensitivity, peak $P_{ET}CO_2$, and peak V_E/Vco_2 ratio are independently associated with the presence of CSA and correlate with CSA severity.[7] These observations suggest the presence of abnormal ventilatory control in patients with HF with hyperventilation at rest, during exercise, and with sleep, and may promote recognition of the CSA phenotype during CPET.[7]

Abnormalities in the ventilatory control system are commonly found in advanced chronic HF: these derangements are exacerbated in physiologic situations in which afferent stimulation is strongly influenced by metabolism; for example, exercise and sleep.

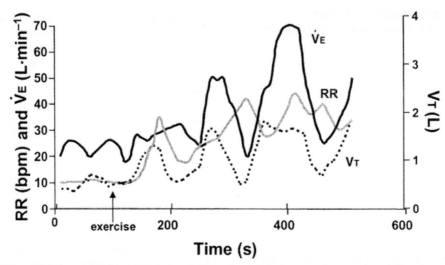

Fig. 3. Exercise oscillatory ventilation is a consequence of respiratory control system instability characterized by waxing and waning of V_T, breathing frequency (respiration rate [RR]), and V_E without interposed apnea caused by oscillations of central respiratory drive. (*Reprinted from* Olson TP, Snyder EM, Johnson BD. Exercise-disordered breathing in chronic heart failure. Exerc Sport Sci Rev 2006;34(4):200. Figure 10; with permission.)

SPECIAL CONSIDERATIONS FOR HEART FAILURE WITH PRESERVED EJECTION FRACTION

HFpEF is frequent and accounts for more than half of HF cases.[95] Moreover, HFpEF is associated with increased risk of hospitalization and death.[96,97] Guazzi and colleagues[79] showed V_E/V_{CO_2} but not peak V_{O_2} to be associated with all-cause and cardiac-related mortality and hospitalization in patients with HFpEF.[98] These result were supported by Yan and colleagues,[99] who also showed V_E/V_{CO_2} but not peak V_{O_2} to be associated with all-cause mortality in patients with HFpEF. In contrast, Shafiq and colleagues[100] showed an association of peak V_{O_2} but not V_E/V_{CO_2} with all-cause mortality and cardiac transplant. In addition, Nadruz and colleagues[101] showed both V_E/V_{CO_2} and peak V_{O_2} to be independent prognostic tools in HFpEF.

SPECIAL CONSIDERATIONS FOR PULMONARY ARTERY HYPERTENSION

Chronically increased cardiac filling pressure is a common cause of PAH in both patients with HFrEF and HFpEF.[20] The prevalence of this comorbidity is high in patients with HFrEF (up to 72%)[102] and in patients with HFpEF (up to 83%).[103] PAH is associated with exercise dyspnea, increased V_E/V_{CO_2} slope, and poor prognosis.[104] Physiologically, V_E/V_{CO_2} decreases and $P_{ET}CO_2$ increases from rest to peak exercise.[105] This physiologic pattern may also be observed in patients with HF.[7,106] In contrast, in patients with moderate to severe PAH, V_E/V_{CO_2} increased[107] and $P_{ET}CO_2$ decreased during exercise because of poor pulmonary perfusion.[108] In patients with PAH, ventilatory response to exercise seems to be more closely related to ventilatory-perfusion mismatch and increased ventilatory drive than altered pulmonary mechanics (further discussion the topic is provided in Pulmonary Hypertension and Exercise).[109]

SUMMARY

Ultimately in the pathogenesis of HF, the disease becomes a systemic illness with a marked impact on the respiratory system. This impact creates a significant codependence between organ systems that is accentuated as the disease progresses and is further enhanced during exercise, with the respiratory system becoming a major contributor to exertional symptoms and an important marker to track disease severity and prognosis.

REFERENCES

1. Ceridon M, Wanner A, Johnson BD. Does the bronchial circulation contribute to congestion in heart failure? Med Hypotheses 2009;73(3): 414–9.
2. Olson TP, Beck KC, Johnson JB, et al. Competition for intrathoracic space reduces lung capacity in patients with chronic heart failure*a radiographic study. Chest 2006;130(1):164–71.
3. Guazzi M. Alveolar gas diffusion abnormalities in heart failure. J Card Fail 2008;14(8):695–702.

4. Siegel JL, Miller A, Brown LK, et al. Pulmonary diffusing capacity in left ventricular dysfunction. Chest 1990;98(3):550–3.

5. Arena R, Myers J, Abella J, et al. The partial pressure of resting end-tidal carbon dioxide predicts major cardiac events in patients with systolic heart failure. Am Heart J 2008;156(5):982–8.

6. Woods PR, Olson TP, Frantz RP, et al. Causes of breathing inefficiency during exercise in heart failure. J Card Fail 2010;16(10):835–42.

7. Cundrle I, Somers VK, Johnson BD, et al. Exercise end-tidal CO2 predicts central sleep apnea in patients with heart failure. Chest 2015;147(6): 1566–73.

8. Johnson BD, Beck KC, Olson LJ, et al. Ventilatory constraints during exercise in patients with chronic heart failure. Chest 2000;117(2):321–32.

9. Ceridon ML, Morris NR, Hulsebus ML, et al. Influence of bronchial blood flow and conductance on pulmonary function in stable systolic heart failure. Respir Physiol Neurobiol 2011;177(3):256–64.

10. Johnson BD, Beck KC, Olson LJ, et al. Pulmonary function in patients with reduced left ventricular function: influence of smoking and cardiac surgery. Chest 2001;120(6):1869–76.

11. Agostoni PG, Doria E, Bortone F, et al. Systemic to pulmonary bronchial blood flow in heart failure. Chest 1995;107(5):1247–52.

12. Wagner EM, Mitzner WA. Effect of left atrial pressure on bronchial vascular hemodynamics. J Appl Physiol (1985) 1990;69(3):837–42.

13. Agostoni P, Cattadori G, Bussotti M, et al. Cardiopulmonary interaction in heart failure. Pulm Pharmacol Ther 2007;20(2):130–4.

14. Long WM, Yerger LD, Martinez H, et al. Modification of bronchial blood flow during allergic airway responses. J Appl Physiol 1988;65(1):272–82.

15. Lorenzi-Filho G, Azevedo ER, Parker JD, et al. Relationship of carbon dioxide tension in arterial blood to pulmonary wedge pressure in heart failure. Eur Respir J 2002;19(1):37–40.

16. Ceridon ML, Snyder EM, Olson TP, et al. Influence of acute graded hypoxia on the bronchial circulation in healthy humans. FASEB J 2008;22(1_ supplement):1150.15.

17. King LS, Nielsen S, Agre P, et al. Decreased pulmonary vascular permeability in aquaporin-1-null humans. Proc Natl Acad Sci USA 2002;99(2): 1059–63.

18. Ceridon ML, Snyder EM, Strom NA, et al. Influence of rapid fluid loading on airway structure and function in healthy humans. J Card Fail 2010;16(2): 175–85.

19. Bucca CB, Brussino L, Battisti A, et al. Diuretics in obstructive sleep apnea with diastolic heart failure. Chest 2007;132(2):440–6.

20. Shin JT, Semigran MJ. Heart failure and pulmonary hypertension. Heart Fail Clin 2010;6(2): 215–22.

21. Meyer FJ, Ewert R, Hoeper MM, et al. Peripheral airway obstruction in primary pulmonary hypertension. Thorax 2002;57(6):473–6.

22. Rastogi D, Ngai P, Barst RJ, et al. Lower airway obstruction, bronchial hyperresponsiveness, and primary pulmonary hypertension in children. Pediatr Pulmonol 2004;37(1):50–5. https://doi.org/10.1002/ppul.10363.

23. Rothman A, Kulik TJ. Pulmonary hypertension and asthma in two patients with congenital heart disease. Am J Dis Child 1989;143(8):977–9.

24. Miller WW, Park CD, Waldhausen JA. Bronchial compression from enlarged, hypertensive right pulmonary artery with corrected transposition of great arteries, dextrocardia, and ventricular septal defect. Diagnosis and surgical treatment. J Thorac Cardiovasc Surg 1970;60(2):233–6.

25. Haworth SG, Hall SM, Panja M, et al. Peripheral pulmonary vascular and airway abnormalities in adolescents with rheumatic mitral stenosis. Int J Cardiol 1988;18(3):405–16.

26. Leeds SE, Uhley HN, Teleszky LB. Direct cannulation and injection lymphangiography of the canine cardiac and pulmonary efferent mediastinal lymphatics in experimental congestive heart failure. Invest Radiol 1981;16(3):193–200.

27. Agostoni P, Cattadori G, Guazzi M, et al. Cardiomegaly as a possible cause of lung dysfunction in patients with heart failure. Am Heart J 2000;140(5): A17–21.

28. McCormack DG. Increase in vital capacity after cardiac transplantation. Am J Med 1991;90(5): 660–1.

29. Puri S, Baker BL, Dutka DP, et al. Reduced alveolar-capillary membrane diffusing capacity in chronic heart failure. Its pathophysiological relevance and relationship to exercise performance. Circulation 1995;91(11):2769–74.

30. Robertson HT, Pellegrino R, Pini D, et al. Exercise response after rapid intravenous infusion of saline in healthy humans. J Appl Physiol (1985) 2004; 97(2):697–703.

31. Mutlu GM, Factor P. Alveolar epithelial beta2-adrenergic receptors. Am J Respir Cell Mol Biol 2008;38(2):127–34.

32. Guazzi M, Pontone G, Brambilla R, et al. Alveolar-capillary membrane gas conductance: a novel prognostic indicator in chronic heart failure. Eur Heart J 2002;23(6):467–76.

33. Lalande S, Yerly P, Faoro V, et al. Pulmonary vascular distensibility predicts aerobic capacity in healthy individuals. J Physiol 2012;590(17): 4279–88.

34. Agostoni PG, Marenzi GC, Pepi M, et al. Isolated ultrafiltration in moderate congestive heart failure. J Am Coll Cardiol 1993;21(2):424–31.

35. Mettauer B, Lampert E, Charloux A, et al. Lung membrane diffusing capacity, heart failure, and heart transplantation. Am J Cardiol 1999;83(1): 62–7.

36. Cundrle I, Johnson BD, Somers VK, et al. Effect of cardiac resynchronization therapy on pulmonary function in patients with heart failure. Am J Cardiol 2013;112(6):838–42.

37. Agostoni P, Swenson ER, Fumagalli R, et al. Acute high-altitude exposure reduces lung diffusion: data from the HIGHCARE Alps project. Respir Physiol Neurobiol 2013;188(2):223–8.

38. Banfi C, Agostoni P. Surfactant protein B: from biochemistry to its potential role as diagnostic and prognostic marker in heart failure. Int J Cardiol 2016;221:456–62.

39. De Pasquale CG, Arnolda LF, Doyle IR, et al. Plasma surfactant protein-B: a novel biomarker in chronic heart failure. Circulation 2004;110(9):1091–6.

40. Gargiulo P, Banfi C, Ghilardi S, et al. Surfactant-derived proteins as markers of alveolar membrane damage in heart failure. PLoS One 2014;9(12): e115030.

41. Magrì D, Banfi C, Maruotti A, et al. Plasma imma-ture form of surfactant protein type B correlates with prognosis in patients with chronic heart failure. A pilot single-center prospective study. Int J Cardiol 2015;201:394–9.

42. Fanfulla F, Mortara A, Maestri R, et al. The develop-ment of hyperventilation in patients with chronic heart failure and Cheyne-Strokes respiration: a possible role of chronic hypoxia. Chest 1998; 114(4):1083–90.

43. Arena R, Myers J, Aslam SS, et al. Peak VO2 and VE/VCO2 slope in patients with heart failure: a prognostic comparison. Am Heart J 2004;147(2): 354–60.

44. Johnson RL. Gas exchange efficiency in conges-tive heart failure. Circulation 2000;101(24):2774–6.

45. Roberts AM, Bhattacharya J, Schultz HD, et al. Stimulation of pulmonary vagal afferent C-fibers by lung edema in dogs. Circ Res 1986;58(4): 512–22.

46. Lloyd TCJ. Effect of increased left atrial pressure on breathing frequency in anesthetized dog. J Appl Physiol (1985) 1990;69(6):1973–80.

47. Olson TP, Frantz RP, Snyder EM, et al. Effects of acute changes in pulmonary wedge pressure on periodic breathing at rest in heart failure patients. Am Heart J 2007;153(1):104.e1-7.

48. Olson TP, Joyner MJ, Johnson BD. Influence of lo-comotor muscle metaboreceptor stimulation on the ventilatory response to exercise in heart failure. Circ Heart Fail 2010;3(2):212–9.

49. Olson LJ, Arruda-Olson AM, Somers VK, et al. Ex-ercise oscillatory ventilation. Chest 2008;133(2): 474–81.

50. Massie BM, Simonini A, Sahgal P, et al. Relation of systemic and local muscle exercise capacity to skeletal muscle characteristics in men with congestive heart failure. J Am Coll Cardiol 1996; 27(1):140–5.

51. Wilson JR, Mancini DM. Factors contributing to the exercise limitation of heart failure. J Am Coll Cardiol 1993;22(4 Suppl A):93A–8A.

52. Wensel R, Francis DP, Georgiadou P, et al. Exercise hyperventilation in chronic heart failure is not caused by systemic lactic acidosis. Eur J Heart Fail 2005;7(7):1105–11.

53. Wasserman K, Zhang YY, Gitt A, et al. Lung func-tion and exercise gas exchange in chronic heart failure. Circulation 1997;96(7):2221–7.

54. Banning AP, Lewis NP, Northridge DB, et al. Perfu-sion/ventilation mismatch during exercise in chronic heart failure: an investigation of circulatory determinants. Br Heart J 1995;74(1):27–33.

55. Reindl I, Wernecke K-D, Opitz C, et al. Impaired ventilatory efficiency in chronic heart failure: possible role of pulmonary vasoconstriction. Am Heart J 1998;136(5):778–85.

56. Francis DP, Shamim W, Davies LC, et al. Cardiopul-monary exercise testing for prognosis in chronic heart failure: continuous and independent prog-nostic value from VE/VCO2slope and peak VO2. Eur Heart J 2000;21(2):154–61.

57. Arena R, Humphrey R. Comparison of ventilatory expired gas parameters used to predict hospitali-zation in patients with heart failure. Am Heart J 2002;143(3):427–32.

58. Corrà U, Mezzani A, Bosimini E, et al. Ventilatory response to exercise improves risk stratification in patients with chronic heart failure and intermediate functional capacity. Am Heart J 2002;143(3): 418–26.

59. Chua TP, Ponikowski P, Harrington D, et al. Clinical correlates and prognostic significance of the venti-latory response to exercise in chronic heart failure. J Am Coll Cardiol 1997;29(7):1585–90.

60. Kleber FX, Vietzke G, Wernecke KD, et al. Impair-ment of ventilatory efficiency in heart failure prog-nostic impact. Circulation 2000;101(24):2803–9.

61. Myers J, Gujja P, Neelagaru S, et al. End-tidal CO2 pressure and cardiac performance during exercise in heart failure. Med Sci Sports Exerc 2009;41(1): 19–25.

62. Arena R, Peberdy MA, Myers J, et al. Prognostic value of resting end-tidal carbon dioxide in patients with heart failure. Int J Cardiol 2006;109(3):351–8.

63. Seguchi O, Hisamatsu E, Nakano A, et al. Low par-tial pressure of end-tidal carbon dioxide predicts left ventricular assist device implantation in

patients with advanced chronic heart failure. Int J Cardiol 2017;230:40–6.

64. Ingle L, Rigby AS, Sloan R, et al. Development of a composite model derived from cardiopulmonary exercise tests to predict mortality risk in patients with mild-to-moderate heart failure. Heart 2014; 100(10):781–6.

65. Myers J, Arena R, Dewey F, et al. A cardiopulmonary exercise testing score for predicting outcomes in patients with heart failure. Am Heart J 2008;156(6):1177–83.

66. Cundrle I, Johnson BD, Rea RF, et al. Modulation of ventilatory reflex control by cardiac resynchronization therapy. J Card Fail 2015;21(5): 367–73.

67. Bradley TD. The ups and downs of periodic breathing. Implications for mortality in heart failure*. J Am Coll Cardiol 2003;41(12):2182–4.

68. Leung RST, Douglas Bradley T. Sleep apnea and cardiovascular disease. Am J Respir Crit Care Med 2001;164(12):2147–65.

69. Francis DP, Willson K, Davies LC, et al. Quantitative general theory for periodic breathing in chronic heart failure and its clinical implications. Circulation 2000;102(18):2214–21.

70. Bradley TD, Phillipson EA. Central sleep apnea. Clin Chest Med 1992;13(3):493–505.

71. Clark AL, Piepoli M, Coats AJ. Skeletal muscle and the control of ventilation on exercise: evidence for metabolic receptors. Eur J Clin Invest 1995;25(5): 299–305.

72. Khoo MC, Kronauer RE, Strohl KP, et al. Factors inducing periodic breathing in humans: a general model. J Appl Physiol (1985) 1982;53(3):644–59.

73. Leite JJ, Mansur AJ, de Freitas HFG, et al. Periodic breathing during incremental exercise predicts mortality in patients with chronic heart failure evaluated for cardiac transplantation. J Am Coll Cardiol 2003;41(12):2175–81.

74. Steens RD, Millar TW, Su X, et al. Effect of inhaled 3% CO2 on Cheyne-Stokes respiration in congestive heart failure. Sleep 1994;17(1):61–8.

75. Murphy RM, Shah RV, Malhotra R, et al. Exercise oscillatory ventilation in systolic heart failure: an indicator of impaired hemodynamic response to exercise. Circulation 2011;124(13):1442–51.

76. Agostoni P, Apostolo A, Albert RK. Mechanisms of periodic breathing during exercise in patients with chronic heart failure. Chest 2008;133(1):197–203.

77. Balady Gary J, Ross A, Kathy S, et al. Clinician's guide to cardiopulmonary exercise testing in adults. Circulation 2010;122(2):191–225.

78. Olson TP, Snyder EM, Johnson BD. Exercise-disordered breathing in chronic heart failure. Exerc Sport Sci Rev 2006;34(4):194–201.

79. Guazzi M, Myers J, Peberdy MA, et al. Exercise oscillatory breathing in diastolic heart failure:

80. prevalence and prognostic insights. Eur Heart J 2008;29(22):2751–9.

80. Ponikowski P, Anker SD, Chua TP, et al. Oscillatory breathing patterns during wakefulness in patients with chronic heart failure: clinical implications and role of augmented peripheral chemosensitivity. Circulation 1999;100(24):2418–24.

81. Sun X-G, Hansen JE, Beshai JF, et al. Oscillatory breathing and exercise gas exchange abnormalities prognosticate early mortality and morbidity in heart failure. J Am Coll Cardiol 2010;55(17): 1814–23.

82. Guazzi M, Arena R, Pellegrino M, et al. Prevalence and characterization of exercise oscillatory ventilation in apparently healthy individuals at variable risk for cardiovascular disease: a subanalysis of the EURO-EX trial. Eur J Prev Cardiol 2016;23(3): 328–34.

83. Corrà U, Pistono M, Mezzani A, et al. Sleep and exertional periodic breathing in chronic heart failure. Circulation 2006;113(1):44–50.

84. Roche F, Maudoux D, Jamon Y, et al. Monitoring of ventilation during the early part of cardiopulmonary exercise testing: the first step to detect central sleep apnoea in chronic heart failure. Sleep Med 2008;9(4):411–7.

85. Wolk R, Kara T, Somers VK. Sleep-disordered breathing and cardiovascular disease. Circulation 2003;108(1):9–12.

86. Bradley TD, Floras JS. Sleep apnea and heart failure part II: central sleep apnea. Circulation 2003; 107(13):1822–6.

87. Caples SM, Wolk R, Somers VK. Influence of cardiac function and failure on sleep-disordered breathing: evidence for a causative role. J Appl Physiol (1985) 2005;99(6):2433–9.

88. Eckert DJ, Jordan AS, Merchia P, et al. Central sleep apnea: pathophysiology and treatment. Chest 2007;131(2):595–607.

89. Olson LJ, Somers VK. Sleep apnea: implications for heart failure. Curr Heart Fail Rep 2007;4(2): 63–9.

90. Javaheri S. Heart failure and sleep apnea: emphasis on practical therapeutic options. Clin Chest Med 2003;24(2):207–22.

91. Mansfield D, Kaye DM, Brunner La Rocca H, et al. Raised sympathetic nerve activity in heart failure and central sleep apnea is due to heart failure severity. Circulation 2003;107(10):1396–400.

92. Naughton MT, Benard DC, Liu PP, et al. Effects of nasal CPAP on sympathetic activity in patients with heart failure and central sleep apnea. Am J Respir Crit Care Med 1995;152(2):473–9.

93. Khayat R, Abraham W, Patt B, et al. Central sleep apnea is a predictor of cardiac readmission in hospitalized patients with systolic heart failure. J Card Fail 2012;18(7):534–40.

94. Naughton MT, Bradley TD. Sleep apnea in congestive heart failure. Clin Chest Med 1998;19(1): 99–113.

95. Owan TE, Hodge DO, Herges RM, et al. Trends in prevalence and outcome of heart failure with preserved ejection fraction. N Engl J Med 2006; 355(3):251–9.

96. Burkhoff D. Mortality in heart failure with preserved ejection fraction: an unacceptably high rate. Eur Heart J 2012;33(14):1718–20.

97. Smith GL, Masoudi FA, Vaccarino V, et al. Outcomes in heart failure patients with preserved ejection fraction: mortality, readmission, and functional decline. J Am Coll Cardiol 2003;41(9):1510–8.

98. Guazzi M, Myers J, Arena R. Cardiopulmonary exercise testing in the clinical and prognostic assessment of diastolic heart failure. J Am Coll Cardiol 2005;46(10):1883–90.

99. Yan J, Gong S-J, Li L, et al. Combination of B-type natriuretic peptide and minute ventilation/carbon dioxide production slope improves risk stratification in patients with diastolic heart failure. Int J Cardiol 2013;162(3):193–8.

100. Shafiq A, Brawner CA, Aldred HA, et al. Prognostic value of cardiopulmonary exercise testing in heart failure with preserved ejection fraction. The Henry Ford HosplTal CardioPulmonary EXercise Testing (FIT-CPX) project. Am Heart J 2016;174:167–72.

101. Nadruz W, West E, Sengeløv M, et al. Prognostic value of cardiopulmonary exercise testing in heart failure with reduced, midrange, and preserved ejection fraction. J Am Heart Assoc 2017;6(11). https://doi.org/10.1161/JAHA.117.006000.

102. Butler J, Chomsky DB, Wilson JR. Pulmonary hypertension and exercise intolerance in patients with heart failure. J Am Coll Cardiol 1999;34(6): 1802–6.

103. Lam CSP, Roger VL, Rodeheffer RJ, et al. Pulmonary hypertension in heart failure with preserved ejection fraction: a community-based study. J Am Coll Cardiol 2009;53(13):1119–26.

104. Rausch CM, Taylor AL, Ross H, et al. Ventilatory efficiency slope correlates with functional capacity, outcomes, and disease severity in pediatric patients with pulmonary hypertension. Int J Cardiol 2013;169(6):445–8.

105. Faisal A, Webb KA, Guenette JA, et al. Effect of age-related ventilatory inefficiency on respiratory sensation during exercise. Respir Physiol Neurobiol 2015;205:129–39.

106. Matsumoto A, Itoh H, Eto Y, et al. End-tidal CO_2 pressure decreases during exercise in cardiac patients: association with severity of heart failure and cardiac output reserve. J Am Coll Cardiol 2000; 36(1):242–9.

107. Sun XG, Hansen JE, Oudiz RJ, et al. Exercise pathophysiology in patients with primary pulmonary hypertension. Circulation 2001;104(4):429–35.

108. O'Donnell DE, Elbehairy AF, Berton DC, et al. Advances in the evaluation of respiratory pathophysiology during exercise in chronic lung diseases. Front Physiol 2017;8. https://doi.org/10.3389/fphys.2017.00082.

109. Aguggini G, Clement MG, Widdicombe JG. Lung reflexes affecting the larynx in the pig, and the effect of pulmonary microembolism. Q J Exp Physiol 1987;72(1):95–104.

Exertional Periodic Breathing in Heart Failure
Mechanisms and Clinical Implications

Piergiuseppe Agostoni, MD, PhD[a,b,*],
Elisabetta Salvioni, PhD[b]

KEYWORDS

- Periodic breathing • Cardiopulmonary exercise test • Ventilation • Heart failure

KEY POINTS

- Exercise-induced periodic breathing (PB) is a relatively frequent observation in male, but not in female individuals, with chronic heart failure.
- It is associated with a negative prognosis, particularly if concomitant with PB during sleep.
- The physiology of PB is still unclear, but increased sympathetic activity, low cardiac output, and cerebrovascular reactivity to CO_2 all have a definite role.

Exertional periodic breathing (PB) is a fascinating event characterized by a cyclic fluctuation of minute ventilation (VE), tidal volume, oxygen uptake (VO_2), carbon dioxide production (VCO_2), and end-tidal pressure for O_2 and CO_2 (**Fig. 1**). In a few cases, also heart and respiratory rates show some fluctuation. However, the most striking fluctuation is observed on the Respiratory Exchange Ratio (RER), which is VCO_2/VO_2 (**Fig. 2**). PB during exercise has been originally described as anecdotal,[1–3] but nowadays it is frequently observed, and is considered as a marker of disease severity and of worse prognosis.[4,5] PB is a slow, prominent, consistent fluctuation in VE and derived parameters, that may be persistent for the entire exercise or present only in the early phases of exercise usually up to the anaerobic threshold. PB is mainly reported in patients with severe heart failure (HF), with an overall incidence ranging from 7% to 51% (further discussion the topic is provided in Pulmonary Limitations in Heart Failure; Clinical and Physiological Implications of Negative Cardiopulmonary Interactions in Coexisting COPD-Heart Failure).[6–14]

There are 3 main attributes for defining PB: amplitude and interval (length) of the single VE oscillation, and duration of the abnormal VE phenomenon during exercise. The wide variability of PB patterns is mystified by assessment methods, which include manual scoring and/or visual interpretation. Several description about cycle length, amplitude of single VE oscillation, and duration of oscillatory phenomenon during exercise have been reported. Concerning cycle length, many descriptions are given, such as the distance between 2 nadirs, the period of observed oscillation divided by the number of oscillations, and the interval from peak to peak for each cycle at rest expressed as mean value.[15] Regarding the duration of the VE cycle, definitions vary significantly: approximately 60 s, 40–140 s, 30–60 s, or it is calculated as a percentage of the average.[15] Furthermore, the amplitude of the VE oscillations is described using several approaches: (1) it is calculated as the difference between the peak of the oscillation of VE and the average of the VE of the 2 surrounding nadirs, (2) it is calculated

---

Disclosure Statement: Nothing to disclose.
[a] Department of Clinical Sciences and Community Health, Cardiovascular Section, University of Milano, Via Parea 4, Milano 20138, Italy; [b] Centro Cardiologico Monzino, IRCCS, Via Parea 4, Milano 20138, Italy
* Corresponding author. Via Parea 4, Milano 20138, Italy.
E-mail address: piergiuseppe.agostoni@ccfm.it

Clin Chest Med 40 (2019) 449–457
https://doi.org/10.1016/j.ccm.2019.02.016
0272-5231/19/© 2019 Elsevier Inc. All rights reserved.

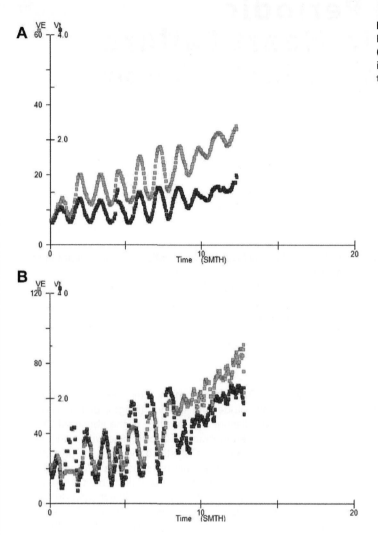

Fig. 1. Example of exercise-induced PB that lasts for the entire exercise (*A*) and example of exercise-induced PB that disappears during the exercise (*B*).

by the variation coefficient of VE, (3) it is calculated by assessing the correlation coefficient of VE, or (4) it is calculated as a percentage of the mean of the rest VE.[15] Finally, the total duration of the PB also varies. For the definition of PB presence, a duration $\geq$ 66% of the exercise protocol, or $\geq$60%, or $\geq$50% have been proposed.[15] Therefore, no gold standard has been proposed so far and an accepted PB definition is still lacking, making comparison between studies difficult, if not impossible in some cases.[16]

PB refers to a slow, prominent, consistent fluctuation in ventilation that may be persistent throughout exercise or present only in its early phases. It is reported (but not exclusively) in patients with severe HF, carrying important negative prognostic implications.

PREVALENCE OF EXERCISE-INDUCED PERIODIC BREATHING (EXERCISE-INDUCED EXERTIONAL OSCILLATORY VENTILATION)

Few data are available regarding the prevalence of exercise-induced PB in patients with HF.[8,9,17,18] In approximately 6000 patients with systolic HF who underwent a maximal cardiopulmonary exercise test, followed by the MECKI (Metabolic Exercise Cardiac Kidney Index) score research group,[19,20] PB was present in 17.5% of cases, and mainly in those with the most impaired exercise capacity. **Table 1** shows the incidence of exercise-induced PB according to the severity of exercise limitation in the MECKI score population, which is a cardiopulmonary exercise test (CPET)-based register of systolic HF. Notably, the number of female patients with exercise-induced PB is low, being in the MECKI score HF population, exercise-induced

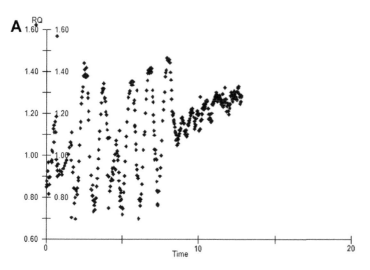

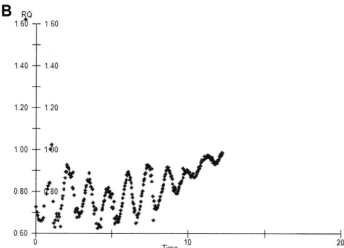

Fig. 2. Oscillations of respiratory quotient (RQ) of the 2 cases shown in **Fig. 1**. *Panel A*: PB that lasts for the entire exercise. *Panel B*: PB that disappears during the exercise.

PB is present in 13.5% of female and 18.4% of male individuals. This gender-specific PB behavior is present in all the severity groups analyzed. The same observation was made with regard to PB in patients with HF during sleep and in healthy subjects at high altitude.[9,21,22] In a recent report by Lombardi and colleagues,[21] the occurrence of PB during sleep at high altitude has been evaluated at different altitudes and up to 5400 m (Mount Everest South Base Camp). Female gender was associated with a lower presence of PB during sleep regardless of altitude and acclimatization time. Indeed, sleep studies were performed at different altitudes (Manche Bazar, 3450 m, and Mount Everest Base Camp, 5500 m) and after different acclimatization periods (after 1 and 3 weeks sojourn at Mount Everest Base Camp). Lombardi and colleagues[21] proposed that differences in peripheral muscle CO_2 production, apneic CO_2 threshold, or in the chemoreflex response to Po_2 and Pco_2 (related to the effect of sex hormones) are possibly responsible for the observed gender differences in high altitude regarding PB, but clearly those are only hypotheses: no definite cause-effect relationship has been proven.

Table 1			
Heart failure population grouped by Vo_2 class			
HF Patients	Vo_2 <50% (2199, m = 1955 f = 244)	Vo_2 50%–80% (2926, m = 2314 f = 612)	Vo_2 >80% (541, m = 362 f = 179)
All	528 (24)	419 (14.3)	45 (8.3)
Male	488 (25)	336 (14.5)	28 (7.7)
Female	40 (16.4)	83 (13.6)	17 (9.5)

Values are n (%).

Abbreviations: f, female; m, male; Vo_2, oxygen consumption expressed by % of predicted value.

PHYSIOLOGY OF EXERCISE-INDUCED PERIODIC BREATHING IN HEART FAILURE

Little is known about exercise-induced PB physiology. The main concepts have been derived from central sleep apneas in HF, but it is unknown whether these concepts apply also to exercise-induced PB. It has been reported that at least 3 factors have a pivotal role in exercise-induced PB in HF, specifically hyperventilation, low cardiac output leading to increased circulatory delay, and cerebrovascular reactivity to CO_2[23] (**Box 1**). Hyperventilation is part of the increased sympathetic activity frequently observed in HF, and it is due to increased stimulation of intrapulmonary receptors and of chemoreceptors and metaboreceptors (further discussion in the topic is provided in Update on Chemoreception: Influence on Cardiorespiratory Regulation and Patho-Physiology).[24] Due to hyperventilation, $Paco_2$ falls below the respiratory threshold, so that breath stops due to temporary absence of central drive to respiratory muscles, which ends when an increase of $Paco_2$ promotes ventilation with a further period of hyperventilation. Moreover, patients with HF have a reduced cerebrovascular reactivity to CO_2, further increasing breathing instability.[23] The increased circulatory delay, which is due to

a low cardiac output, is considered as another factor responsible of exercise-induced PB occurrence. Indeed circulatory delay leads to a temporary misalignment of the chemical signals (low or high $Paco_2$) to the respiratory response (increased or reduced ventilation).[23,25] Notably, albeit frequently suggested, the role of low cardiac output in the pathogenesis of exercise-induced PB has at present almost no scientific evidence. Indeed, no significant differences in cardiac output or in the circulatory delay from lungs to peripheral receptors have been found between patients with HF with and without exercise-induced PB.[26,27] Similarly, no correlation exists between cardiac output and circulatory delay at rest in patients with severe HF. However, no data of the relationship between circulatory delay and cardiac output exists during physical activity. In a recent series of patients with HF who successfully underwent implantation of a left ventricle assisting device (LVAD) (the Jarvik 2000), resting cardiac output and circulatory delay resulted unrelated to each other both at low LVAD pump speed and at high pump speed, but again at rest (**Fig. 3**). Interestingly, in a group of 15 patients with HF with LVAD, exercise-induced PB occurred in 9 cases with LVAD at pump speed = 2 and in 5 patients at pump speed = 4. Moreover, the presence of exercise-induced PB in this series of patients was associated with a lower cardiac output at rest. A reduction of exercise-induced PB due to HF improvement has been reported by Ribeiro and colleagues,[2] who showed that exercise-induced PB disappeared after HF improvement in a series of 5 patients.

Box 1
Mechanisms underlying central sleep apnea in heart failure

Chronic hyperventilation

1. Pulmonary interstitial congestion due to rostral fluid displacement.

2. Exaggerated peripheral chemoreceptor activity.

3. Upper airway resistance.

Circulatory delay (it delays detection of changes in blood gases between the peripheral and the central chemoreceptors)

1. Low cardiac output.

Cerebrovascular reactivity

1. Respiratory-induced changes in the $Paco_2$ do alter the regulatory circulation of the cerebral district.

2. The normal buffering action to changes in central hydrogen ion concentration is impaired (as a consequence).

3. Depressed ability of the central respiratory control center to dampen ventilatory undershoots or overshoots, such as those seen during apnea or at apnea termination.

At least 3 factors have a pivotal role in exercise-induced PB in HF: hyperventilation, low cardiac output leading to increased circulatory delay, and heightened cerebrovascular reactivity to CO_2.

In approximately 60% of cases, PB disappears during a progressive effort before exhaustion. Cardiac output increase during exercise has been suggested as the cause of the disappearance of exercise-induced PB. In this regard, Schmid and colleagues[28] showed that, in 52% of patients in whom exercise-induced PB ceased during the exercise, the Vo_2 versus work relationship increased after PB cessation, it was still present in 24% of cases, and it decreased in 24% of cases (see **Fig. 3**; **Fig. 4**). Notably, the evaluation of the Vo_2 versus work relationship allows understanding of the amount of O_2 delivery to the working muscle,

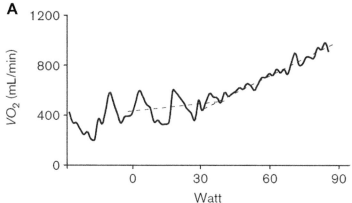

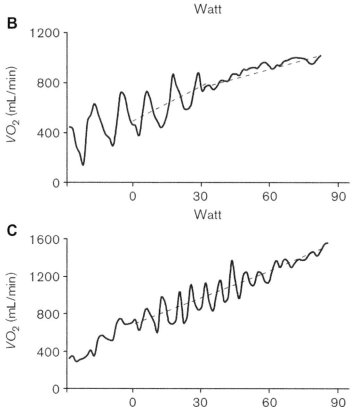

Fig. 3. Examples of an increase (*A*), a decrease (*B*), and a lack of change (*C*) of the V_{O_2}/workload slope in patients with PB disappearing during the exercise test. Dashed lines indicate the change of V_{O_2}/workload slope from the PB phase to the phase after PB disappearance. (*From* Schmid JP, Apostolo A, Antonioli L, et al. Influence of exertional oscillatory ventilation on exercise performance in heart failure. Eur J Cardiovasc Prev Rehabil 2008;15(6):688–92.)

because a reduction of this relationship during exercise is suggestive of a reduction of cardiac output, either due to exercise-induced cardiac ischemia or to mitral insufficiency.[29,30] An increase of the V_{O_2} versus work relationship during exercise is a rare event and it has been reported only in patients in whom PB ceased during exercise and specifically in approximately 50% of cases. This implies a higher O_2 delivery to the working muscles, possibly due to a reduction of the work of breathing. In other PB cases it seems to be associated with an increased work of breathing and its disappearance allows an increase of V_{O_2} delivery to the exercising muscles. However, it is still unclear why exercise-induced PB persists throughout a progressive exercise session in some and not in other patients.

One of the major unsolved question is what oscillates first; whether it is ventilation or circulation that leads oscillation. A few pieces of evidence suggest that oscillation in blood flow is the first initiating mechanism. Pioneering studies by Ben

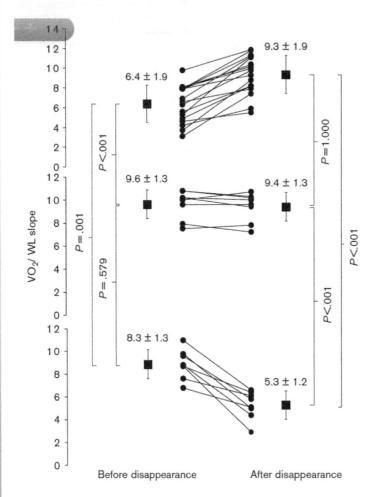

Fig. 4. Individual behavior of V_{O_2}/ workload slope in 33 patients in which PB disappeared. During exercise, the disappearance of PB was accompanied by an increase of V_{O_2}/workload slope in 17 patients, a decrease in 8 patients, and no change in 8 patients. (*From* Schmid JP, Apostolo A, Antonioli L, et al. Influence of exertional oscillatory ventilation on exercise performance in heart failure. Eur J Cardiovasc Prev Rehabil 2008;15(6):691; with permission.)

Dov and colleagues[3] demonstrated that, when aligning V_{O_2}, VCO_2, and VE, V_{O_2} oscillation anticipates VCO_2 and VE oscillations (**Fig. 5**). However, we reevaluated this finding in our population of patients with HF and found that this specific behavior was present in some, but not in all of the studied patients. Moreover, Francis and colleagues[31] showed that exercise-induced PB can be voluntarily induced by acting on ventilation.

Further relevant, albeit spotty, information about the physiology of exercise-induced PB have been reported, but the complete physiologic image of

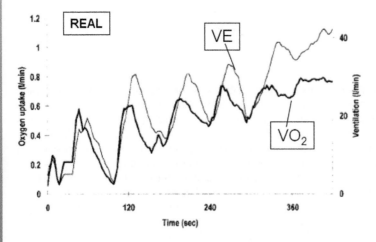

Fig. 5. When aligning V_{O_2}, VCO_2 and VE, V_{O_2} oscillation anticipates VCO_2 and VE oscillations. (*Reprinted* with permission of the American Thoracic Society. Copyright © 2018 American Thoracic Society. Ben-Dov I, Sietsema KE, Casaburi R, et al. Evidence that circulatory oscillations accompany ventilatory oscillations during exercise in patients with heart failure. Am Rev Respir Dis 1992;145(4 Pt 1):778. The American Journal of Respiratory and Critical Care Medicine is an official journal of the American Thoracic Society.)

this mosaic is still unknown. As reported previously, we do know that exercise-induced PB is mainly associated with severe HF, and that it disappears if severe HF is successfully treated. This seems to link the disappearance of exercise-induced PB to both an improvement in lung mechanics and in cardiac function. The temporal relationship between the disappearance of PB and the improvement of HF is, however, not defined, so that the disappearance of exercise-induced PB may possibly occur later than the hemodynamic improvement. In other words, it is possible that some sort of PB memory persist for some time after clinical improvement.

> Based on the knowledge that exercise-induced PB is mainly associated with severe HF, and that it disappears if the disease is successfully treated, it is conceivable that both cardiac function and lung mechanics are mechanistically linked to this phenomenon.

Besides the reduction of PB through treatment or its spontaneous disappearance during exercise, there are several pieces of evidence that exercise-induced PB can be eliminated by adding a further ventilation stimulus. For example, if a hypoxic stimulus is suddenly added during constant low workload, exercise PB disappears. Similarly, Apostolo and colleagues[32] showed that when 2% CO_2 is added into the breathing air during constant workload exercise in a subject with exercise-induced PB, PB ceases. However, if the added respiratory stimulus is lower, like with 1% CO_2 instead of 2% CO_2, PB persists. A rather complicated interplay between O_2-dependent and CO_2-dependent chemoreceptors is likely the basis of this finding. Indeed, the tendency to PB may arise from an augmentation in the summed chemoreceptor inputs to respiratory drive, which are O_2-dependent (peripheral) and CO_2-dependent (peripheral and central). Although the slight rise in Pco_2 stimulates the ventilatory drive, the concurrent rise in Po_2 (higher with 2% CO_2 and lower with 1% CO_2) may exert a counterinhibitory effect via withdrawal of peripheral chemoreceptor afferent signaling. Although O_2-sensitive carotid body output is not generally thought to be important when Pao_2 is greater than 70 mm Hg due to the very hyperbolic nature of the hypoxic ventilatory response, some peripheral chemoreceptor activity is still present at normal physiologic Pao_2 (and more so in patients with HF), and it can be suppressed with further elevation of Pao_2 beyond 100 mm Hg.[33] However, other explanations are

possible, like the direct role of lactic acid on the chemoreceptors. Indeed, lactic acid production may fluctuate with O_2 delivery (cardiac output) fluctuation and in the carotid body many lactic acid receptors have been described.[34]

Finally, when an external dead space is added, PB disappears early during exercise, or it does not appear at all, according to the amount of added dead space, 250 and 500 mL, respectively.[35]

> There are several pieces of evidence that exercise-induced PB can be eliminated by adding an additional stimulus to ventilation, such as CO_2 and an external dead space.

PROGNOSTIC ROLE OF EXERCISE-INDUCED PERIODIC BREATHING

PB is a robust CPET risk index in distinct HF cohorts,[7–14,18] including heart transplantation candidates, and in patients chronically treated with beta-blockers. PB and several CPET-derived parameters have proven to be predictive in HF,[36] but most have been studied in a binary analysis, considering risk indexes in isolation, disregarding the potential value of combining variables. In addition, few observations have been validated yet. So far, only peak Vo_2, VE/VCO_2 slope, and PB (representing the so-called 2008 ESC [European Society of Cardiology] model) have been validated[37]: the 2008 ESC multiparametric model was superior to other predictive prototypes, created by adding, in isolation, predicted peak Vo_2, peak oxygen pulse, peak RER, peak circulatory power, peak VE/VCO_2, VE/VCO_2 slope normalized by peak Vo_2, Vo_2 efficiency slope, ventilatory anaerobic threshold detection, peak end-tidal CO_2 partial pressure, peak heart rate, and peak systolic arterial blood pressure. Hence, although difficult to properly compute, PB should always be taken into account during CPET, if evident at visual or analytical inspection.

> Collectively, a low peak Vo_2, a high VE/VCO_2 slope, and the presence of PB are the key exercise-related parameters that can reliably predict poor prognosis in patients with HF.

SUMMARY

Exercise-induced PB is a relatively frequent observation in male, but not in female individuals, with chronic HF. It is associated with a negative prognosis, particularly if concomitant with PB during sleep. The physiology behind it is complex and still not clearly defined. However, hyperventilation is likely due to an increased sympathetic activity combined with an enhanced stimulation of intrapulmonary, chemoreceptors and metaboreceptors, low cardiac output leading to increased circulatory delay, and cerebrovascular reactivity to CO_2, all have a definite role.

REFERENCES

1. Kremser CB, O'Toole MF, Leff AR. Oscillatory hyperventilation in severe congestive heart failure secondary to idiopathic dilated cardiomyopathy or to ischemic cardiomyopathy. Am J Cardiol 1987; 59(8):900–5.

2. Ribeiro JP, Knutzen A, Rocco MB, et al. Periodic breathing during exercise in severe heart failure. Reversal with milrinone or cardiac transplantation. Chest 1987;92(3):555–6.

3. Ben-Dov I, Sietsema KE, Casaburi R, et al. Evidence that circulatory oscillations accompany ventilatory oscillations during exercise in patients with heart failure. Am Rev Respir Dis 1992;145(4 Pt 1):776–81.

4. Dickstein K, Cohen-Solal A, Filippatos G, et al. ESC guidelines for the diagnosis and treatment of acute and chronic heart failure 2008: the task force for the diagnosis and treatment of acute and chronic heart failure 2008 of the European Society of Cardiology. Developed in collaboration with the Heart Failure Association of the ESC (HFA) and endorsed by the European Society of Intensive Care Medicine (ESICM). Eur Heart J 2008;29(19):2388–442.

5. Cornelis J, Taeymans J, Hens W, et al. Prognostic respiratory parameters in heart failure patients with and without exercise oscillatory ventilation—a systematic review and descriptive meta-analysis. Int J Cardiol 2015;182:476–86.

6. Feld H, Priest S. A cyclic breathing pattern in patients with poor left ventricular function and compensated heart failure: a mild form of Cheyne-Stokes respiration? J Am Coll Cardiol 1993;21(4):971–4.

7. Leite JJ, Mansur AJ, de Freitas HF, et al. Periodic breathing during incremental exercise predicts mortality in patients with chronic heart failure evaluated for cardiac transplantation. J Am Coll Cardiol 2003; 41(12):2175–81.

8. Corra U, Giordano A, Bosimini E, et al. Oscillatory ventilation during exercise in patients with chronic heart failure: clinical correlates and prognostic implications. Chest 2002;121(5):1572–80.

9. Corra U, Pistono M, Mezzani A, et al. Sleep and exertional periodic breathing in chronic heart failure: prognostic importance and interdependence. Circulation 2006;113(1):44–50.

10. Guazzi M, Arena R, Ascione A, et al. Exercise oscillatory breathing and increased ventilation to carbon dioxide production slope in heart failure: an unfavorable combination with high prognostic value. Am Heart J 2007;153(5):859–67.

11. Guazzi M, Raimondo R, Vicenzi M, et al. Exercise oscillatory ventilation may predict sudden cardiac death in heart failure patients. J Am Coll Cardiol 2007;50(4):299–308.

12. Guazzi M, Boracchi P, Arena R, et al. Development of a cardiopulmonary exercise prognostic score for optimizing risk stratification in heart failure: the (P)e(R)i(O)dic (B)reathing during (E)xercise (PROBE) study. J Card Fail 2010;16(10):799–805.

13. Arena R, Myers J, Abella J, et al. Prognostic value of timing and duration characteristics of exercise oscillatory ventilation in patients with heart failure. J Heart Lung Transplant 2008;27(3):341–7.

14. Corra U, Mezzani A, Giordano A, et al. Exercise haemodynamic variables rather than ventilatory efficiency indexes contribute to risk assessment in chronic heart failure patients treated with carvedilol. Eur Heart J 2009;30(24):3000–6.

15. Cornelis J, Beckers P, Vanroy C, et al. An overview of the applied definitions and diagnostic methods to assess exercise oscillatory ventilation–a systematic review. Int J Cardiol 2015;190:161–9.

16. Dhakal BP, Murphy RM, Lewis GD. Exercise oscillatory ventilation in heart failure. Trends Cardiovasc Med 2012;22(7):185–91.

17. Francis DP, Davies LC, Piepoli M, et al. Origin of oscillatory kinetics of respiratory gas exchange in chronic heart failure. Circulation 1999;100(10): 1065–70.

18. Sun XG, Hansen JE, Beshai JF, et al. Oscillatory breathing and exercise gas exchange abnormalities prognosticate early mortality and morbidity in heart failure. J Am Coll Cardiol 2010;55(17): 1814–23.

19. Agostoni P, Corra U, Cattadori G, et al. Metabolic exercise test data combined with cardiac and kidney indexes, the MECKI score: a multiparametric approach to heart failure prognosis. Int J Cardiol 2013;167(6):2710–8.

20. Carubelli V, Metra M, Corra U, et al. Exercise performance is a prognostic indicator in elderly patients with chronic heart failure—application of metabolic exercise cardiac kidney indexes score. Circ J 2015;79(12):2608–15.

21. Lombardi C, Meriggi P, Agostoni P, et al. High-altitude hypoxia and periodic breathing during sleep: gender-related differences. J Sleep Res 2013; 22(3):322–30.

22. Sin DD, Fitzgerald F, Parker JD, et al. Risk factors for central and obstructive sleep apnea in 450 men and women with congestive heart failure. Am J Respir Crit Care Med 1999;160(4):1101–6.

23. Costanzo MR, Khayat R, Ponikowski P, et al. Mechanisms and clinical consequences of untreated central sleep apnea in heart failure. J Am Coll Cardiol 2015;65(1):72–84.

24. Yu J, Zhang JF, Fletcher EC. Stimulation of breathing by activation of pulmonary peripheral afferents in rabbits. J Appl Physiol (1985) 1998;85(4):1485–92.

25. Pryor WW. Cheyne-Stokes respiration in patients with cardiac enlargement and prolonged circulation time. Circulation 1951;4(2):233–8.

26. Javaheri S, Parker TJ, Liming JD, et al. Sleep apnea in 81 ambulatory male patients with stable heart failure. Types and their prevalences, consequences, and presentations. Circulation 1998;97(21):2154–9.

27. Bradley TD, Floras JS. Sleep apnea and heart failure: Part II: central sleep apnea. Circulation 2003; 107(13):1822–6.

28. Schmid JP, Apostolo A, Antonioli L, et al. Influence of exertional oscillatory ventilation on exercise performance in heart failure. Eur J Cardiovasc Prev Rehabil 2008;15(6):688–92.

29. Bussotti M, Apostolo A, Andreini D, et al. Cardiopulmonary evidence of exercise-induced silent ischaemia. Eur J Cardiovasc Prev Rehabil 2006; 13(2):249–53.

30. Belardinelli R, Lacalaprice F, Carle F, et al. Exercise-induced myocardial ischaemia detected by cardiopulmonary exercise testing. Eur Heart J 2003; 24(14):1304–13.

31. Francis DP, Davies LC, Willson K, et al. Impact of periodic breathing on measurement of oxygen uptake and respiratory exchange ratio during cardiopulmonary exercise testing. Clin Sci (Lond) 2002;103(6): 543–52.

32. Apostolo A, Agostoni P, Contini M, et al. Acetazolamide and inhaled carbon dioxide reduce periodic breathing during exercise in patients with chronic heart failure. J Card Fail 2014;20(4):278–88.

33. Schultz HD, Marcus NJ. Heart failure and carotid body chemoreception. In: Nurse C, editor. Arterial chemoreception: from molecules to systems. Heidelberg (Germany): Adv Exp Med Bio; 2012. p. 387–95.

34. Parati G, Lombardi C, Castagna F, et al. Heart failure and sleep disorders. Nat Rev Cardiol 2016;13: 389–403.

35. Agostoni P, Apostolo A, Albert RK. Mechanisms of periodic breathing during exercise in patients with chronic heart failure. Chest 2008;133(1):197–203.

36. Corra U, Piepoli MF, Adamopoulos S, et al. Cardiopulmonary exercise testing in systolic heart failure in 2014: the evolving prognostic role: a position paper from the committee on exercise physiology and training of the heart failure association of the ESC. Eur J Heart Fail 2014;16(9):929–41.

37. Corra U, Giordano A, Mezzani A, et al. Cardiopulmonary exercise testing and prognosis in heart failure due to systolic left ventricular dysfunction: a validation study of the European Society of Cardiology Guidelines and Recommendations (2008) and further developments. Eur J Prev Cardiol 2012; 19(1):32–40.

Pulmonary Hypertension and Exercise

James R. Vallerand, PhD[a], Jason Weatherald, MD[b,c,d,1],
Pierantonio Laveneziana, MD, PhD[e,f,*,1]

KEYWORDS

- Pulmonary vascular disease • Pulmonary arterial hypertension
- Chronic thromboembolic pulmonary hypertension • Cardiopulmonary exercise testing • Dyspnea

KEY POINTS

- Cardiopulmonary exercise testing (CPET) helps magnify the aberrant physiology in pulmonary hypertension (PH) including reduced cardiac output, aerobic capacity, anaerobic threshold, inefficient ventilation, dynamic hyperinflation, and dyspnea.
- Important CPET variables in PH include peak oxygen consumption, peak work rate, oxygen pulse, peak systolic blood pressure, exercise duration and 6-minute walk distance.
- Additional important CPET variables include ratio of physiologic dead space to tidal volume, ratio of minute ventilation to CO_2 production, end-tidal and arterial partial pressures of CO_2.
- Clinical trials have used variables from CPET as primary efficacy outcomes, yet few trials evaluate the efficacy of exercise training as adjuvant therapy in PH.
- Exercise training with light-intensity endurance, strength, and respiratory training is safe and beneficial in PH, and merits further consideration.

INTRODUCTION

Pulmonary hypertension (PH) is a condition wherein the resting mean pulmonary artery pressure (mPAP) is pathologically elevated greater than or equal to 25 mm Hg.[1] Several physiologic processes can produce PH, and these are reflected in the 5 different classes of PH (**Table 1**).[2] For example, pulmonary arterial hypertension (PAH) and chronic thromboembolic PH (CTEPH) represent 2 distinct classes of PH affecting precapillary sites within the pulmonary vasculature. In addition to idiopathic causes, PAH can result from genetic mutations, drugs and toxins, connective tissue disorders, infections (eg, HIV and schistosomiasis), portal hypertension, and congenital heart abnormalities. In contrast, CTEPH is a consequence of a proinflammatory remodeling in response to pulmonary thromboembolism, which causes persistent structural changes that obstruct pulmonary vasculature. Altogether, PH

Disclosure Statement: The authors have no disclosures.
[a] Undergraduate Medical Education, Cumming School of Medicine, University of Calgary, 3330 Hospital Drive Northwest G702, Calgary, Alberta T2N 4N1, Canada; [b] Division of Respiratory Medicine, Department of Medicine, Cumming School of Medicine, University of Calgary, Calgary, Alberta, Canada; [c] Libin Cardiovascular Institute of Alberta, Calgary, Alberta, Canada; [d] Peter Lougheed Centre, 3500 26 Avenue Northeast, Calgary, Alberta T1Y 6J4, Canada; [e] Sorbonne Universés, Université Pierre et Marie Curie Université Paris 06, Institut National de la Santé et de la Recherche Médicale, Unité Mixte de Recherche S_1158 Neurophysiologie Respiratoire Expérimentale et Clinique, Paris, France; [f] Service des Explorations Fonctionnelles de la Respiration, de l'Exercice et de la Dyspnée Hôpital Universitaire Pitié-Salpêtrière (AP-HP), Département Respiration, Réanimation, Sommeil, Pôle PRAGUES, Groupe Hospitalier Pitié-Salpêtrière Charles Foix, Assistance Publique-Höpitaux de Paris, Paris, France
[1] J. Weatherald and P. Laveneziana contributed equally.
* Corresponding author. Service d'Explorations Fonctionnelles de la Respiration, de l'Exercice et de la Dyspnée Hôpital Universitaire Pitié-Salpêtrière (AP-HP), 47-83 Boulevard de l'Hôpital, Paris 75013, France.
E-mail address: pierantonio.laveneziana@psl.aphp.fr

Clin Chest Med 40 (2019) 459–469
https://doi.org/10.1016/j.ccm.2019.02.003

Table 1
Groupings of the different classes of pulmonary hypertension

Pulmonary Hypertension Classification	Description
Group 1	PAH
Group 2	PH due to left-sided heart disease
Group 3	PH due to lung diseases and/or chronic hypoxia
Group 4	CTEPH and other pulmonary artery obstructions
Group 5	PH with unclear and/or multifactorial mechanisms

is rare but its prevalence continues to increase.[3] A diagnosis of PH, irrespective of the underlying cause (ie, groups 1–4 inclusively), presents an especially unfavorable prognosis of a 7-fold increase in 1-year mortality.[3]

Exercise intolerance is an ominous early warning sign common in, but not specific for, PH.[1] The added demand placed on the cardiopulmonary system during exercise magnifies the aberrant pathophysiology in PH,[4] and, accordingly, PH patients report significantly greater levels of physical inactivity, dyspnea, and sedentary time.[5–7] Together, the pairing of physiologic limitations and behavioral limitations produces a debilitating spiral of deconditioning that ultimately leads to even greater levels of fatigue[8] and much poorer quality of life.[9,10] This article discusses the cardiorespiratory manifestations of PH, reviews the potential diagnostic and prognostic utility of cardiopulmonary exercise testing (CPET), and looks toward the potential role of exercise training as adjuvant therapy for PH.

EXERCISE PATHOPHYSIOLOGY IN PULMONARY HYPERTENSION
General Hallmarks

The physiologic derangements of PH result in characteristic abnormalities observed during dynamic exercise and often lead to dyspnea and exercise intolerance, which are summarized in **Fig. 1** and are discussed in other articles in this issue (including The Pathophysiology of Dyspnea and Exercise Intolerance in COPD and Unraveling the Causes of Unexplained Dyspnea: The Value of Exercise Testing). Impaired cardiac function results in reductions in aerobic capacity,

anaerobic threshold (AT), and oxygen consumption (VO_2).[11–16] Both high physiologic dead space (V_D) (ie, as measured by the ratio of V_D to tidal volume [V_T] [V_D/V_T]) and chemosensitivity contribute to an elevated ratio of minute ventilation (V_E) to carbon dioxide production (VCO_2), expressed as V_E/VCO_2, during CPET.[17–25] Consequently, resting hypocapnia with low end-tidal PCO_2 ($P_{et}CO_2$) throughout exercise is typically observed and related to the severity of disease.[18,26–29] Exertional hypoxemia also is a common finding during exercise, which can be related to ventilation-perfusion heterogeneity, low mixed venous oxygen content from impaired cardiac output, and right-to-left shunting through a patent foramen ovale.[30] Even in the absence of significant resting airflow obstruction, dynamic hyperinflation can occur in pulmonary vascular diseases, which contributes to exertional dyspnea and exercise intolerance.[31–33] Peripheral muscle dysfunction is another common component of exercise pathophysiology in these conditions (further discussion in the topic is provided in The Relevance of Limb Muscle Dysfunction In COPD: A Review for Clinicians).[34–37]

> Low cardiac output, ventilatory inefficiency, abnormal lung mechanics, hypoxemia, and skeletal (peripheral and respiratory) muscle dysfunction contribute, to varying degrees, to decreased exercise tolerance in patients with PH.

Cardiovascular Anomalies

Elevated mPAP from increased pulmonary vascular resistance (PVR) has profound deleterious effects on the cardiovascular system. Early in PH, the distensibility of the pulmonary vasculature is compromised,[38] impairing right ventricular outflow and thus increasing its afterload.[39] As such, left atrial filling (ie, preload) is limited by a reduction in blood flow through the lungs from the right heart,[12,40–42] and even further restricted by a leftward shift in the interventricular septum due to the overloaded right ventricle.[11,12] Ultimately, this decompensated cardiac morphology limits cardiac output and stroke volume, which has functional and prognostic implications (see also Clinical and Physiological Implications of Negative Cardiopulmonary Interactions in Coexisting COPD-Heart Failure).[13,14]

Stroke volume impairments become problematic during exercising conditions, as increased metabolic demands of active peripheral muscles require proportional increases in cardiac output,

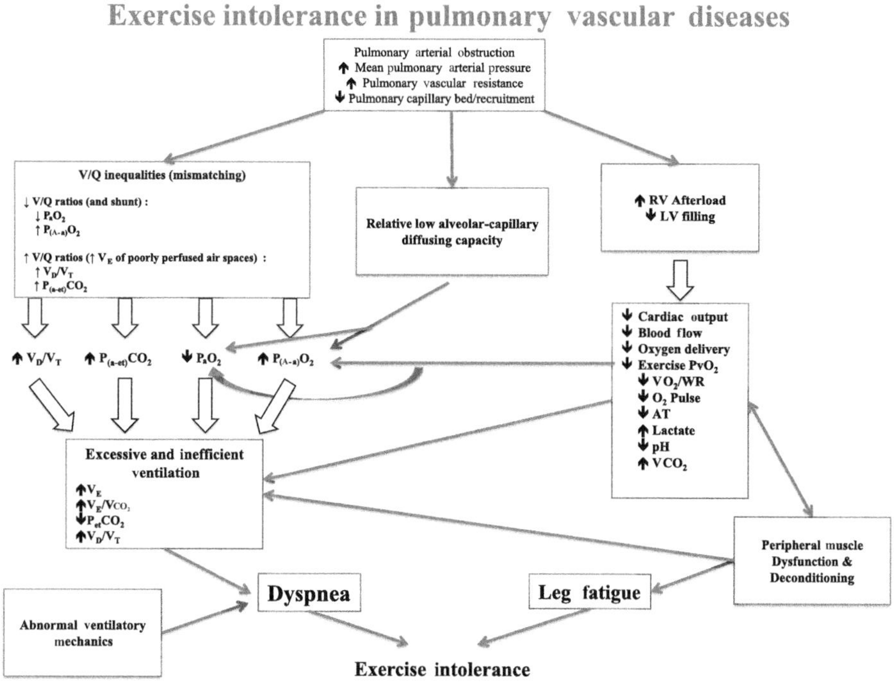

Exercise intolerance in pulmonary vascular diseases

Fig. 1. Pathophysiology and mechanisms of exercise intolerance in pulmonary hypertension. Pulmonary vascular obstruction results in high ventilation-perfusion ratios and impaired cardiac output and can result in hypoxemia due to right to left shunting through a patent foramen ovale. Inefficient ventilation proposes high ventilatory demand, high V_E/VCO_2 and V_D/V_T, and low $P_{et}CO_2$. Cardiac limitation and peripheral muscle abnormalities result in a low AT, early-onset lactic acidosis, and increased VCO_2, which provide further stimulation for excessive ventilation. Ventilatory mechanical constraints on V_T expansion also contribute to dyspnea during exercise. $P_{(A-a)}O_2$, alveolar-arterial difference in partial pressure of oxygen; LV, left ventricle; O_2 pulse, VO_2 to heart rate ratio; PvO_2, venous pressure of oxygen; RV, right ventricle; V/Q, ventilation-perfusion ratio. This is an original figure; no permission is required.

which then must inefficiently hinge on changes in heart rate to a much greater degree.[43] A blunted cardiac output response during exercise that relies heavily on changes in heart rate has several consequences, including a reduced aerobic capacity (peak VO_2 [VO_{2peak}]) and flattened oxygen pulse (VO_2/HR) during CPET.[15,16] Conformational abnormalities in the microcirculation of skeletal muscles and lower type 1 muscle fiber density in PH further impairs peripheral oxygen use and limits overall muscle strength.[34–37] As such, the peak work rate (WR_{peak}) is reduced in PH but usually the ratio of VO_2/WR also remains low (**Fig. 2**),[44] indicative of impaired cardiovascular function and/or abnormal oxygen utilization peripherally.[15,16,18] Therefore, PH patients rely on anaerobic metabolism to a greater degree and at lower levels of work than healthy individuals, reflected in a reduced AT.[15] Collectively, these abnormal responses to exercise help explain the cardiovascular determinants of why PH patients report disproportionally elevated levels of work-related dyspnea (**Fig. 3**A).[19]

> Impaired cardiac function in PH is reflected in reduced VO_{2peak}, WR, VO_2/WR, and AT. Abnormal skeletal musculature is superimposed on impaired cardiac function, resulting in disproportionally higher levels of ventilation and work-related dyspnea.

Ventilatory Anomalies

A mismatch between low capillary perfusion and well-ventilated alveoli is characteristically found in PH; thus, the volume of ventilated lung not involved in gas exchange (ie, physiologic dead space; V_D/V_T) is increased.[17–20] To compensate for this ventilation-perfusion mismatch, patients must increase their V_E, which contributes to inefficient ventilation for a given VCO_2 (high V_E/VCO_2) (further discussion in the topic is provided in Respiratory Determinants of Exercise Limitation: Focus on Phrenic Afferents and The Lung Vasculature).[15,21,45] Unfortunately, respiratory

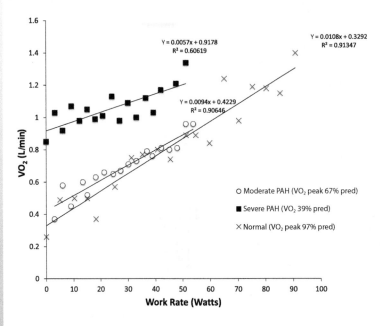

Fig. 2. Comparison of oxygen consumption (VO_2) to WR relationships. A normal individual with peak VO_2 of 97% has a VO_2/WR slope of 10.8 mL/W. A patient with PAH (PVR 9.3 Wood units) and a preserved cardiac index (2.7 L.min⁻¹.m⁻²) and moderately reduced peak VO_2 of 67% predicted has a borderline reduction in the VO_2/WR slope of 9.4 mL/W. The patient with PAH and severe reduction in VO_{2peak} (39% predicted) demonstrates a reduced VO_2/WR slope of 5.7 mL/W. Note that the difference in Y intercept (VO_2) at WR of 0 W is largely related to variability in body mass between these individuals. (*Reproduced* with permission of the © ERS 2018. *From* Weatherald J, Laveneziana P. Patterns of cardiopulmonary response to exercise in pulmonary vascular diseases. Eur Respir Monogr 2018;80:162.)

muscle weakness is also common in PH and results in reduced maximal inspiratory and expiratory strength.[32,46,47] Therefore, patients often rely on rapid and shallow breathing during exercise. A rapid shallow breathing pattern also may be observed as a consequence of sympathetic hyperstimulation from chemoreflexes and metaboreflexes (further discussion in the topic is provided in Update on Chemoreception: Influence on Cardiorespiratory Regulation and Patho-Physiology).[21] Still, some PH patients demonstrate dynamic reductions in inspiratory capacity (**Fig. 4**)[19] in the absence of respiratory muscle fatigue, suggestive of true dynamic hyperinflation, likely a consequence of mild expiratory airflow limitation that may be undetectable at rest but becomes pronounced during rapid breathing.[31–33] This dynamic hyperinflation likely further intensifies perceptions of excessive dyspnea during exercise,[33] beyond what would be expected at given V_E (see **Fig. 3**B).[19]

A consequence of increased V_E is a low $P_{et}CO_2$, but during incremental exercise, the body metabolically produces more carbon dioxide (higher VCO_2), so normally $P_{et}CO_2$ increases. In PAH, however (**Fig. 5**),[44] patients increase their V_E disproportionally to the rise in VCO_2,[16,27,28,48–51] resulting in decreasing $P_{et}CO_2$.[18,26–29] Similarly, this abnormality can be seen when comparing the P_aCO_2 to $P_{et}CO_2$ ($P_{[a–et]}CO_2$), whereby $P_{et}CO_2$ in patients with pulmonary vascular disease are lower than the P_aCO_2 (resulting in positive $P_{[a–et]}CO_2$ difference) versus the inverse (a negative $P_{[a–et]}CO_2$ difference) in healthy individuals.[19,29,52] Although

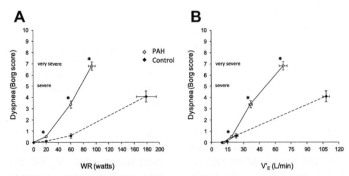

Fig. 3. Exertional dyspnea intensity as measured by Borg score is displayed in response to (*A*) increasing work rate (WR) and (*B*) increasing minute ventilation (V_E) during symptom limited CPET in 25 patients with PAH and 10 healthy control subjects. *$p<.05$, PAH versus health control at rest and standardized exercise WRs (20 W and 60 W) and peak exercise. (*Reproduced* with permission of the © ERS 2018. *From* Laveneziana P, Garcia G, Joureau B, et al. Dynamic respiratory mechanics and exertional dyspnoea in pulmonary arterial hypertension. Eur Respir J 2013;41(3):582.)

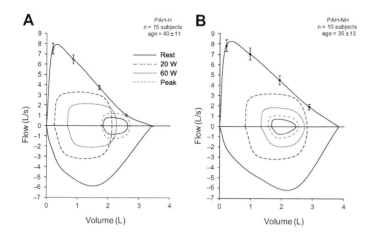

Fig. 4. Maximal and tidal flow-volume loops (averaged data) are shown during CPET in patients with PAH who (*A*) develop dynamic hyperinflation (PAH-H, n = 15) and (*B*) do not develop hyperinflation (PAH-NH, n = 10). Tidal flow-volume loops provided are at rest, early exercise (20 W), late exercise (60 W), and peak exercise. Note the significant decrease in dynamic inspiratory capacity and increase in end-expiratory lung volume in PAH-H in comparison to PAH-NH. (*From* Laveneziana P, Garcia G, Joureau B, et al. Dynamic respiratory mechanics and exertional dyspnoea in pulmonary arterial hypertension. Eur Respir J 2013;41(3):582; with permission of the © ERS 2018.)

patients are hypocapnic at rest and during exercise, the $P_{[a-et]}CO_2$ is positive at peak because of the characteristic rapid shallow breathing pattern (low V_T, high breathing rate) that results from sympathetic over-stimulation, so there is less expiratory time for the $P_{et}CO_2$ to rise relative to the reduction in P_aCO_2 from alveolar hyperventilation.[21] Although this exercise hyperventilation and hypocapnia are likely in part due to a compensation for the increased V_D/V_T, PH patients also may possess altered lower arterial carbon dioxide setpoints and exaggerated chemoreflexes, which inappropriately increase V_E despite already low carbon dioxide levels (further discussion in the topic is provided in Update on Chemoreception: Influence on Cardiorespiratory Regulation and Patho-Physiology).[21–25]

> Increased exertional ventilation on exercise (high V_E/VCO_2) is a key abnormality in PH, reflecting increased wasted ventilation, enhanced chemoreflexes, and a decrease in the arterial CO_2 set point, the latter 2 consequences of increase afferent sympathetic stimuli.

DIAGNOSTIC UTILITY OF CARDIOPULMONARY EXERCISE TESTING

Although right heart catheterization serves as the gold standard diagnostic test for PH,[1] CPET unveils the magnification of the aberrant physiology during exercise to provide additional noninvasive metrics that can be used diagnostically or for prognostication (**Fig. 6**) (see case # 4 in Unraveling the Causes of Unexplained Dyspnea: The Value of Exercise Testing).[44] For

example, CPET can be useful in distinguishing PH patients from those with other cardiopulmonary abnormalities or even between the different types of PH. Although several abnormal parameters are shared between PAH and chronic left heart failure patients, their magnitude of dysfunction can help separate the 2 patient groups. For example, higher V_E/VCO_2 slopes and V_D/V_T as well as lower $P_{et}CO_2$ and O_2 pulse are found in PAH versus those in left heart failure.[16,53] Furthermore, PAH patients also frequently experience exertional hypoxemia whereas stable left heart failure patients do not.[16,53] Despite similar presentations of high V_E/VCO_2 and chemosensitivity in both PAH and left heart failure patients, a pattern of oscillatory breathing during exercise may be observed in left heart disease that does not occur in PAH (further discussion in the topic is provided in Exertional periodic breathing in heart failure: mechanisms and clinical implications).[49]

CPET can also be useful in distinguishing between precapillary PH subgroups. Specifically, CTEPH patients have more pronounced vascular obstruction than PAH and thus higher dead space. This leads to greater ventilatory demand (V_E peak and at the AT) and more inefficient ventilation ($V_E - VCO_2$ slope and V_E/VCO_2 ratio at the AT) on CPET.[27] Moreover, a $P_{[a-et]}CO_2$ greater than 7 mm Hg discriminated patients with CTEPH from PAH, with a sensitivity of 88% and specificity of 90%.[29] Similarly, a composite score factoring $V_E - VCO_2$ slope, $P_{et}CO_2$ at the AT, alveolar–arterial oxygen pressure gradient at peak exercise, and $P_{[a-et]}CO_2$ identified CTEPH, with a sensitivity of 83% and specificity of 92%, despite patients having normal or undetectable right ventricular dysfunction on echocardiogram.[54]

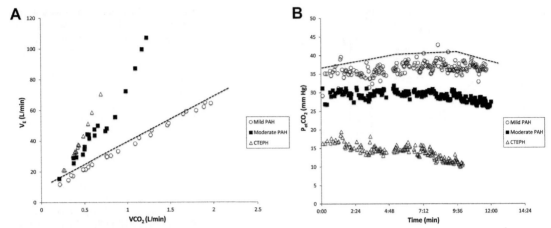

Fig. 5. (*A*) V_E plotted against VCO_2 for patients with mild PAH (*circles*) moderate PAH (*solid squares*), and CTEPH (*triangles*). The dashed line represents the upper limit of normal. Note that in the patient with mild PAH, the V_E/VCO_2 slope is only mildly abnormal (V_E/VCO_2 slope = 30), whereas the patients with moderate PAH and severe CTEPH have significantly elevated V_E/VCO_2 slopes of 84 and 115, respectively. (*B*) $P_{et}CO_2$, plotted against time for the same patients in (*A*). Note that the patient with mild PAH (*circles*) exhibits a slight increase in $P_{et}CO_2$ during early exercise, similar to the predicted normal response (*dashed line*). The patient with moderate PAH exhibits a flat $P_{et}CO_2$ during early exercise with a terminal decline coinciding with hyperventilation after the AT. The patient with severe CTEPH demonstrates a progressive decrease in $P_{et}CO_2$ characteristic of severe pulmonary vascular disease. (*From* Weatherald J, Laveneziana P. Patterns of cardiopulmonary response to exercise in pulmonary vascular diseases. Eur Respir Monogr 2018;80:165; with permission of the © ERS 2018.)

CARDIOPULMONARY EXERCISE TESTING FOR PROGNOSTIC EVALUATION

Results from CPET also can be useful indicators of disease severity and prognosis. For example, low peak systolic blood pressures ($\leq$120 mm Hg) during exercise and reduced peak aerobic capacity (VO_{2peak} $\leq$10.4 mL/kg/min) are indicators of poorer survival in PH.[55] Although similar studies have echoed the relationship between poor aerobic capacity and survival,[56] others have added that inefficient ventilation (eg, elevated V_E − VCO_2 slope and V_E/VCO_2 ratio at the AT) and delayed postexercise heart rate recovery also portend a higher risk of mortality.[18,57–59] CPET may be particularly useful in identifying exercise-induced right-to-left shunt through a patent foramen ovale. These conditions of significantly elevated right atrial pressures leading to patency of a shunt can be seen when $P_{et}CO_2$ and oxygen saturations drop precipitously during exercise, a finding that carries a 65% increased risk of 5-year mortality.[30]

> CPET is a valuable tool for prognostic assessment in PH. Low peak systolic blood pressure, low VO_{2peak}, a very high V_E/VCO_2, and identification of exercise-induced shunt are common worrisome findings that relate to reduced patient survival.

EXERCISE VARIABLES AS CLINICAL TRIAL EFFICACY ENDPOINTS

Because of their link with important clinical outcomes, exercise variables serve as common efficacy endpoints for clinical trials. In PAH, for example, intravenous prostacyclin dramatically improves $\dot{V}O_{2peak}$,[60] and sildenafil showed promise in improving $\dot{V}O_{2peak}$, O_2 pulse, V_E/VCO_2 and $P_{et}CO_2$.[61] In CTEPH, pulmonary endarterectomy serves as the preferred definitive treatment option because it improves survival and coincidingly, numerous CPET variables as well (eg, $\dot{V}O_{2peak}$, V_E − VCO_2 slope, V_E/VCO_2 ratio at the AT, V_D/V_T, and P_aCO_2.[62] CPET has also shown that inoperable CTEPH patients may benefit from balloon pulmonary angioplasty (eg, improved $\dot{V}O_{2peak}$, WR_{peak}, O_2 pulse, V_D/V_T, V_E − VCO_2 slope, and exercise duration) or pharmacotherapy with phosphodiesterase-5 inhibitors or endothelin receptor antagonists (eg, improved VO_{2peak}, WR_{peak}, O_2 pulse, and V_D/V_T).[63,64] Despite guidelines now recommending supervised exercise training for deconditioned patients receiving medical therapies,[1] few trials have examined the potential synergistic effects of pharmacotherapy plus structured exercise training,[65] perhaps due to safety concerns or lack of specific recommendations detailing targeted exercise programming.

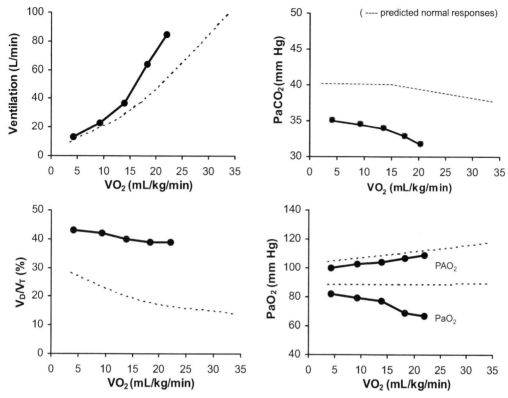

Fig. 6. Gas exchange abnormalities for a patient with PAH. Dashed lines represent predicted normal responses. Note the excessive ventilation for a given VO_2 (*upper left panel*) with high V_D/V_T at rest and throughout exercise (*lower left panel*). The P_aCO_2 is low at rest and decreases early during exercise to a greater extent than in a normal individual (*upper right panel*). The arterial oxygen pressure (P_aO_2) decreases abnormally during exercise despite a normal increase in alveolar oxygen pressure (P_AO_2), resulting in a wide and increasing alveolar-arterial O_2 difference at peak exercise (*lower right panel*). (*From* Weatherald J, Laveneziana P. Patterns of cardiopulmonary response to exercise in pulmonary vascular diseases. Eur Respir Monogr 2018;80:168; with permission of the © ERS 2018.)

EXERCISE TRAINING IN PULMONARY HYPERTENSION
Safety Considerations for Programming

Prior to the availability of effective therapies for PAH, it was recommended that strenuous physical activity be avoided due to a perceived risk of syncope, sudden death, and worsening right heart failure.[65,66] The safety of exercise training in PH, however, has now been well established. A meta-analysis of 16 trials, including 469 patients, found an overall risk of adverse events during exercise training at 4.7% and syncope a rare occurrence (<1%).[65] Furthermore, no deaths and no episodes of worsening right heart failure occurred during these studies. The potential risks of exercise can be mitigated by taking appropriate precautions.[67] For example, the risk of exertional presyncope and syncope can be minimized by ensuring patients with PH are stable and on optimal medical therapies. Weight

training that focuses on single muscle groups (rather than complex movements using multiple muscle groups) using low weights and high repetitions dampens the effect of Valsalva maneuvers on right heart filling and function. The risk of syncope, arrhythmia, and palpitations can be minimized by avoidance of high-intensity exercise, maintaining effort at less than 80% of the maximal work load or heart rate. During initial exercise training sessions, supervision and frequent monitoring of vital signs are essential to detect hypotension and oxygen desaturation.

> Exercise training in PH can be safe when patients are stable on optimal medical therapies, avoid high-intensity training regimens, and are supervised while they acclimate to the program during their initial sessions.

Preliminary Efficacy of Exercise Trials

Exercise training programs have the potential to improve muscle strength, endurance, peak exercise capacity, quality of life, and pulmonary hemodynamics in PH patients. In a study of 19 stable idiopathic PAH patients, a 12-week program of cycle endurance and quadriceps strength training led to 34% and 13% improvements in endurance time and quadriceps strength, respectively.[68] These improvements were mediated by an increase in capillary density and oxidative capacity in muscle biopsies. A meta-analysis of controlled trials involving exercise training found that such programs improve performance on the 6-minute walk distance (6MWD), a key endpoint in most pivotal pharmaceutical trials in PAH and CTEPH, by 60.1 m and $\dot{V}O_{2peak}$ by 2.41 mL/kg/min.[69] For comparison, pharmaceutical trials in PAH improve the 6MWD on average by 31 m.[70] Improvements in 6MWD are consistent regardless of the severity of impairment at baseline (ie, similar improvements for patients in World Health Organization functional classes II, III, and IV at baseline) and across types of PH.[71] Some of the improvements in exercise capacity and $\dot{V}O_{2peak}$ may be related to the effects of exercise training on hemodynamics. This was shown in a randomized trial of PAH and inoperable CTEPH patients that were already on stable PAH therapies for 2 months. After undergoing a 15-week training program, patients had a decrease in mPAP by 8 mm Hg, a decrease in PVR by 2.1 Wood units, and an increase in cardiac of 0.5 L/min/m² compared with a control group.[72] Performance during exercise training can be optimized by using supplemental oxygen during incremental WR exercise and constant load endurance exercise. Ulrich and colleagues[73] performed a randomized sham-controlled crossover trial of oxygen (fraction of inspired oxygen 0.50) versus ambient air in PAH and inoperable CTEPH patients. By diminishing the effects of arterial desaturation on chemoreceptor-induced hyperventilation, hyperoxia improved maximal work load by 19.7 W and cycle endurance time by 11.2 minutes.

> Exercise training programs might help PH patients by improving hemodynamics (cardiac index, mPAP, and PVR) and muscle function (strength and endurance) and may improve exercise capacity above and beyond pharmaceutical interventions.

Table 2
Recommendations for supervised exercise programming in patients with pulmonary hypertension

Exercise Modality	Frequency of Exercise (Sessions per week)	Duration per Session (min)	Intensity	Additional Comment
Endurance	2–3	10–25	60%–80% of symptom-free capacity	Low-intensity interval exercise recommended (for example, low workloads for 30s followed by higher workload for 1 min)
Strength training	1–2	15–30	4–5/10 on Borg scale (somewhat strong/strong)	Strength devices or dumbbells, single muscle groups (eg, quadriceps leg extensions), 1–2 sets. Avoid complex, multiple muscle group exercises (eg, squats).
Respiratory muscle training	5–7	10–15	—	Specific techniques, stretching exercises for respiration-related muscles, body perception improvement, yoga breathing techniques
Activities of daily living	Daily	Whenever possible	Low intensity	Walking, cycling, gardening, stairs

Reproduced from Richter MJ, Grimminger J, Krüger B, et al. Effects of exercise training on pulmonary hemodynamics, functional capacity and inflammation in pulmonary hypertension. Pulm Circ 2017;7:33; with permission from SAGE Publications.

Exercise Programming Recommendations

The key components of a supervised exercise program for PH patients are shown in **Table 2**.[74] Regular endurance training, strength training, and respiratory muscle training should be performed in addition to activities of daily living. Respiratory training may include breathing techniques, stretching exercises, inspiratory threshold loading devices, and activities, such as yoga.[75,76]

SUMMARY

PH patients demonstrate numerous indicators of decompensated cardiopulmonary physiology during exercise, which can help point clinicians toward a diagnosis of PH. Specifically, the presence of high V_E/VCO_2 with a low $P_{et}CO_2$ during CPET in a patient with unexplained dyspnea should prompt consideration of pulmonary vascular disease in the differential diagnosis and further diagnostic investigations. CPET is also well established for assessing the degree of exercise intolerance and dyspnea, providing important prognostic information for patients with PAH and CTEPH. Furthermore, with exercise training deemed safe and feasible and several clinical trials using exercise variables as primary efficacy outcomes, the emerging field of research examining the therapeutic benefits of exercise training in PH merits additional consideration. Future clinical trials are needed to evaluate the efficacy of exercise programs focusing on light-intensity endurance, strength, and respiratory training.

REFERENCES

1. Galie N, Humbert M, Vachiery JL, et al. 2015 ESC/ERS guidelines for the diagnosis and treatment of pulmonary hypertension: the joint task force for the diagnosis and treatment of pulmonary hypertension of the European Society of Cardiology (ESC) and the European Respiratory Society (ERS): endorsed by: Association for European Paediatric and Congenital Cardiology (AEPC), International Society for Heart and Lung Transplantation (ISHLT). Eur Heart J 2016;37(1):67–119.
2. Simonneau G, Gatzoulis MA, Adatia I, et al. Updated clinical classification of pulmonary hypertension. J Am Coll Cardiol 2013;62(25 Suppl):D34–41.
3. Wijeratne DT, Lajkosz K, Brogly SB, et al. Increasing incidence and prevalence of world health organization groups 1 to 4 pulmonary hypertension: a population-based cohort study in Ontario, Canada. Circ Cardiovasc Qual Outcomes 2018;11(2):e003973.
4. Weatherald J, Farina S, Bruno N, et al. Cardiopulmonary exercise testing in pulmonary hypertension. Ann Am Thorac Soc 2017;14(Supplement_1):S84–92.
5. Pugh ME, Buchowski MS, Robbins IM, et al. Physical activity limitation as measured by accelerometry in pulmonary arterial hypertension. Chest 2012; 142(6):1391–8.
6. Mainguy V, Provencher S, Maltais F, et al. Assessment of daily life physical activities in pulmonary arterial hypertension. PLoS One 2011;6(11):e27993.
7. Matura LA, Shou H, Fritz JS, et al. Physical activity and symptoms in pulmonary arterial hypertension. Chest 2016;150(1):46–56.
8. Tartavoulle TM, Karpinski AC, Aubin A, et al. Multidimensional fatigue in pulmonary hypertension: prevalence, severity and predictors. ERJ Open Res 2018; 4(1) [pii:00079-2017].
9. Delcroix M, Howard L. Pulmonary arterial hypertension: the burden of disease and impact on quality of life. Eur Respir Rev 2015;24(138):621–9.
10. Mathai SC, Ghofrani HA, Mayer E, et al. Quality of life in patients with chronic thromboembolic pulmonary hypertension. Eur Respir J 2016;48(2):526–37.
11. Naeije R, Badagliacca R. The overloaded right heart and ventricular interdependence. Cardiovasc Res 2017;113(12):1474–85.
12. Nootens M, Wolfkiel CJ, Chomka EV, et al. Understanding right and left ventricular systolic function and interactions at rest and with exercise in primary pulmonary hypertension. Am J Cardiol 1995;75(5):374–7.
13. Weatherald J, Boucly A, Chemla D, et al. Prognostic value of follow-up hemodynamic variables after initial management in pulmonary arterial hypertension. Circulation 2018;137(7):693–704.
14. Hasler ED, Muller-Mottet S, Furian M, et al. Pressure-flow during exercise catheterization predicts survival in pulmonary hypertension. Chest 2016;150(1):57–67.
15. Sun XG, Hansen JE, Oudiz RJ, et al. Exercise pathophysiology in patients with primary pulmonary hypertension. Circulation 2001;104(4):429–35.
16. Deboeck G, Niset G, Lamotte M, et al. Exercise testing in pulmonary arterial hypertension and in chronic heart failure. Eur Respir J 2004;23(5):747–51.
17. D'Alonzo GE, Gianotti LA, Pohil RL, et al. Comparison of progressive exercise performance of normal subjects and patients with primary pulmonary hypertension. Chest 1987;92(1):57–62.
18. Riley MS, Porszasz J, Engelen MP, et al. Gas exchange responses to continuous incremental cycle ergometry exercise in primary pulmonary hypertension in humans. Eur J Appl Physiol 2000;83(1):63–70.
19. Laveneziana P, Garcia G, Joureau B, et al. Dynamic respiratory mechanics and exertional dyspnoea in pulmonary arterial hypertension. Eur Respir J 2013;41(3):578–87.
20. American Thoracic Society. ATS/ACCP statement on cardiopulmonary exercise testing. Am J Respir Crit Care Med 2003;167(2):211–77.

21. Weatherald J, Sattler C, Garcia G, et al. Ventilatory response to exercise in cardiopulmonary disease: the role of chemosensitivity and dead space. Eur Respir J 2018;51(2) [pii:1700860].

22. Velez-Roa S, Ciarka A, Najem B, et al. Increased sympathetic nerve activity in pulmonary artery hypertension. Circulation 2004;110(10):1308–12.

23. Naeije R, van de Borne P. Clinical relevance of autonomic nervous system disturbances in pulmonary arterial hypertension. Eur Respir J 2009;34(4): 792–4.

24. Wensel R, Jilek C, Dorr M, et al. Impaired cardiac autonomic control relates to disease severity in pulmonary hypertension. Eur Respir J 2009;34(4): 895–901.

25. Farina S, Bruno N, Agalbato C, et al. Physiological insights of exercise hyperventilation in arterial and chronic thromboembolic pulmonary hypertension. Int J Cardiol 2018;259:178–82.

26. Yasunobu Y, Oudiz RJ, Sun XG, et al. End-tidal PCO2 abnormality and exercise limitation in patients with primary pulmonary hypertension. Chest 2005; 127(5):1637–46.

27. Zhai Z, Murphy K, Tighe H, et al. Differences in ventilatory inefficiency between pulmonary arterial hypertension and chronic thromboembolic pulmonary hypertension. Chest 2011;140(5):1284–91.

28. Godinas L, Sattler C, Lau EM, et al. Dead-space ventilation is linked to exercise capacity and survival in distal chronic thromboembolic pulmonary hypertension. J Heart Lung Transplant 2017;36(11): 1234–42.

29. Scheidl SJ, Englisch C, Kovacs G, et al. Diagnosis of CTEPH versus IPAH using capillary to end-tidal carbon dioxide gradients. Eur Respir J 2012;39(1): 119–24.

30. Oudiz RJ, Midde R, Hovenesyan A, et al. Usefulness of right-to-left shunting and poor exercise gas exchange for predicting prognosis in patients with pulmonary arterial hypertension. Am J Cardiol 2010; 105(8):1186–91.

31. Richter MJ, Voswinckel R, Tiede H, et al. Dynamic hyperinflation during exercise in patients with precapillary pulmonary hypertension. Respir Med 2012; 106(2):308–13.

32. Manders E, Bonta PI, Kloek JJ, et al. Reduced force of diaphragm muscle fibers in patients with chronic thromboembolic pulmonary hypertension. Am J Physiol Lung Cell Mol Physiol 2016;311(1): L20–8.

33. Laveneziana P, Humbert M, Godinas L, et al. Inspiratory muscle function, dynamic hyperinflation and exertional dyspnoea in pulmonary arterial hypertension. Eur Respir J 2015;45(5):1495–8.

34. Mainguy V, Maltais F, Saey D, et al. Peripheral muscle dysfunction in idiopathic pulmonary arterial hypertension. Thorax 2010;65(2):113–7.

35. Bauer R, Dehnert C, Schoene P, et al. Skeletal muscle dysfunction in patients with idiopathic pulmonary arterial hypertension. Respir Med 2007;101(11): 2366–9.

36. Dimopoulos S, Tzanis G, Manetos C, et al. Peripheral muscle microcirculatory alterations in patients with pulmonary arterial hypertension: a pilot study. Respir Care 2013;58(12):2134–41.

37. Tolle J, Waxman A, Systrom D. Impaired systemic oxygen extraction at maximum exercise in pulmonary hypertension. Med Sci Sports Exerc 2008; 40(1):3–8.

38. Lau EMT, Chemla D, Godinas L, et al. Loss of vascular distensibility during exercise is an early hemodynamic marker of pulmonary vascular disease. Chest 2016;149(2):353–61.

39. Naeije R, Vanderpool R, Dhakal BP, et al. Exercise-induced pulmonary hypertension: physiological basis and methodological concerns. Am J Respir Crit Care Med 2013;187(6):576–83.

40. Groepenhoff H, Westerhof N, Jacobs W, et al. Exercise stroke volume and heart rate response differ in right and left heart failure. Eur J Heart Fail 2010; 12(7):716–20.

41. Holverda S, Gan CT, Marcus JT, et al. Impaired stroke volume response to exercise in pulmonary arterial hypertension. J Am Coll Cardiol 2006;47(8): 1732–3.

42. Kasner M, Westermann D, Steendijk P, et al. Left ventricular dysfunction induced by nonsevere idiopathic pulmonary arterial hypertension: a pressure-volume relationship study. Am J Respir Crit Care Med 2012;186(2):181–9.

43. Chemla D, Castelain V, Hoette S, et al. Strong linear relationship between heart rate and mean pulmonary artery pressure in exercising patients with severe precapillary pulmonary hypertension. Am J Physiol Heart Circ Physiol 2013;305(5): H769–77.

44. Weatherald J, Laveneziana P. Patterns of cardiopulmonary response to exercise in pulmonary vascular diseases. Eur Respir Monogr 2018;80:160–74.

45. McCabe C, Deboeck G, Harvey I, et al. Inefficient exercise gas exchange identifies pulmonary hypertension in chronic thromboembolic obstruction following pulmonary embolism. Thromb Res 2013; 132(6):659–65.

46. de Man FS, van Hees HW, Handoko ML, et al. Diaphragm muscle fiber weakness in pulmonary hypertension. Am J Respir Crit Care Med 2011;183(10): 1411–8.

47. Meyer FJ, Lossnitzer D, Kristen AV, et al. Respiratory muscle dysfunction in idiopathic pulmonary arterial hypertension. Eur Respir J 2005;25(1):125–30.

48. Theodore J, Robin ED, Morris AJ, et al. Augmented ventilatory response to exercise in pulmonary hypertension. Chest 1986;89(1):39–44.

49. Vicenzi M, Deboeck G, Faoro V, et al. Exercise oscillatory ventilation in heart failure and in pulmonary arterial hypertension. Int J Cardiol 2016;202:736–40.

50. Reybrouck T, Mertens L, Schulze-Neick I, et al. Ventilatory inefficiency for carbon dioxide during exercise in patients with pulmonary hypertension. Clin Physiol 1998;18(4):337–44.

51. Liu WH, Luo Q, Liu ZH, et al. Pulmonary function differences in patients with chronic right heart failure secondary to pulmonary arterial hypertension and chronic left heart failure. Med Sci Monit 2014;20:960–6.

52. Laveneziana P, Montani D, Dorfmuller P, et al. Mechanisms of exertional dyspnoea in pulmonary veno-occlusive disease with EIF2AK4 mutations. Eur Respir J 2014;44(4):1069–72.

53. Liu WH, Luo Q, Liu ZH, et al. Differences in pulmonary function and exercise capacity in patients with idiopathic dilated cardiomyopathy and idiopathic pulmonary arterial hypertension. Heart Lung 2014;43(4):317–21.

54. Held M, Grun M, Holl R, et al. Cardiopulmonary exercise testing to detect chronic thromboembolic pulmonary hypertension in patients with normal echocardiography. Respiration 2014;87(5):379–87.

55. Wensel R, Opitz CF, Anker SD, et al. Assessment of survival in patients with primary pulmonary hypertension: importance of cardiopulmonary exercise testing. Circulation 2002;106(3):319–24.

56. Grunig E, Tiede H, Enyimayew EO, et al. Assessment and prognostic relevance of right ventricular contractile reserve in patients with severe pulmonary hypertension. Circulation 2013;128(18):2005–15.

57. Schwaiblmair M, Faul C, von Scheidt W, et al. Ventilatory efficiency testing as prognostic value in patients with pulmonary hypertension. BMC Pulm Med 2012;12:23.

58. Deboeck G, Scoditti C, Huez S, et al. Exercise testing to predict outcome in idiopathic versus associated pulmonary arterial hypertension. Eur Respir J 2012;40(6):1410–9.

59. Ramos RP, Arakaki JS, Barbosa P, et al. Heart rate recovery in pulmonary arterial hypertension: relationship with exercise capacity and prognosis. Am Heart J 2012;163(4):580–8.

60. Wax D, Garofano R, Barst RJ. Effects of long-term infusion of prostacyclin on exercise performance in patients with primary pulmonary hypertension. Chest 1999;116(4):914–20.

61. Oudiz RJ, Roveran G, Hansen JE, et al. Effect of sildenafil on ventilatory efficiency and exercise tolerance in pulmonary hypertension. Eur J Heart Fail 2007;9(9):917–21.

62. Charalampopoulos A, Gibbs JS, Davies RJ, et al. Exercise physiological responses to drug treatments in chronic thromboembolic pulmonary hypertension. J Appl Physiol (1985) 2016;121(3):623–8.

63. Andreassen AK, Ragnarsson A, Gude E, et al. Balloon pulmonary angioplasty in patients with inoperable chronic thromboembolic pulmonary hypertension. Heart 2013;99(19):1415–20.

64. Fukui S, Ogo T, Goto Y, et al. Exercise intolerance and ventilatory inefficiency improve early after balloon pulmonary angioplasty in patients with inoperable chronic thromboembolic pulmonary hypertension. Int J Cardiol 2015;180:66–8.

65. Pandey A, Garg S, Khunger M, et al. Efficacy and safety of exercise training in chronic pulmonary hypertension: systematic review and meta-analysis. Circ Heart Fail 2015;8(6):1032–43.

66. Gaine SP, Rubin LJ. Primary pulmonary hypertension. Lancet 1998;352(9129):719–25.

67. Keusch S, Turk A, Saxer S, et al. Rehabilitation in patients with pulmonary arterial hypertension. Swiss Med Wkly 2017;147:w14462.

68. de Man FS, Handoko ML, Groepenhoff H, et al. Effects of exercise training in patients with idiopathic pulmonary arterial hypertension. Eur Respir J 2009;34(3):669–75.

69. Morris NR, Kermeen FD, Holland AE. Exercise-based rehabilitation programmes for pulmonary hypertension. Cochrane Database Syst Rev 2017;(1):CD011285.

70. Liu HL, Chen XY, Li JR, et al. Efficacy and safety of pulmonary arterial hypertension-specific therapy in pulmonary arterial hypertension: a meta-analysis of randomized controlled trials. Chest 2016;150(2):353–66.

71. Grunig E, Lichtblau M, Ehlken N, et al. Safety and efficacy of exercise training in various forms of pulmonary hypertension. Eur Respir J 2012;40(1):84–92.

72. Ehlken N, Lichtblau M, Klose H, et al. Exercise training improves peak oxygen consumption and haemodynamics in patients with severe pulmonary arterial hypertension and inoperable chronic thrombo-embolic pulmonary hypertension: a prospective, randomized, controlled trial. Eur Heart J 2016;37(1):35–44.

73. Ulrich S, Hasler ED, Saxer S, et al. Effect of breathing oxygen-enriched air on exercise performance in patients with precapillary pulmonary hypertension: randomized, sham-controlled cross-over trial. Eur Heart J 2017;38(15):1159–68.

74. Richter MJ, Grimminger J, Kruger B, et al. Effects of exercise training on pulmonary hemodynamics, functional capacity and inflammation in pulmonary hypertension. Pulm Circ 2017;7(1):20–37.

75. Kabitz HJ, Bremer HC, Schwoerer A, et al. The combination of exercise and respiratory training improves respiratory muscle function in pulmonary hypertension. Lung 2014;192(2):321–8.

76. Saglam M, Arikan H, Vardar-Yagli N, et al. Inspiratory muscle training in pulmonary arterial hypertension. J Cardiopulm Rehabil Prev 2015;35(3):198–206.

Unraveling the Causes of Unexplained Dyspnea
The Value of Exercise Testing

Denis E. O'Donnell, MD, FRCPI, FRCPC, FERS[a],*,
Kathryn M. Milne, MD, FRCPC[a,b], Sandra G. Vincent, BScH[a],
J. Alberto Neder, MD, PhD, FRCPC, FERS[a]

KEYWORDS

- Dyspnea of unknown origin • Unexplained dyspnea • Disproportionate dyspnea
- Cardiopulmonary exercise testing • Dyspnea physiology

KEY POINTS

- Dyspnea that is unexplained after thorough clinical assessment presents a significant burden for patients and a significant challenge for caregivers.
- Cardiopulmonary exercise testing (CPET) can identify physiologic abnormalities of the integrated cardiopulmonary, neuromuscular and sensory systems that contribute to exertional dyspnea and are not uncovered by other investigations.
- CPET interpretation requires a systematic integrated physiologic approach to measurement of respiratory sensation, ventilatory control, dynamic respiratory mechanics and cardio-circulatory responses to exercise.
- CPET identifies patterns of physiologic impairment in unexplained dyspnea that can provide critical guidance for further diagnostic investigations and management.

INTRODUCTION

Persistent unexplained dyspnea is a relatively common reason for referral to specialized respiratory centers and pulmonary function laboratories. There are very sparse epidemiologic data on the prevalence of unexplained dyspnea in the general population. In one study of patients referred to a specialty clinic, approximately 15% had previously unexplained chronic dyspnea.[1] Dyspnea is an important symptom that impacts quality of life and results in progressive functional limitation and disability.[2] Although specific studies of the negative impact of unexplained dyspnea are lacking, there is general agreement that persistent breathing discomfort can present a significant diagnostic challenge. Dyspnea, reduced peak oxygen uptake ($\dot{V}O_2$) and physical inactivity are closely interrelated but independently predict mortality in chronic lung diseases. Clearly, there is need to develop better investigative and management strategies for this troublesome symptom than currently exist.[3–7]

According to the most recent American Thoracic Society statement, dyspnea is defined as "a subjective experience of breathing discomfort that consists of qualitatively distinct sensations that vary in intensity."[8] Dyspnea of unknown origin is more likely to be identified in patients who are older and often, the root of the problem is multifactorial,

Disclosure Statement: Dr D.E. O'Donnell has received research funding via Queen's University from Canadian Institutes of Health Research, Canadian Respiratory Research Network, AstraZeneca, and Boehringer Ingelheim and has served on speaker bureaus, consultation panels and advisory boards for AstraZeneca, Boehringer Ingelheim, and Novartis. There are no conflicts of interest to declare in the publication of this article.

[a] Department of Medicine, Queen's University, Kingston Health Sciences Centre, 102 Stuart Street, Kingston, Ontario K7L 2V6, Canada; [b] Department of Medicine, Clinician Investigator Program, University of British Columbia, Vancouver, British Columbia, Canada
* Corresponding author. 102 Stuart Street, Kingston, Ontario K7L 2V6, Canada.
E-mail address: odonnell@queensu.ca

chestmed.theclinics.com

presenting unique diagnostic challenges. Comprehensive evaluation and diagnosis become important to validate and explain to the patient the cause of the symptom and to guide caregivers by providing diagnostic clarity and individualized management strategies. Patients with unexplained dyspnea frequently undergo multiple expensive investigations in their clinical evaluation.[1] Given the widespread availability of cardiovascular testing and radiographic imaging, many patients are referred for assessment of unexplained dyspnea only after the results of cardiovascular stress tests and echocardiograms are negative. The overarching objective of the current review was to demonstrate the clinical utility of exercise testing in the evaluation of dyspnea by presenting illustrative case studies. We hope to demonstrate that cardiopulmonary exercise testing (CPET) can identify specific physiologic abnormalities of the integrated cardiopulmonary, neuromuscular, and sensory systems that contribute to persistent perceived respiratory discomfort.

DEFINITIONS AND ETIOLOGY

There is no consensus on a definition of *unexplained dyspnea* (sometimes referred to as *dyspnea of unknown origin*). For the purpose of this review, we defined it as persistent dyspnea (of at least 3 months' duration), of clinically significant severity (Medical Research Council Questionnaire [MRC] $\geq$3) that remains unexplained after a thorough clinical assessment, basic pulmonary function tests (eg, pre and post bronchodilator spirometry) and radiographic studies (eg, chest radiograph). Similarly, there is no consensus definition for *disproportionate dyspnea*. It has been suggested that dyspnea becomes disproportionate when a patient has only minor abnormalities of resting physiologic or radiographic tests (eg, pulmonary function test, echocardiogram, stress echocardiogram) that do not adequately explain the severity of dyspnea. However, resting physiologic tests poorly predict exertional dyspnea and exercise intolerance and this endorses the notion that, in many instances, exercise tests are required to uncover potential causes.[1]

Recognized physiologic causes of unexplained dyspnea are presented in **Box 1** and include (1) impaired pulmonary gas exchange, (2) mechanical abnormalities (airways, lung parenchyma, chest wall), (3) neuromuscular disorders, (4) cardio-circulatory abnormalities, (5) endocrine disorders, (6) metabolic diseases, (7) hematologic diseases, and (8) psychogenic dyspnea, unexplained by physiologic impairment. Exercise testing allows identification of specific physiologic contributors, either

---

Box 1
Etiologies of unexplained dyspnea

1. Pulmonary gas exchange abnormalities
2. Respiratory mechanical abnormalities:
   - Airway (eg, COPD)
   - Lung parenchyma (eg, ILD)
   - Chest wall disease (eg, kyphoscoliosis)
3. Neuromuscular disorders
4. Cardio-circulatory abnormalities
5. Endocrine disorders
6. Metabolic disorders
7. Hematologic disorders
8. Psychogenic unexplained by physiologic impairment

Abbreviations: COPD, chronic obstructive pulmonary disease; ILD, interstitial lung disease.

---

singly or in highly variable combinations, that ultimately, can help to explain persistent dyspnea in the individual. It is important to recognize that a variety of other factors including body mass index (BMI), effects of natural aging, deconditioning, musculoskeletal disorders, anemia, and anxiety are common confounders that must be considered when investigating the origins of unexplained dyspnea.

The clinical causes of unexplained dyspnea have not been widely studied and vary with population selection and include bronchial asthma, chronic obstructive pulmonary disease (COPD) (discussed in detail in The Pathophysiology of Dyspnea and Exercise Intolerance in COPD), interstitial lung disease (ILD) (discussed in detail in Exercise Pathophysiology in Interstitial Lung Disease), and cardiomyopathy.[9] Skeletal muscle deconditioning accounted for dyspnea in as many as 50% of patients in one study (see The Relevance of Limb Muscle Dysfunction In COPD: A Review for Clinicians).[10] In a recent retrospective study, causes of unexplained dyspnea included (1) pulmonary arterial hypertension present only during exercise (see Pulmonary Hypertension and Exercise), (2) heart failure with preserved ejection fraction present only during exercise (see Pulmonary Limitations in Heart Failure), (3) dysregulation of the autonomic nervous system, (4) oxidative myopathy, (5) primary alveolar hyperventilation, (6) shunt, (7) cardiac chronotropic incompetence, (8) alveolar hypoventilation and (9) deconditioning.[1] In many cases, CPET per se is not diagnostic, but can uncover patterns of physiologic impairment and guide further investigations that lead to a diagnosis and management plan.

Importantly, a normal CPET provides reassurance for both the patient and clinician by excluding significant cardiopulmonary and other underlying organic disease implicated in dyspnea causation.

INTEGRATING PHYSIOLOGY AND CLINICAL APPROACH
Diagnostic Evaluation

Evaluation of a patient presenting with unexplained dyspnea must first include a thorough clinical assessment (**Table 1**). The clinician should perform a detailed physical examination of the cardiovascular, respiratory, musculoskeletal, and neurologic systems. Pulmonary function tests: spirometry, body plethysmography and diffusing capacity for carbon dioxide (DLCO) (further discussion in this topic is provided in Incorporating Lung Diffusing Capacity for Carbon Monoxide to Clinical Decision Making in Chest Medicine), should be scrutinized to determine if there is evidence of obstructive or restrictive ventilatory impairment. Bronchodilator reversibility studies and methacholine challenge may be indicated in patients suspected of having asthma. Pulmonary gas exchange should be assessed by resting oxygen saturation using pulse oximetry (SpO_2). SpO_2 consistently less than 88% while walking might require arterial blood gas sampling to assess arterial partial pressure of oxygen (Pao_2) and can also provide assessment of carbon dioxide ($Paco_2$) as well as acid-base status. Reduced static respiratory muscle strength using maximum inspiratory (MIP) and maximum expiratory pressures (MEP), should prompt more comprehensive tests of neuromuscular disease (see Michael I. Polkey's article, "Respiratory Muscle assessment in Clinical Practice," elsewhere in this issue). Evaluation of hematologic and endocrine disorders that can lead to unexplained dyspnea, such as anemia and thyroid disease, should be investigated with appropriate laboratory testing.

Mechanisms of Dyspnea

Fundamentally, dyspnea during activity occurs when the central respiratory drive from bulbopontine and cortical motor centers in the brain to

Table 1
Clinical approach to unexplained dyspnea

History	• Symptom onset, chronology and fluctuation (frequency of crisis dyspnea events)
	• Gradation of dyspnea severity using a validated score (MRC, OCD, BDI)
	• Diurnal variation
	• Triggers, exacerbating and alleviating factors
	• Relationship to and impact of physical activity
	• Functional limitation
	• Current and previous physical activity level
	• Association with body position (orthopnea, platypnea, bendopnea)
	• Associated symptoms (wheeze, cough, sputum production, chest pain, pre-syncope/syncope, palpitations, paroxysmal nocturnal dyspnea, peripheral edema, anxiety/panic, peri-oral and peripheral paresthesia)
	• Manifestations of systemic disease (eg, endocrine disorders, neurologic disease)
	• Comorbidities
	• Smoking history
	• Occupation and environment exposures
	• Medication and illicit drug use history
Physical examination	• Detailed cardiorespiratory, neurologic, musculoskeletal examination for evidence of disease suspected to cause dyspnea
Investigations	• Pulmonary function testing: spirometry, body plethysmography, diffusing capacity for carbon dioxide, pre-bronchodilator and post- bronchodilator testing, methacholine challenge testing
	• Chest imaging: radiograph, computed tomography, ventilation/perfusion scan
	• Cardiology testing: resting 12-lead electrocardiogram, echocardiogram, stress testing (eg, exercise stress test, dobutamine stress echocardiogram)
	• Laboratory work for investigation of hematologic, endocrine and other disease as appropriate: complete blood count, TSH

Abbreviations: BDI, baseline dyspnea index; COPD, chronic obstructive pulmonary disease; ILD, interstitial lung disease; MRC, Medical Research Council; OCD, oxygen cost diagram; TSH, thyroid-stimulating hormone.

the respiratory muscles is excessively increased relative to maximum. Unpleasant respiratory sensations that result from increased chemoreflex activation are known to be perceived directly (likely via central corollary discharge to the somatosensory cortex). There is experimental evidence that breathing difficulty can be provoked by chemo-stimulation alone in the absence of attendant respiratory muscle activity.[11] However, in spontaneously breathing humans, the experience of dyspnea is profoundly influenced by simultaneous afferent feedback from sensory receptors throughout the respiratory system. It is impossible to directly measure descending efferent output from the respiratory control centers in the brain or indeed from ascending afferent feedback inputs. Moreover, it is not precisely known how these efferent and afferent inputs are centrally integrated to induce unpleasant respiratory sensations. Nevertheless, there is compelling evidence in health and in lung diseases (using surrogate markers of central drive, muscular and mechanical responses) that dyspnea occurs in the context of *demand-capacity imbalance* of the respiratory system. In neurophysiological terms this is referred to as neuro-muscular, neuro-mechanical, or efferent-afferent dissociation of the respiratory system (further discussion in the topic is provided in The Pathophysiology of Dyspnea and Exercise Intolerance in COPD).

Crude indirect measures of increased central drive include overall ventilatory output (ventilation relative to maximal ventilatory capacity [$\dot{V}_E$/MVC]), magnitude of forces generated by the muscles of respiration during tidal breathing (esophageal pressure relative to maximum [Pes/Pes,max]) or inspiratory neural drive (IND) to the diaphragm (diaphragm activation relative to maximum [EMGdi/EMGdi,max]). The underlying causes of increased IND in a dyspneic individual can generally be deduced from assessment of pulmonary gas exchange, acid-base, metabolic and cardio-circulatory responses to exercise. The mechanical response of the respiratory system to increased IND can be evaluated by measuring breathing pattern, ventilation, operating lung volumes and tidal/maximal flow-volume loop analysis. In select cases, esophageal manometry and diaphragm electromyography (EMGdi) can be very useful.

CARDIOPULMONARY EXERCISE TESTING FOR INVESTIGATION OF DYSPNEA OF UNKNOWN ORIGIN

We suggest a simple ordered interrogation of perceptual and physiologic responses to incremental exercise (**Table 2**).

Table 2
Integrated approach to cardiopulmonary exercise testing (CPET)

Interpretation Step	Key Variables to Assess
1. General test overview	• Review indication for CPET • Assess test quality • Assess maximal test criteria • Determine degree of exercise limitation and reason for exercise cessation
2. Baseline resting data	• Demographic data (age, sex, BMI) • Resting vital signs (BP, HR, SpO_2, breathing frequency) • Resting spirometry • Resting 12-lead ECG
3. Perceptual response	• Assessment of dyspnea and leg fatigue using standardized scale (eg, Borg scale) • Dyspnea/WR; dyspnea/$\dot{V}O_2$; dyspnea/$\dot{V}_E$
4. Ventilatory control	• $\dot{V}_E$ • $\dot{V}_E$-$\dot{V}CO_2$ (nadir, slope and intercept) • SpO_2 • $P_{ET}CO_2$ • $Paco_2$ • AT • RER
5. Dynamic respiratory mechanics	• Exercise flow-volume loops relative to maximal resting flow-volume loops • IC • IRV • VT • Fb
6. Cardio vascular	• $\dot{V}O_2$/WR • HR • O_2 pulse
7. Integration and interpretation	• Review of pattern of physiologic limitation considering the degree of exercise impairment, perceptual, ventilatory, respiratory mechanical and cardiovascular responses

Abbreviations: AT, anaerobic threshold; BMI, body mass index; BP, blood pressure; CPET, cardiopulmonary exercise test; ECG, electrocardiogram; Fb, breathing frequency; HR, heart rate; IC, inspiratory capacity; IRV, inspiratory reserve volume; $Paco_2$, arterial carbon dioxide; $P_{ET}CO_2$, end-tidal carbon dioxide; RER, respiratory exchange ratio; SpO_2, oxygen saturation measured by pulse oximetry; $\dot{V}CO_2$, carbon dioxide production; $\dot{V}E$, minute ventilation; $\dot{V}E$-$\dot{V}CO_2$, ventilatory equivalent for carbon dioxide; $\dot{V}O2$, oxygen consumption; V_T, tidal volume.

Perceptual Responses

Incremental CPET allows an assessment of dyspnea intensity (measured by Borg or visual analogue scales)[12,13] during graduated physiologic stress (increasing work rate [WR], oxygen uptake [$\dot{V}O_2$] or ventilation [$\dot{V}_E$]) relative to age-matched and sex-matched healthy controls.[14–20] Generally, in patients with persistent unexplained activity-related dyspnea, intensity ratings are uniformly higher than healthy controls at any given submaximal WR, $\dot{V}O_2$, or $\dot{V}_E$. However, in some situations, dyspnea intensity may be increased as a function of increased $\dot{V}O_2$ or WR (compared with healthy control) but not as a function of increasing ventilation: dyspnea/$\dot{V}_E$ slopes are similar in the dyspneic patient and healthy control subject (**Fig. 1**). This suggests that increasing IND is the main source of dyspnea and that respiratory mechanics and muscle strength are reasonably preserved. In this circumstance, the predominant source of the increased drive may include pulmonary gas exchange, acid-base, and metabolic abnormalities. Other conditions that can present as unexplained dyspnea with dominant increased IND and relatively normal respiratory mechanics include pulmonary hypertension or any cause of high physiologic dead space in which respiratory mechanical abnormalities are nonexistent or relatively mild (early or mild COPD and ILD), thyrotoxicosis, anemia, right to left shunt, pregnancy and metabolic abnormalities including mild obesity.

An assessment of the qualitative dimensions of respiratory discomfort experienced at the limits of tolerance can be obtained using a validated questionnaire,[21] although the diagnostic specificity and sensitivity of this approach in the exercise setting are still uncertain. Importantly, a careful evaluation of the affective dimensions of dyspnea (fear, anxiety, distress, panic) is integral to assessing the impact and personal burden of this chronic symptom.[8,22–25]

Ventilatory Control

In most cases of increased exertional dyspnea, $\dot{V}_E$ is increased at any given $\dot{V}O_2$ or WR with notable exceptions being: coexistent severe respiratory mechanical limitations, profound inspiratory muscle weakness, or high $Paco_2$ set point that dampen the normal ventilatory response to increasing carbon dioxide production ($\dot{V}CO_2$).

Ventilation-carbon dioxide production ratio

The ventilation-carbon dioxide production ratio ($\dot{V}_E/\dot{V}CO_2$) is influenced by the physiologic dead space (dead space to tidal volume ratio [V_D/V_T]) and the $Paco_2$ set point (see Jerome A. Dempsey's article "Update on Chemoreception: Influence on cardiorespiratory regulation and pathophysiology", elsewhere in this issue). High $\dot{V}_E/\dot{V}CO_2$ values identify a potentially important source of ventilatory stimulation of IND and dyspnea.[17,19,20] The $\dot{V}_E/\dot{V}CO_2$ slope provides a useful surrogate for physiologic dead space when respiratory mechanics are intact or only mildly impaired. $\dot{V}_E/\dot{V}CO_2$ is increased when there are areas of the lungs in which perfusion is reduced relative to alveolar ventilation. Normal population reference values have been generated by Neder and colleagues.[26] Examples of high $\dot{V}_E/\dot{V}CO_2$ include normal aging effects, syndromes of increased pulmonary artery resistance, high ventilation/perfusion ratios and wasted ventilation in COPD, ILD, congestive heart failure (CHF), pulmonary hypertension, primary alveolar hyperventilation, extraneous sources of ventilatory stimulation (muscle ergoreceptor activation),

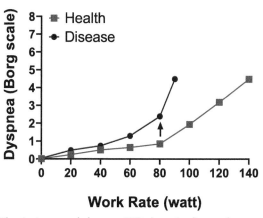

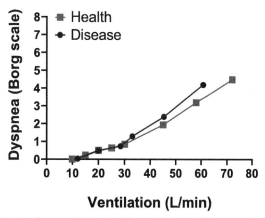

Fig. 1. Increased dyspnea/WR slope in disease however similar dyspnea/V_E in health and disease. This scenario suggests that increased IND is the main source of dyspnea and that respiratory mechanics and muscle strength are relatively preserved.

pulmonary c-receptor activation, and increased cardiovascular mechanoreceptor activation.[27,28]

Hypoxemia

Low SpO_2 <88% (or PaO_2 <60 mm Hg) stimulate peripheral chemoreceptor activation and increase IND and dyspnea. The magnitude of stimulation is strongly influenced by $PaCO_2$. Low O_2 saturation usually signifies a preponderance of alveolar units with low ventilation/perfusion ratios in the setting of low systemic mixed venous O_2 saturation. Other less common causes of arterial O_2 desaturation during exercise are right to left shunts or alveolar hypoventilation.

Carbon dioxide

Low arterialized capillary or $PaCO_2$ can indicate alveolar hyperventilation, which may be primary or secondary. Exclusive reliance on end-tidal carbon dioxide ($P_{ET}CO_2$) measurements may lead to erroneous conclusions about pulmonary gas exchange impairment because of the known disparity between $P_{ET}CO_2$ and actual $PaCO_2$ measurements.[19] The $\dot{V}CO_2$ provides information on the metabolic costs of physical work and is increased in obesity and hypermetabolic states (thyrotoxicosis). In these situations, increased ventilatory demand of physical exertion contributes to dyspnea.

Anaerobic threshold

A low anaerobic threshold (AT) represents reduced O_2 delivery/utilization at the peripheral muscle level. Early accumulation of lactic acid at relatively low WRs causes powerful stimulation of central chemoreceptors and severe exertional dyspnea. A low AT signifies early metabolic acidosis during exercise in conditions where there is low O_2 delivery/utilization such as heart failure or severe skeletal muscle deconditioning.

Dynamic Respiratory Mechanics

Operating lung volumes

Inspiratory capacity (IC) is a simple and useful mechanical measurement that indicates the proximity of tidal volume (V_T) to total lung capacity (TLC). Serial IC measurements (every 2 minutes) throughout exercise are used to track the behavior of end-expiratory lung volume (EELV) on the assumption that TLC remains unchanged.[29] The difference between end-inspiratory lung volume (EILV) and TLC (inspiratory reserve volume [IRV], [IRV = IC − V_T]) dictates the position of V_T on the S-shaped pressure-volume relationship of the respiratory system (**Fig. 2**). Accordingly, the prevailing operating lung volumes relative to TLC inform us about possible dissociation between IND and the

mechanical/muscular response of the dynamic respiratory system, a fundamental mechanism of exertional dyspnea.

A reduced IC can reflect restrictive or obstructive lung disease (with lung hyperinflation) or inspiratory muscle weakness. A progressive decline in IC as exercise progresses in obstructive airway disease suggests dynamic lung hyperinflation as a result of the combined effects of expiratory flow limitation (EFL) and excessive ventilation.[15] This can occur in the presence of coexistent small airways disease and high physiologic dead space even when forced expiratory volume in 1 second (FEV_1) is preserved.[16,17,19] Increased resistive and/or elastic loading of the inspiratory muscles together with functional inspiratory muscle weakness necessitate high cortical motor command output, which is thought to give rise to perceived increased breathing effort. A rapid shallow breathing pattern generally reflects restrictive ventilatory impairment that can result from lung or chest wall restriction, severe lung hyperinflation constraining IC and IRV, or profound inspiratory muscle weakness. When the V_T/IC ratio reaches approximately 0.7 (or the IRV reaches <0.5–1.0 L below TLC) during exercise at relatively low $\dot{V}_E$, critical mechanical constraints or even frank ventilatory limitation is present and usually marks the point at which dyspnea rises abruptly to intolerable levels.[17]

Flow-volume loop analysis

Examination of tidal exercise flow-volume loops relative to maximal resting flow-volume loops provides a qualitative "at-a-glance" assessment of dynamic respiratory mechanics (**Fig. 3**). It is critically important however that V_T be anchored on the volume axis relative to TLC by accurate IC measurements during exercise. The size and configuration of the maximal flow-volume envelope provides information on the underlying mechanical condition and ventilatory capacity. Reduction of IC and IRV as well as increase in EELV (dynamic hyperinflation) can readily be identified on flow-volume loops. Flow-volume loops allow for a crude assessment of the degree of EFL when there is greater than 25% apposition of the V_T expiratory loop with the maximal resting expiratory envelope.[15] Inspiratory flow limitation can similarly be identified when the V_T inspiratory loop encroaches on greater than 50% to 70% of the maximal resting inspiratory flow envelope.[15] Maximal flow-volume loop configuration can change with exercise (for example, intrinsic bronchodilation or bronchoconstriction) and the postexercise maximal loop may therefore be the

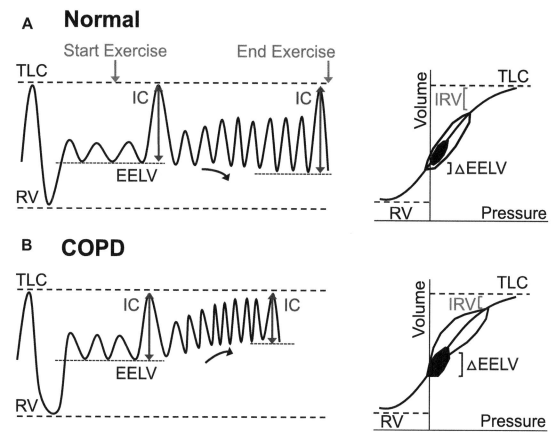

Fig. 2. Change in EELV, IC, and IRV during exercise in (*A*) normal and (*B*) COPD demonstrating change in position of V_T relative to TLC on pressure-volume curve of the respiratory system. (*Reprinted* with permission of the American Thoracic Society. Copyright © 2019 American Thoracic Society. O'Donnell DE. Hyperinflation, dyspnea, and exercise intolerance in chronic obstructive pulmonary disease. Proc Am Thorac Soc 2006;3:180–4. The Annals of the American Thoracic Society is an official journal of the American Thoracic Society.)

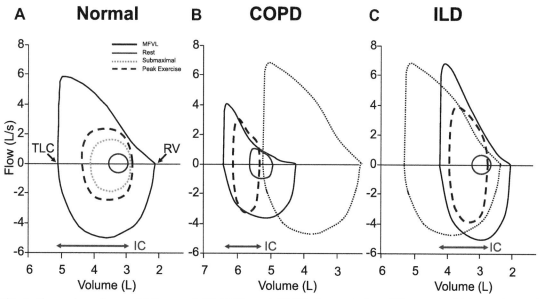

Fig. 3. Flow-volume loops of (*A*) normal, (*B*) COPD, and (*C*) ILD demonstrating difference in tidal, exercise, and maximal resting flow-volume loops. (*Adapted from* O'Donnell DE, Chau LK, Webb KA. Qualitative aspects of exertional dyspnea in patients with interstitial lung disease. J Appl Physiol (1985) 1998;84(6):2000–9; with permission.)

best comparator. Flow-volume loop analysis is best undertaken in the context of examining simultaneous changes in breathing pattern and operating lung volumes. Quantitative values for the volume and flow components of the maximal flow-volume loop at peak exercise (**Fig. 4**) have been developed by Johnson and colleagues[15] (**Box 2**).

Cardio-Circulatory Responses

Traditional CPET provides only limited evaluation of cardio-circulatory function. Cardiac measurements (and their derivations) include heart rate (HR) relative to predicted maximal HR, systemic blood pressure and O_2 pulse ($\dot{V}O_2$/HR), which provides a crude assessment of stroke volume (provided the arterial-venous O_2 content difference is

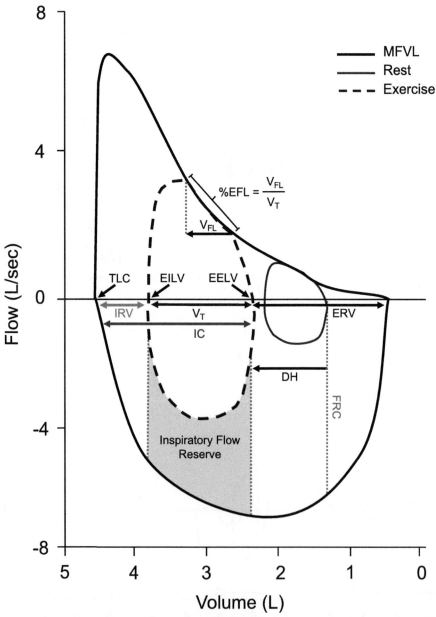

Fig. 4. Tidal, exercise, and maximal resting flow-volume loops of patient with COPD illustrating dynamic hyperinflation, EFL, and inspiratory flow reserve. DH, dynamic hyperinflation; MFVL, maximal flow-volume loop at rest; TLC, total lung capacity; V_{FL}, volume of tidal breath that is flow limited; V_T, tidal volume. (*Adapted from* Johnson BD, Weisman IM, Zeballos RJ, et al. Emerging concepts in the evaluation of ventilatory limitation during exercise: the exercise tidal flow-volume loop. Chest 1999;116(2):488–503; with permission.)

stable). A high $\dot{V}_E/\dot{V}CO_2$ may point to reduced pulmonary perfusion and increased wasted ventilation, which can occur when cardiac output is diminished or when pulmonary artery resistance is increased. A low $\dot{V}O_2$/WR slope and an early AT are also nonspecific indicators of poor systemic O_2 delivery, which can indicate cardio-circulatory dysfunction. A low $\dot{V}O_2$/WR slope is also seen in conditions of low O_2 utilization such as anorexia or malnutrition.

ILLUSTRATIVE CARDIOPULMONARY EXERCISE TESTING CASE EXAMPLES
Normal Healthy Subject

Fig. 5 demonstrates average values obtained during CPET for several healthy control male and female subjects (n = 50), mean age 66 years, studied at the Respiratory Investigation Unit, Kingston Health Sciences Center. The normal response to exercise is briefly outlined as follows.

Test description
Control subjects performed an incremental CPET that met maximal test criteria based on peak HR greater than 90% predicted (panel not shown) and respiratory exchange ratio (RER) >1.1. On average, control subjects exercised for 14 minutes to a peak WR of 140 W reaching a peak $\dot{V}O_2$ greater than 95% predicted (see **Fig. 5**A).[30]

Perceptual response
Subjects experienced an increase in dyspnea (see **Fig. 5**B, C) and leg fatigue (peak Borg 5) during exercise. The predominant symptom limiting exercise was leg fatigue.

Ventilatory response
$\dot{V}_E$ increased throughout exercise (see **Fig. 5**D), initially with an increase in both V_T and breathing frequency (see **Fig. 5**I, J). At higher submaximal WRs, an inflection in V_T was discernible (close to 70% of IC)[31] and increase in $\dot{V}_E$ was achieved by further increase in breathing frequency.

Ventilatory control
As the metabolic demands of exercise increase $\dot{V}O_2$, $\dot{V}CO_2$ and $\dot{V}_E$ increase. As exercise progresses following AT (see **Fig. 5**E), production of lactic acid stimulates further increase in $\dot{V}_E$ relative to $\dot{V}CO_2$ (inflection point of further increase in $\dot{V}_E$ identified by arrow in **Fig. 5**B, D, I, J). Increased ventilation leads to a decrease in $P_{ET}CO_2$ and increase in $\dot{V}_E/\dot{V}CO_2$ (see **Fig. 5**H, F). There is no decrease in SpO_2 (see **Fig. 5**G). At peak WR there is significant breathing reserve (37 L/min).

Ventilatory mechanics
V_T expansion during exercise is recruited from both the IRV and expiratory reserve volume (ERV) (see **Fig. 5**L). This pattern of V_T expansion maintains tidal breathing during exercise at a favorable position on the pressure-volume curve of the respiratory system relative to TLC, evidenced by the absence of decline in IC (see **Fig. 5**K).[31] There is no evidence of EFL from assessment of the flow-volume loops (see **Fig. 4**A).

Cardiovascular response
The normal cardio-circulatory response to exercise is characterized by a linear increase in $\dot{V}O_2$/WR as cardiac output increases to meet increasing metabolic demands (see **Fig. 5**A). Early in exercise cardiac output increases due to increase in both HR and stroke volume (estimated during CPET by the surrogate O_2 pulse [O_2 pulse = $SV(Ca\text{-}vO_2)$]). At higher submaximal WRs, O_2 pulse plateaus and subsequent increases in cardiac output are met by increased HR (see control values in case 4 **Fig. 12**H, I).

Conclusion
Exercise capacity in these healthy subjects was normal. The perceptual, ventilatory, pulmonary gas exchange, respiratory mechanical and cardiovascular responses to exercise were normal.

Case 1

A 31-year-old woman with suspected asthma reported progressive exertional dyspnea over the previous 8 months. She experienced moderate dyspnea while walking 500 m from the parking lot to her workplace and had to stop briefly 2 to 3 times to recover (MRC 4). She noticed "wheezy

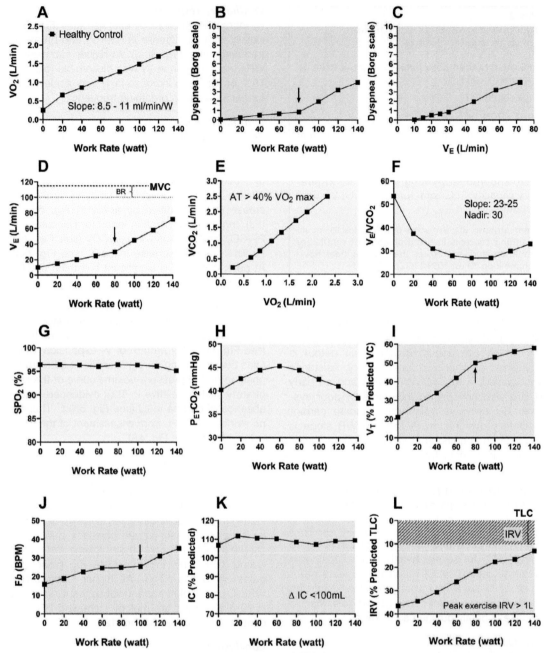

Fig. 5. Selected panels from incremental cardiopulmonary exercise tests performed by 50 healthy control male and female subjects (mean age 66 years). Inflection points corresponding to compensatory increase in ventilation at submaximal exercise are indicated by an arrow. Colored panels highlight the following important groups of CPET variables: (A) V_{O_2}/WR relationship, (B, C) perceptual response to exercise, (D) ventilatory response to exercise, (E–H) variables of ventilatory control, and (I–L) dynamic ventilatory mechanical variables. BPM, breaths per minute; BR, estimated breathing reserve; Fb, breathing frequency; VCO_2, carbon dioxide production; V_E, minute ventilation; V_E/VCO_2, ventilatory equivalent for carbon dioxide; V_{O_2}, oxygen consumption; V_T, tidal volume.

breathing" during activity on an episodic basis. She had no history of atopy and her dyspnea was provoked only by exercise. She was a lifelong nonsmoker.

Her BMI was 36 kg/m^2, resting blood pressure (BP) 115/80 mm Hg, HR 85 beats per minute, SpO$_2$ 97% on room air. Expiratory wheeze was audible with forced expiration bilaterally on examination. The remainder of her physical examination demonstrated thoraco-abdominal obesity.

Initial investigations before referral included peak expiratory flow rate (73% predicted). Pulmonary function tests were consistent with a nonspecific pattern (FEV$_1$/forced vital capacity [FVC] 0.75, FEV$_1$ 80% predicted, FVC 75% predicted, no evidence of bronchodilator reversibility, TLC 99% predicted, ERV 65% predicted, functional residual capacity [FRC] 70% predicted, residual volume [RV] 80% predicted and DLCO 84% predicted). A methacholine challenge test was normal. Her family physician prescribed a short-acting beta-2 agonist bronchodilator, high-dose inhaled corticosteroid plus long-acting beta-2 agonist bronchodilator. There was no improvement in her symptoms with this treatment and this prompted a referral to the Dyspnea Clinic.

Case interpretation

Test description The patient performed an incremental CPET that met maximal test criteria based on peak HR greater than 90% predicted. She exercised for 12 minutes and 10 seconds to a peak WR of 90 W. The peak $\dot{V}O_2$ was 79% predicted (**Fig. 6**A), but adjusted for weight was greater than 90% predicted.[32,33]

Perceptual response Dyspnea ratings were increased at standardized WR (**Fig. 6**B) but were not increased for $\dot{V}_E$ compared with control (**Fig. 6**C). Leg discomfort also increased during exercise (peak Borg 3). The predominant symptom limiting exercise was dyspnea.

Ventilatory response Assessment of ventilatory response to exercise demonstrated elevated $\dot{V}_E$ throughout exercise with preservation of a normal $\dot{V}_E$/WR slope (**Fig. 6**D).

Ventilatory control $\dot{V}O_2$ (see **Fig. 6**A) and $\dot{V}CO_2$ (**Fig. 6**E) were similarly elevated as a function of increasing WR throughout exercise compared with healthy control with preservation of normal slopes. This reflected the higher metabolic cost of physical work and consequent higher $\dot{V}CO_2$ stimulating increased IND and $\dot{V}_E$ during exercise in obesity. The normal $\dot{V}_E/\dot{V}CO_2$ nadir at AT (**Fig. 6**G) and AT at 45% predicted $\dot{V}O_2$ max (**Fig. 6**F), suggests these factors did not contribute to increased $\dot{V}_E$ early in exercise. In addition, there was no evidence of decreased SpO$_2$ (**Fig. 6**H).

Ventilatory mechanics V$_T$ was slightly more shallow than normal throughout exercise (**Fig. 6**I) with compensatory tachypnea (**Fig. 6**J), in the absence of significant mechanical constraints (IRV was well preserved at peak exercise, see

Fig. 6L). However, decreased chest wall and lung (micro-atelectasis) compliance due to the effects of thoraco-abdominal obesity may play a role in producing the observed rapid shallow breathing pattern. The presence of EFL in the setting of a relatively high submaximal $\dot{V}_E$ resulted in increased EELV from baseline (**Fig. 7**), which in turn, gave rise to "pseudo-normalization" of EELV (FRC) and decrease in IC (**Fig. 6**K), a mechanical advantage for the muscles of inspiration.[33] Another possibility is that the patient "chose" not to expand V$_T$ to mitigate unpleasant respiratory sensation associated with increased elastic loading.

Cardiovascular response Cardiovascular response to exercise was normal (not shown).

Conclusion The patient's low peak $\dot{V}O_2$ normalized when adjusted for ideal body weight, an important consideration when assessing cardiorespiratory fitness in obesity. Ventilatory demand was increased and mainly reflected the high metabolic cost of physical work. Dyspnea/$\dot{V}_E$ slopes were similar in the patient and control suggesting that the increased $\dot{V}CO_2$ and resultant increased IND and $\dot{V}_E$ were important contributors to dyspnea, particularly in the absence of significant pulmonary gas exchange and acid-base abnormalities. In keeping with previous studies in moderate obesity, the recruitment of IC at rest and small increases in EELV during exercise provided a mechanical advantage that attenuated the expected neuro-mechanical dissociation of the respiratory system in mild to moderate obesity.[33] Based on these results, all asthma medications were stopped; the patient successfully lost weight through diet and exercise with disappearance of her high ventilatory requirements and exertional dyspnea (related discussion in the topic is provided in The Pathophysiology of Dyspnea and Exercise Intolerance in COPD).

Case 2

A 50-year-old man presented with progressive exertional dyspnea that remained unexplained after initial investigations by his family physician and medical internist. He developed progressive dyspnea over 6 months to the point that he had breathing discomfort after walking only a few minutes: he had to abandon playing golf, his main recreational past time (MRC 4). He reported a persistent nonproductive cough. He had no symptoms to suggest heart failure. He had no identified adverse occupational or environmental exposures. He was an ex-smoker with a remote 10-pack-year smoking history.

His BMI was 34 kg/m^2, resting BP 128/76 mm Hg, HR 76 beats per minute and SpO2 94% on

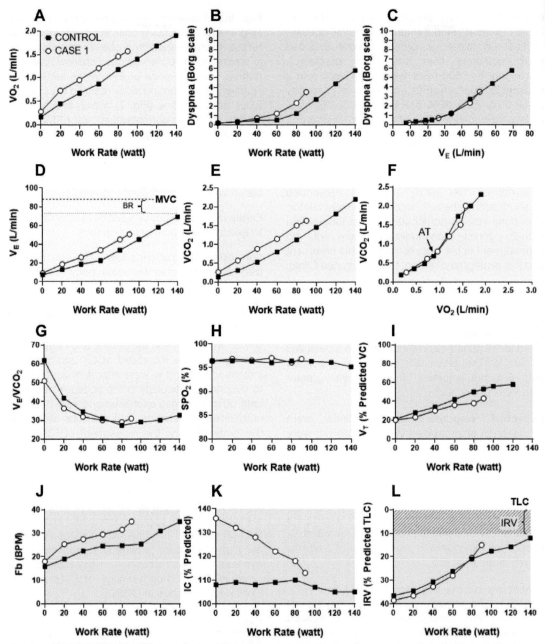

Fig. 6. Selected panels from incremental cardiopulmonary exercise test for case 1 and normal control subjects. Colored panels highlight the following important groups of CPET variables: (A) Vo₂/WR relationship, (B, C) perceptual response to exercise, (D) ventilatory response to exercise, (E–H) variables of ventilatory control, and (I–L) dynamic ventilatory mechanical variables. BPM, breaths per minute; BR, estimated breathing reserve; Fb, breathing frequency; VCO₂, carbon dioxide production; Vₑ, minute ventilation; Vₑ/VCO₂, ventilatory equivalent for carbon dioxide; Vo₂, oxygen consumption; Vₜ, tidal volume.

room air. On auscultation, sparse, intermittent, soft inspiratory crackles were noted at his left lung base. There was no digital clubbing, stigmata of connective tissue disease or chest wall deformity. The remainder of his physical examination was normal.

Initial investigations before referral to the Dyspnea Clinic included a normal chest radiograph,

no ischemic changes on treadmill cardiac stress test, and normal echocardiogram. Pulmonary function tests showed a normal FEV₁/FVC ratio with proportionate mild reduction in FEV₁ (81% predicted) and FVC (77% predicted). TLC and ERV were mildly reduced (75% and 60% predicted, respectively) consistent with his high BMI.

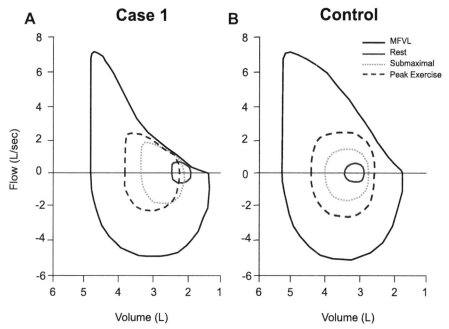

Fig. 7. Flow-volume loop of (*A*) case 1 and (*B*) normal control demonstrating maximal flow-volume loop, tidal breathing at rest, submaximal exercise and peak exercise. MFVL, maximal flow-volume loop at rest.

There was a mild reduction in DLCO (74% predicted). Static maximal inspiratory and expiratory pressures were normal. Finally, a high-resolution computed tomography (CT) chest was reported as normal but the radiologist commented on localized subtle reticular changes in the lower lobes, which were nonspecific and of uncertain clinical significance.

Persistence of progressive, severe exertional dyspnea, which remained unexplained after this comprehensive evaluation, prompted referral to the Dyspnea Clinic.

Case interpretation
Test description The patient performed an incremental CPET that met maximal test criteria based on development of severe dyspnea limiting exercise with a Borg score of 6 and RER greater than 1.1. He exercised for a total of 5 minutes and 18 seconds to a peak WR of 50 W. The $\dot{V}O_2$ peak was 36% predicted (**Fig. 8**A).

Perceptual response Dyspnea/$\dot{V}O_2$ (**Fig. 8**B) and dyspnea/$\dot{V}_E$ increased throughout exercise. The predominant symptom limiting exercise was dyspnea, qualitatively described as "I *can't get enough air in*."

Ventilatory response Ventilatory demand was increased: $\dot{V}_E/\dot{V}O_2$ slope was increased throughout exercise compared with control (**Fig. 8**C). The breathing reserve was 28 L/min at peak exercise.

Ventilatory control Increased physiologic dead space was suggested by elevated $\dot{V}_E/\dot{V}CO_2$ nadir and intercept (**Fig. 8**D). Using arterial blood gas analysis, it was determined that V_D/V_T was elevated at rest and did not decrease normally (expected decrease by ~30%) during exercise (**Fig. 8**E). As $\dot{V}_E$ increased throughout exercise $Paco_2$ decreased (**Fig. 8**F). SpO_2 decreased by greater than 5% from baseline (**Fig. 8**G) and hypoxemia with an increased alveolar-arterial oxygen (A-aPO_2) gradient during exercise was evident (**Fig. 8**H). Significant ventilation/perfusion abnormalities and likely low mixed venous O_2 saturation due to increased O_2 extraction resulted in hypoxemia, a potential source of peripheral and central chemoreceptor stimulation. Collectively, these data point to clinically significant impairment in pulmonary gas exchange, which stimulated high ventilatory demand.

Ventilatory mechanics There was an abnormal rapid shallow breathing pattern (**Fig. 8**I, J) during exercise for a given WR (a hallmark feature of restrictive lung diseases).[34] IC was reduced at rest and throughout exercise (**Fig. 8**K) and expansion of V_T was limited by reduced IRV (see **Fig. 8**L). These abnormalities were also evident on flow-volume loop analysis without evidence of EFL (**Fig. 9**).

Cardiovascular response Cardiovascular response to exercise was normal (not shown).

Conclusion CPET provided important insights into the mechanisms of this patient's exertional

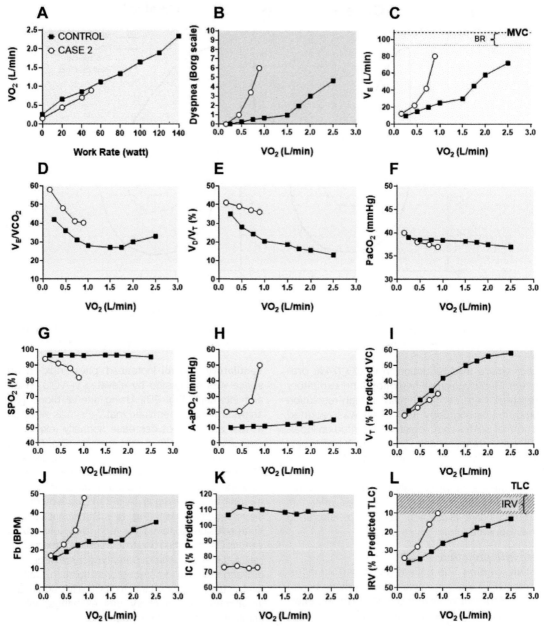

Fig. 8. Selected panels from incremental cardiopulmonary exercise test for case 2 and healthy control subjects. Colored panels highlight the following important groups of CPET variables: (A) Vo_2/WR relationship, (B) perceptual response to exercise, (C) ventilatory response to exercise, (D–H) variables of ventilatory control, and (I–L) dynamic ventilatory mechanical variables. A-aPO$_2$, alveolar-arterial oxygen gradient; BPM, breaths per minute; BR, estimated breathing reserve; Fb, breathing frequency; V_D, dead space; V_E, minute ventilation; V_E/VCO$_2$, ventilatory equivalent for carbon dioxide; Vo_2, oxygen consumption; V_T, tidal volume.

dyspnea that was unexplained after an exhaustive workup. Despite only mild nonspecific resting physiologic and radiographic abnormalities, significant dynamic pulmonary gas exchange and mechanical abnormalities were revealed on CPET. Collectively, these factors contributed to heightened IND to the mechanically overloaded respiratory muscles (due to reduced lung compliance), a powerful source of dyspnea.[20,35,36] The overall pattern is best explained by ILD with physiologic impairment during the stress of physical activity that precedes the development of definitive pulmonary function and CT scan abnormalities. In fact, within a year, this patient developed significant restriction of vital

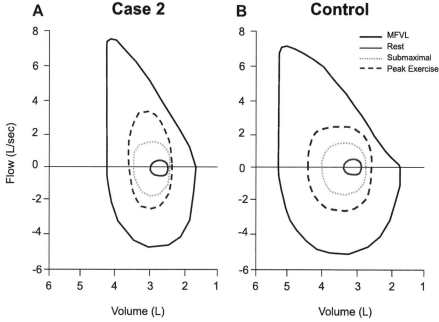

Fig. 9. Flow-volume loop of (*A*) case 2 and (*B*) normal control demonstrating maximal flow-volume loop, tidal breathing at rest, submaximal exercise and peak exercise. MFVL, maximal flow-volume loop at rest.

capacity (VC) and decline in DLCO with rapid evolution of radiographic features of Usual Interstitial Pneumonia (see also Exercise Pathophysiology in Interstitial Lung Disease).

Case 3

A 54-year-old male smoker with a 30-pack-year smoking history presented to his family physician with progressive exertional dyspnea. Over the past 2 years he noticed increasing dyspnea, first on climbing stairs and now on walking 250 m on a level surface at a slow pace before having to stop to recover (MRC 3). He had no known family history of respiratory, cardiovascular, or neurologic disease.

His BMI was 23.7 kg/m^2, resting BP 132/76 mm Hg, HR 82 beats per minute, SpO$_2$ 96% on room air. He had a normal physical examination.

Initial investigations included spirometry that demonstrated mild obstruction of mid-volume flows without bronchodilator reversibility (FEV$_1$/FVC 0.68, FEV$_1$ 81% predicted, FVC 88% predicted). Chest radiograph, resting 12-lead electrocardiogram (ECG) and echocardiogram were normal. A trial of bronchodilator provided little perceived benefit. Concerned about the patient's progressive dyspnea in the setting of unremarkable spirometry, he was referred to the Dyspnea Clinic.

Body plethysmography showed TLC 110% predicted, functional residual capacity (FRC) 128% predicted, RV 129% predicted, RV/TLC ratio 39%. DLCO was normal (86% predicted).

Case interpretation

Test description The patient performed an incremental CPET that met maximal test criteria based on development of very severe dyspnea with a Borg score of 7 and a RER greater than 1.1. He exercised for a total of 10 minutes and 33 seconds to a peak WR of 100 W and peak $\dot{V}O_2$ 54% predicted (**Fig. 10**A).

Perceptual response Dyspnea ratings were higher than control at any given $\dot{V}O_2$, WR and $\dot{V}_E$ throughout exercise (**Fig. 10**B, C). The predominant symptom limiting exercise was dyspnea.

Ventilatory response The ventilatory response to exercise was abnormal. Submaximal $\dot{V}_E$ was elevated throughout exercise and increased slope of $\dot{V}_E$/WR occurred in the setting of apparent adequate breathing reserve (39 L/min) at peak WR (**Fig. 10**D).

Ventilatory control $\dot{V}_E$/$\dot{V}CO_2$ nadir was increased (**Fig. 10**F) suggesting high V$_D$/V$_T$ (wasted ventilation) or reduced Paco$_2$ set point. P$_{ET}$CO$_2$ was lower compared with control (**Fig. 10**G). SpO$_2$ was in the normal range (**Fig. 10**H) and there was no indication of early AT (**Fig. 10**E).

Ventilatory mechanics Compared with control there was an early inflection in V$_T$ response (**Fig. 10**I) with compensatory increase in breathing frequency (**Fig. 10**J). IC progressively decreased with exercise compared with control indicating

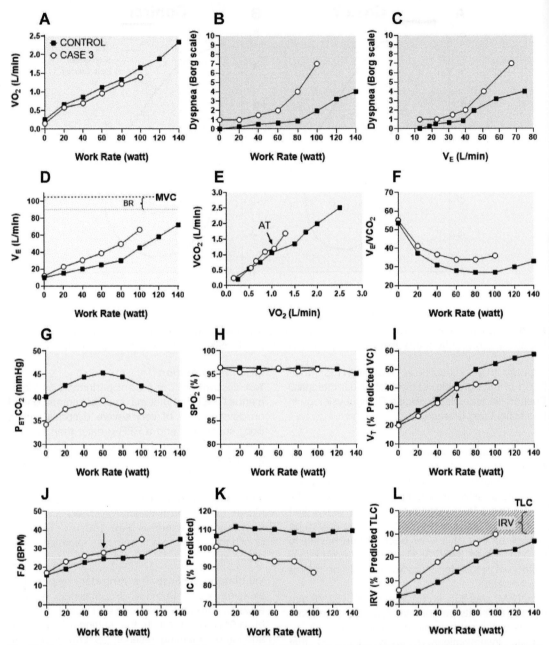

Fig. 10. Selected panels from incremental cardiopulmonary exercise test for case 3 and healthy control subjects. Colored panels highlight the following important groups of CPET variables: (*A*) Vo_2/WR relationship, (*B, C*) perceptual response to exercise, (*D*) ventilatory response to exercise, (*E–H*) variables of ventilatory control, and (*I–L*) dynamic ventilatory mechanical variables. BPM, breaths per minute; BR, estimated breathing reserve; Fb, breathing frequency; VCO_2, carbon dioxide production; V_E, minute ventilation; V_E/VCO_2, ventilatory equivalent for carbon dioxide; Vo_2, oxygen consumption; V_T, tidal volume.

dynamic lung hyperinflation of 0.5 L (**Fig. 10**K). Accordingly, IRV reduction occurred at a faster rate than control (**Fig. 10**L) reaching its minimal value of 0.7 L at a relatively low $\dot{v}_E$. These significant mechanical constraints were corroborated by the relationship between tidal and maximal flow-volume

loops that confirmed both EFL (**Fig. 11**) and critical reduction of IRV (EILV = 0.7 L below TLC) at a relatively low peak $\dot{v}_E$.

Cardiovascular response Cardiovascular response to exercise was normal (not shown).

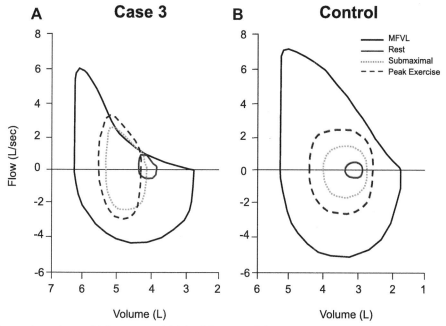

Fig. 11. Flow-volume loop of (*A*) case 3 and (*B*) healthy control demonstrating maximal flow-volume loop, tidal breathing at rest, submaximal exercise and peak exercise. MFVL, maximal flow-volume loop at rest.

Conclusion In this patient who barely met global initiative for chronic obstructive lung disease (GOLD) spirometric criteria for GOLD stage 1 COPD, CPET confirmed significant activity-related dyspnea and exercise intolerance. Ventilatory demand was uniformly increased compared with normal suggesting a high IND due to the combined effects of increased chemo-stimulation (decreased ventilatory efficiency), significant dynamic mechanical loading of the inspiratory muscles and restrictive constraints on ventilation. Recent studies in patients with mild COPD and in smokers at risk for COPD have shown increased diaphragmatic activation and increased elastic and resistive loading to explain increased dyspnea and exercise intolerance.[16–19] This case demonstrates that even in the presence of unremarkable spirometry, normal SpO_2 and apparently adequate breathing reserve (estimated by $\dot{V}_E/MVC$) at peak exercise, symptomatic smokers can have significant physiologic impairment leading to severe exertional dyspnea that, at first glance, seems disproportionate.[37–39] Treatment with a dual long-acting bronchodilator (long-acting beta-2 agonist/muscarinic antagonist) resulted in reduced lung hyperinflation (increased IC) and a delay in reaching critical inspiratory constraints and intolerable dyspnea during exercise (further discussion in the topic is provided in The Pathophysiology of Dyspnea and Exercise Intolerance in COPD).

Case 4

A 23-year-old woman nursing student developed progressive dyspnea over the previous year that advanced to a degree that limited her ability to go grocery shopping (MRC 4). She was a competitive swimmer and was previously able to train at high intensity without symptomatic limitation. She reported occasional palpitations during physical activity but had not noted any other symptoms. She took no medications and was a lifelong nonsmoker.

Her family physician reported that the patient had a BMI of 20.3 kg/m², resting BP 97/56 mm Hg and HR of 92 beats per minute. There was a systolic murmur along the left sternal border. The remainder of her physical examination was normal. Her physician noted that although SpO_2 was 94% at rest on room air it quickly dropped SpO_2 78% on walking the office corridor. Alarmed by her incapacitating dyspnea and exercise hypoxemia, he arranged urgent referral to the Dyspnea Clinic.

Initial investigations included normal spirometry and lung volumes with moderate reduction in DLCO (56% predicted). Her chest radiograph was reported as normal.

A CPET was organized while awaiting further urgent investigations.

Case interpretation
Test description The patient performed an incremental CPET that met maximal test criteria based on very severe dyspnea limiting exercise (Borg score of 7). She exercised for a total of 3 minutes and 50 seconds to a peak WR of 50 W. The peak $\dot{V}O_2$ was 35% predicted (**Fig. 12**A).

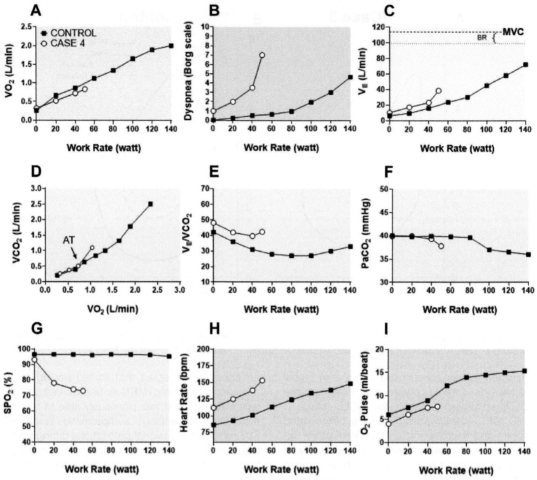

Fig. 12. Selected panels from incremental cardiopulmonary exercise test for case 4 and healthy control subjects. Colored panels highlight the following important groups of CPET variables: (*A*) Vo₂/WR relationship, (*B*) perceptual response to exercise, (*C*) ventilatory response to exercise, (*D–G*) variables of ventilatory control and (*H, I*) cardio-circulatory variables. BPM, beats per minute; BR, estimated breathing reserve; VCO2, carbon dioxide production; V_E, minute ventilation; V_E/VCO_2, ventilatory equivalent for carbon dioxide; Vo₂, oxygen consumption. (*Reprinted* with permission of the American Thoracic Society. Copyright © 2019 American Thoracic Society. Neder JA, Ramos RP, Ota-Arakaki JS, Hirai DM, D'Arsigny CL, O'Donnell D. Exercise Intolerance in Pulmonary Arterial Hypertension. Annals of the American Thoracic Society. 2015;12(4):604–612. The Annals of the American Thoracic Society is an official journal of the American Thoracic Society.)

Perceptual response Submaximal and peak dyspnea Borg scores were uniformly higher than control throughout exercise (**Fig. 12**B). The predominant symptom limiting exercise was dyspnea.

Ventilatory response The $\dot{V}_E$/WR slope was elevated throughout exercise indicating high ventilatory demand compared with control (**Fig. 12**C) with apparent breathing reserve at peak exercise (64 L/min).

Ventilatory control The elevated $\dot{V}_E/\dot{V}CO_2$ nadir (**Fig. 12**E) was in keeping with increased V_D/V_T and low $Paco_2$ set point. Severe hypoxemia likely reflects impaired pulmonary gas exchange and provided a powerful drive to increase $\dot{V}_E$ due to

increased chemo-stimulation (**Fig. 12**G). $Paco_2$ decreased as a result of increased $\dot{V}_E$ at peak exercise (**Fig. 12**F). An early metabolic acidosis (low AT occurring at 23% predicted $\dot{V}O_2$ max) indicated reduced O_2 delivery to the active locomotor muscles (**Fig. 12**D). The very high ventilatory demand helped explain increased breathing discomfort (See James R. Vallerand and colleagues' article, "Pulmonary Hypertension and Exercise," elsewhere in this issue).[40–44]

Ventilatory mechanics No significant abnormalities were seen in breathing pattern or flow-volume loop analysis other than some degree of EFL and minor dynamic hyperinflation, which is sometimes seen in the setting of high ventilatory demand (**Fig. 13**).[28,45,46]

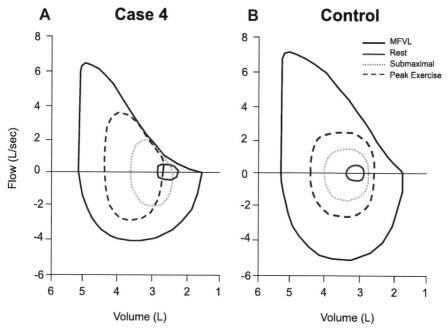

Fig. 13. Flow-volume loop of (*A*) case 4 and (*B*) healthy control demonstrating maximal flow-volume loop, tidal breathing at rest, submaximal exercise and peak exercise. MFVL, maximal flow-volume loop at rest.

Cardiovascular response The cardiovascular response to exercise was abnormal with early plateau in O_2 pulse (**Fig. 12**I) and significant increase in HR/WR slope (**Fig. 12**H). There was a normal BP response to exercise. Peak HR was reduced at 153 beats per minute (83% predicted) as was AT (AT occurring at 23% predicted $\dot{V}O_2$ max) (see **Fig. 12**D). As impairment in O_2 delivery worsened with increasing WR, the $\dot{V}O_2$/WR slope was reduced compared with normal (see **Fig. 12**A).

Conclusion CPET confirmed very severe dyspnea and reduced exercise capacity. Pulmonary gas exchange and cardio-circulatory responses to exercise were markedly abnormal and underpin the high ventilatory requirements and severe dyspnea. The pattern of gas exchange abnormalities strongly suggested pulmonary vascular disease. An echocardiogram was later performed and confirmed pulmonary hypertension with a pulmonary artery systolic pressure of 65 mm Hg, mild dilation of the right ventricle and right atrium, normal left ventricular size and function and a large atrial septal defect (ASD). The pattern of precipitous arterial O_2 desaturation with mild exercise in patients with evidence of pulmonary hypertension is suggestive of a right to left intracardiac shunt, in this case a reversed shunt through an ASD.[47–49] The early plateau of O_2 pulse, increase in HR slope, reduced AT and low $\dot{V}O_2$/WR slope point to significant dynamic cardio-circulatory

impairment that could not be appreciated from resting echocardiogram alone (further discussion in the topic is provided in Pulmonary Hypertension and Exercise).[48]

Case 5

A 29-year-old woman presented with progressive unexplained exertional dyspnea despite thorough assessment by respirology and cardiology specialists. She reported intermittent childhood dyspnea during strenuous activity but this became progressively more troublesome in the 3 years before referral to the Dyspnea Clinic. At presentation she reported that dyspnea limited her ability to walk more than 100 m at a time (MRC 4). She had occasional chest tightness and tachycardia associated with dyspnea on exertion. She experienced leg muscle cramps since age 9, usually following episodes of intense activity, most often affecting the quadriceps and accompanied by perceived muscle fatigue. She had no significant past medical history and took no medications. There was no family history of cardiorespiratory or neurologic disease. She was an ex-smoker with <5-pack-year history.

Her BMI was 23.8 kg/m², resting BP 102/76 mm Hg, HR 88 beats per minute, SpO2 96% on room air. She had a normal respiratory, cardiovascular, neurologic, and musculoskeletal physical examination.

Initial investigations included normal spirometry, chest radiograph, resting 12-lead ECG, 24-h Holter monitoring, echocardiogram, hematology, and endocrine workup. Pulmonary function testing demonstrated a normal FEV_1/FVC ratio, normal FEV_1 and FVC with no evidence of post bronchodilator reversibility. The TLC, subdivisions of lung volumes and DLCO were normal. MIP and MEP were reduced at −61 cmH_2O (69% predicted) and 89 cmH_2O (58% predicted) respectively, suggesting some degree of respiratory muscle weakness.[50] Sniff esophageal pressure at rest measured using esophageal manometry was also reduced at −46 cmH_2O (50% predicted).[51]

Case interpretation

Test description The patient performed an incremental CPET that met maximal test criteria based on peak HR >90% predicted and development of very severe dyspnea with a Borg score of 7. She exercised for a total of 10 minutes and 15 seconds to a peak WR of 90 W and a $\dot{V}O_2$ peak of 67% predicted (not shown).

Perceptual response Dyspnea ratings were greater than control for both $\dot{V}O_2$ and $\dot{V}_E$ (**Fig. 14**A, B). Leg discomfort also increased to Borg 5 at peak exercise, but the predominant symptom limiting exercise was dyspnea.

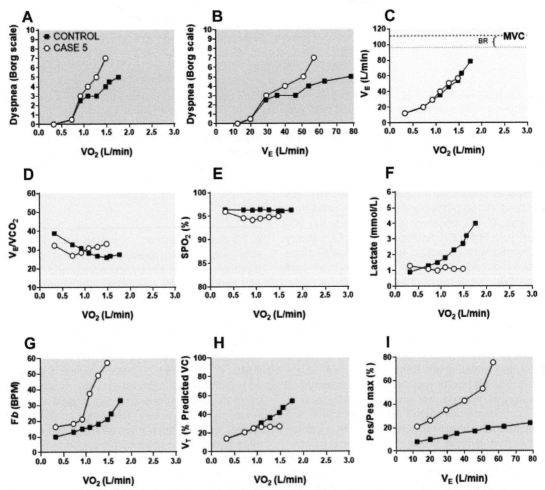

Fig. 14. Selected panels from incremental cardiopulmonary exercise test for case 5 and healthy control subjects. Colored panels highlight the following important groups of CPET variables: (*A, B*) perceptual response to exercise, (*C*) ventilatory response to exercise, (*D–F*) variables of ventilatory control, and (*G–I*) dynamic ventilatory mechanical variables. BR, estimated breathing reserve; BPM, breaths per minute; Fb, breathing frequency; MVC, maximal ventilatory capacity; Pes/Pes,max, esophageal pressure relative to maximum; SpO_2, oxygen saturation measured by pulse oximetry; V_E, minute ventilation; V_E/VCO_2, ventilatory equivalent for carbon dioxide; VC, vital capacity; Vo_2, oxygen consumption; V_T, tidal volume. (*Adapted from* Voduc N, Webb KA, D'Arsigny CL, et al. McArdle's disease presenting as unexplained dyspnea in a young woman. Can Respir J 2004;11(2):163–7; with permission.)

Ventilatory response $\dot{V}_E$ increased normally throughout exercise but peak $\dot{V}_E$ was diminished compared with control (**Fig. 14**C).

Ventilatory control Pulmonary gas exchange ($\dot{V}_E/\dot{V}CO_2$ and SpO_2) was in the normal range during exercise (**Fig. 14**D, E). No AT was detected and notably RER was 0.82. There was absence of an increase in blood lactate with incremental exercise (**Fig. 14**F). Similarly, there was no lactate accumulation during subsequent brachial artery occlusion testing.[52]

Ventilatory mechanics An early inflection in V_T and rapid increase in breathing frequency with exercise (**Fig. 14**H, G) occurred in the absence of mechanical limitation on tidal versus maximal flow-volume loop comparisons and may represent dynamic inspiratory muscle weakness

(**Fig. 15**). Esophageal manometry demonstrated decreased peak inspiratory pressures at rest and throughout exercise, consistent with respiratory muscle weakness. Thus, tidal esophageal pressure relative to maximum (Pes/Pes,max) was relatively increased at any given $\dot{V}_E$ during exercise (**Fig. 14**I), indicating greater contractile effort (and higher cortical motor command output) compared with control which likely contributed to respiratory discomfort.

Cardiovascular response There was a rapid attainment of peak HR greater than 90% predicted at low peak exercise intensity but cardiovascular response was otherwise normal (not shown).

Conclusion Reduced exercise capacity was confirmed. Exercise was limited by development

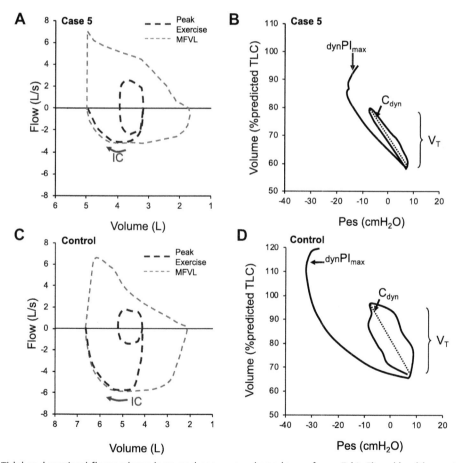

Fig. 15. Tidal and maximal flow-volume loop and pressure-volume loop of case 5 (*A, B*) and healthy control (*C, D*) during peak exercise. Maximal flow-volume loop and pressure-volume loop demonstrated during maximal IC maneuver. Cdyn, dynamic compliance; dynPImax, dynamic maximal inspiratory esophageal pressure; IC, inspiratory capacity; MFVL, maximal flow-volume loop at rest; Pes, esophageal pressure; TLC, total lung capacity; V_T, tidal volume. (*Adapted from* Voduc N, Webb KA, D'Arsigny CL, et al. McArdle's disease presenting as unexplained dyspnea in a young woman. Can Respir J 2004;11(2):163–7; with permission.)

of very severe dyspnea at a relatively low $\dot{V}O_2$. Significant abnormalities of respiratory muscle strength were uncovered at rest and during exercise, which likely explains the abnormal shallow breathing pattern. Pulmonary gas exchange and respiratory mechanics were in the normal range but metabolic abnormalities were clearly present. The lack of increase in blood lactate during exercise and brachial artery occlusion testing was consistent with a diagnosis of myophosphorylase deficiency, a glycogen storage disease V (McArdle disease) which was subsequently confirmed by muscle biopsy and genetic studies. An unusual feature was that of all skeletal muscles, the respiratory muscles were predominantly affected.[53] Functional inspiratory muscle weakness during exercise likely necessitated greater motor command output from cortical centers with resultant perceived increased breathing effort that soon became intolerable (further discussion in the topic is provided in Respiratory Muscle assessment in Clinical Practice).

Case 6

An 18-year-old woman presented to the Dyspnea Clinic with unexplained exertional dyspnea and noisy breathing over a 2-year period. At presentation, activity-related dyspnea was severe (MRC 4). She had a history of audible wheezing that was noticeable over the preceding 6 months and she could no longer tolerate lying supine because of aggravated breathing discomfort. There was no cough, diurnal variation in her symptoms, or atopy. She had no significant past medical history, childhood illness, or family history of respiratory or neuromuscular disease.

Her BMI was 22.5 kg/m^2, resting BP 88/56 mm Hg, HR 78 beats per minute, SpO$_2$ 98% on room air. On examination there was a pronounced inspiratory wheeze on auscultation. Physical examination including neurologic examination was otherwise normal.

Initial investigations included pulmonary function testing, which showed a mixed obstructive and restrictive pattern with normal diffusing capacity (FEV$_1$/FVC 0.63, FEV$_1$ 59% predicted, FVC 73% predicted, no evidence of post bronchodilator reversibility, TLC 77% predicted, IC 69% predicted, RV 85% predicted, DLCO 87% predicted, DLCO/VA 109% predicted). Flow-volume loop showed blunting of the inspiratory and expiratory loops. MIP −30 cmH$_2$O (37% predicted) and MEP 25 cm H$_2$O (26% predicted) were reduced.

Case interpretation
Test description The patient met maximal test criteria with very severe dyspnea (Borg score 9). She exercised for a total of 8 minutes and 9 seconds to a peak WR of 80 W. The $\dot{V}O_2$ peak was 61% predicted (**Fig. 16**A).

Perceptual response Dyspnea was greater than control both at any given $\dot{V}O_2$ and $\dot{V}_E$ (**Fig. 16**B, C). Leg discomfort at peak exercise was Borg 3.

Ventilatory response The ventilatory response to exercise was largely in the normal range with apparent breathing reserve (32 L/min) at peak exercise (**Fig. 16**D).

Ventilatory control $\dot{V}_E/\dot{V}CO_2$ was slightly elevated compared with control early in exercise but reached a normal nadir (**Fig. 16**F). There was no evidence of desaturation with normal SpO$_2$ throughout exercise (**Fig. 16**G). No AT was discernible (**Fig. 16**E).

Ventilatory mechanics Restricted lung volumes and reduced IC throughout exercise (**Fig. 16**J) resulted in relatively low V$_T$ and abnormally increased breathing frequency (**Fig. 16**H, I). IRV became critically reduced early in exercise (**Fig. 16**K). Flow-volume loops indicate critical inspiratory flow limitation at low levels of exercise (**Fig. 17**). Accordingly, esophageal manometry showed tidal inspiratory pressures reached maximal possible values obtained during IC maneuvers at low $\dot{V}_E$ (**Figs. 16**L and **18**, see **Fig. 15**B for comparison) in keeping with the dual effects of increased resistive loading and reduced inspiratory muscle strength. Thus, there were no reserves for further inspiratory flow generation, volume expansion, or force generation by the inspiratory muscles. The widened pressure-volume loop together with truncation of the maximal inspiratory flow loops further endorse these complex physiologic derangements (see **Figs. 17** and **18**).

Cardiovascular response Cardiovascular response to exercise was normal (not shown).

Conclusion This patient had profound exercise intolerance and overwhelming dyspnea due to the combined effects of severe upper airway obstruction and respiratory muscle weakness. In the absence of significant pulmonary gas exchange and metabolic abnormalities, increased motor command output from cortical respiratory centers in the brain was likely the main source of dyspnea. The patient proceeded to undergo comprehensive neurologic evaluation with MRI of the brain, nerve conduction studies,

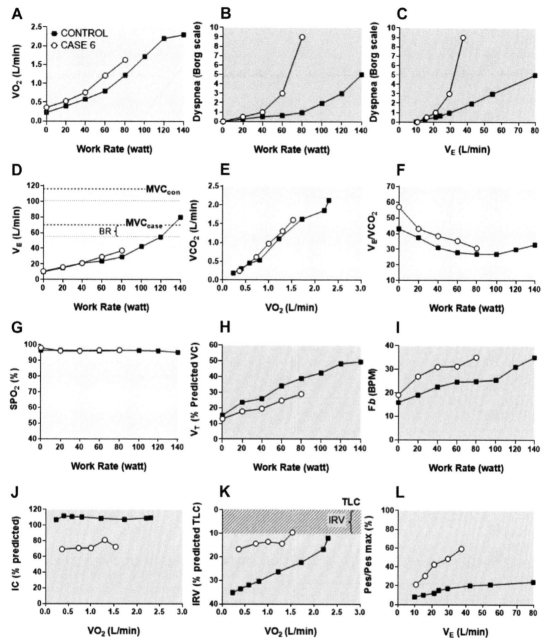

Fig. 16. Selected panels from incremental cardiopulmonary exercise test for case 6 and healthy control subjects. Colored panels highlight the following important groups of CPET variables: (*A*) Vo2/WR relationship, (*B, C*) perceptual response to exercise, (*D*) ventilatory response to exercise, (*E–G*) variables of ventilatory control, and (*H–L*) dynamic ventilatory mechanical variables. BPM, breaths per minute; BR, estimated breathing reserve; Fb, breathing frequency; IC, inspiratory capacity; IRV, inspiratory reserve volume; MVC_case, maximal ventilatory capacity for case; MVC_con, maximal ventilatory capacity for control; Pes/Pes,max, esophageal pressure relative to maximum; SpO2, oxygen saturation measured by pulse oximetry; TLC, total lung capacity; VC, vital capacity; VCO2, carbon dioxide production; V_E, minute ventilation; V_E/VCO2, ventilatory equivalent for carbon dioxide; Vo2, oxygen consumption; V_T, tidal volume. (*Adapted from* Chau LK, Webb KA, Jackson AC, et al. Vocal cord paralysis and respiratory muscle weakness: an unusual presentation of chronic polyneurophathy. Can Respir J 1998;5(2):125–9; with permission.)

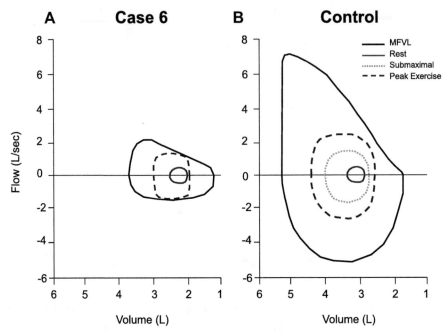

Fig. 17. Flow-volume loop of (*A*) case 6 and (*B*) healthy control demonstrating maximal flow-volume loop, tidal breathing at rest, submaximal exercise and peak exercise. MFVL, maximal flow-volume loop at rest. (*Adapted from* Chau LK, Webb KA, Jackson AC, et al. Vocal cord paralysis and respiratory muscle weakness: an unusual presentation of chronic polyneurophathy. Can Respir J 1998;5(2):125–9; with permission.)

and muscle and nerve biopsy. The patient also underwent largyngoscopy that revealed consistently decreased abduction of the vocal cords during inspiration. The final diagnosis was a variant of Charcot-Marie-Tooth disease (hereditary motor sensory neuropathy) with primary involvement of the upper airway and respiratory muscles in the absence of limb symptoms (see also Respiratory Muscle assessment in Clinical Practice).

Case 7

A 56-year-old woman presented with severe dyspnea and associated light-headedness to the Dyspnea Clinic referred from the emergency department for investigation of her symptoms. Her dyspnea had progressed over the previous 4 months, at times limiting her ability to keep pace with others while walking (MRC 3). Her dyspnea was irregularly associated with exertion and often occurred at rest without identified precipitating or aggravating triggers. She reported anxiety and breathing distress. She had light-headedness and peripheral paresthesia on one occasion culminating in a "dyspnea crisis" and visit to the emergency department. She was a life-long nonsmoker and there was no history of excessive alcohol consumption, illegal drug or medication use.

Her BMI was 26 kg/m^2, resting BP 108/62 mm Hg, HR 65 beats per minute, SpO2 98% on room air. She had a normal physical examination but instruction to voluntarily hyperventilate for more than 1 minute during her clinic visit reproduced a sense of dyspnea and light-headedness reminiscent of her previous attacks.

Prior investigations were all normal and included spirometry, hematology, resting 12-lead ECG, chest radiograph, CT chest, and ventilation/perfusion (V/Q) scan. In addition, a resting and dobutamine stress echocardiogram were normal, as was a stress test for inducible coronary artery ischemia.

Case interpretation

Test description The patient performed an incremental CPET that did not meet met maximal test criteria. Peak dyspnea Borg score was 4. She exercised for a total of 7 minutes and 52 seconds to a peak WR of 80 W and v̇O$_2$ peak 82% predicted.

Perceptual response Dyspnea ratings increased at rest and fluctuated widely during the test with reduction during low-intensity exercise, increasing thereafter (**Fig. 19**A). Peak leg discomfort ratings were Borg 3.

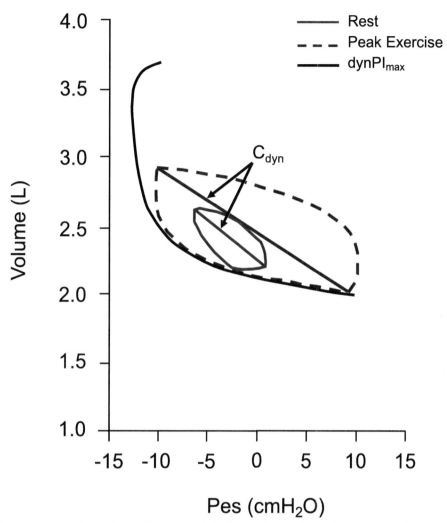

Fig. 18. Pressure-volume loop of case 6 at rest and during peak exercise. Refer to **Fig. 15**B for representative control comparison. Maximal pressure-volume loop demonstrated from esophageal pressure during maximal IC maneuver. Cdyn, dynamic compliance; dynPImax, dynamic maximal inspiratory esophageal pressure; Pes, esophageal pressure. (*Adapted from* Chau LK, Webb KA, Jackson AC, et al. Vocal cord paralysis and respiratory muscle weakness: an unusual presentation of chronic polyneurophathy. Can Respir J 1998;5(2):125–9; with permission.)

Ventilatory response Breathing pattern at rest was chaotic. However the ventilatory response to exercise was surprisingly linear (**Fig. 19**B), matching the metabolic demands of the task despite large variability in V_T and breathing frequency (**Fig. 19**E, F). $\dot{V}_E$/time is used to highlight the irregular pattern of ventilation.

Ventilatory control At rest, irregular episodes of alveolar hyperventilation with elevation of $\dot{V}_E$/$\dot{V}CO_2$ (**Fig. 19**C) with sustained decrease in P_{ET}-CO_2 (**Fig. 19**D) were evident. Clearly, a mismatch was present between relatively low metabolic demand at rest and ventilatory response.

Ventilatory mechanics Mechanics and muscle function were normal at rest (not shown). Under the conditions of irregular breathing pattern and hyperventilation, analysis of operating lung volumes and flow-volume loops are unreliable for the evaluation of dynamic respiratory mechanics.

Cardiovascular response Cardiovascular response to exercise was normal (not shown).

Conclusion Exercise was limited by dyspnea, which had a major affective dimension and was present at rest and throughout exercise in the absence of any concrete evidence of respiratory mechanical, pulmonary gas exchange, or

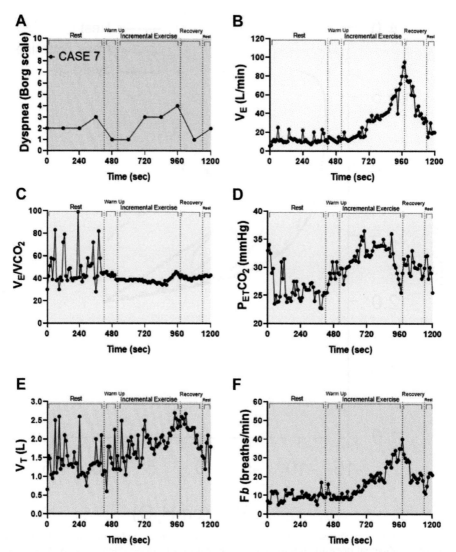

Fig. 19. Selected panels from incremental cardiopulmonary exercise test for case 7. Colored panels highlight the following important groups of CPET variables: (*A*) perceptual response to exercise, (*B*) ventilatory response to exercise, (*C, D*) variables of ventilatory control, and (*E, F*) pattern of breathing variables. Fb, breathing frequency; $P_{ET}CO_2$, end-tidal carbon dioxide; V_E, minute ventilation; V_E/VCO_2, ventilatory equivalent for carbon dioxide; V_T, tidal volume. (*Adapted from* Neder JA, Hirai DM, Jones JH, et al. A 56-year-old, otherwise healthy woman presenting with light-headedness and progressive shortness of breath. Chest 2016;150(1):e23–7; with permission.)

cardiovascular abnormalities. The smoother ventilatory response to exercise compared with rest indicated partial restoration of normal physiologic control mechanisms. The abnormal resting ventilation, irregular breathing pattern, alveolar hyperventilation, and marked anxiety is consistent with a diagnosis of idiopathic hyperventilation.[54] Increased dyspnea in this clinical setting is thought to be related to abnormal central processing of respiratory sensory afferents and increased activation of limbic, paralimbic, sensorimotor, and premotor cortical areas. Decrease in $Paco_2$ of 1 to 2 mm Hg is known to be associated with a 2% to 3% decrease in cerebral blood flow

(**Fig. 20**); in turn this can lead to an increase in hydrogen ion accumulation locally in the brain and provide ongoing stimulation of central bulbo-pontine and medullary chemoreceptors to increase ventilation. Sustained hyperventilation leads to respiratory alkalosis and possibly hypocalcemia, which can cause perioral and peripheral paresthesia. Earlier diagnosis of this condition using CPET could have obviated emergency department visits and multiple expensive investigations (further discussion in the topic is provided in Why Physiology Is Critical to The Practice of Medicine: A 40-Year Personal Perspective).

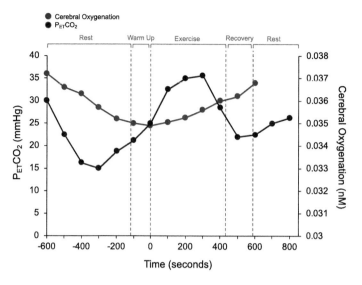

Fig. 20. $P_{ET}CO_2$ and cerebral oxygenation measured using near-infrared spectroscopy during exercise demonstrating decreased cerebral oxygenation with decreased $P_{ET}CO_2$. $P_{ET}CO_2$, end-tidal carbon dioxide. (*Adapted from* Neder JA, Hirai DM, Jones JH, et al. A 56-year-old, otherwise healthy woman presenting with light-headedness and progressive shortness of breath. Chest 2016;150(1):e23–7.)

REFERENCES

1. Huang W, Resch S, Oliverira RKF, et al. Invasive cardiopulmonary exercise testing in the evaluation of unexplained dyspnea: insights from a multidisciplinary dyspnea center. Eur J Prev Cardiol 2017; 24(11):1190–9.
2. Sassi-Dambron DE, Eakin EG, Ries AL, et al. Treatment of dyspnea in COPD. A controlled clinical trial of dyspnea management strategies. Chest 1995; 107(3):724–9.
3. Oga T, Nishimura K, Tsukino M, et al. Analysis of the factors related to mortality in chronic obstructive pulmonary disease: role of exercise capacity and health status. Am J Respir Crit Care Med 2003; 167(4):544–9.
4. Pinto-Plata VM, Cote C, Cabral H, et al. The 6-min walk distance: change over time and value as a predictor of survival in severe COPD. Eur Respir J 2004; 23(1):28–33.
5. Waschki B, Kirsten A, Holz O, et al. Physical activity is the strongest predictor of all-cause mortality in patients with COPD: a prospective cohort study. Chest 2011;140(2):331–42.
6. Ley B, Bradford WZ, Vittinghoff E, et al. Predictors of mortality poorly predict common measures of disease progression in idiopathic pulmonary fibrosis. Am J Respir Crit Care Med 2016;194(6):711–8.
7. Galie N, Humbert M, Vachiery JL, et al. 2015 ESC/ERS guidelines for the diagnosis and treatment of pulmonary hypertension: the Joint Task Force for the Diagnosis and Treatment of Pulmonary Hypertension of the European Society of Cardiology (ESC) and the European Respiratory Society (ERS): endorsed by: Association for European Paediatric and Congenital Cardiology (AEPC), International Society for Heart and Lung Transplantation (ISHLT). Eur Respir J 2015;46(4):903–75.
8. Parshall MB, Schwartzstein RM, Adams L, et al. An official American Thoracic Society statement: update on the mechanisms, assessment, and management of dyspnea. Am J Respir Crit Care Med 2012; 185(4):435–52.
9. Pratter MR, Curley FJ, Dubois J, et al. Cause and evaluation of chronic dyspnea in a pulmonary disease clinic. Arch Intern Med 1989;149(10): 2277–82.
10. Martinez FJ, Stanopoulos I, Acero R, et al. Exercise testing in the evaluation of dyspnea unexplained by routine evaluation. Chest 1994;105(1):168–74.
11. Gandevia SC, Killian K, McKenzie DK, et al. Respiratory sensations, cardiovascular control, kinaesthesia and transcranial stimulation during paralysis in humans. J Physiol 1993;470:85–107.
12. Borg GA. Psychophysical bases of perceived exertion. Med Sci Sports Exerc 1982;14(5):377–81.
13. Noseda A, Carpiaux JP, Schmerber J, et al. Dyspnoea assessed by visual analogue scale in patients with chronic obstructive lung disease during progressive and high intensity exercise. Thorax 1992;47(5):363–8.
14. Weisman IM, Zeballos RJ. An integrated approach to the interpretation of cardiopulmonary exercise testing. Clin Chest Med 1994;15(2):421–45.
15. Johnson BD, Weisman IM, Zeballos RJ, et al. Emerging concepts in the evaluation of ventilatory limitation during exercise: the exercise tidal flow-volume loop. Chest 1999;116(2):488–503.
16. Ofir D, Laveneziana P, Webb KA, et al. Mechanisms of dyspnea during cycle exercise in symptomatic patients with GOLD stage I chronic obstructive pulmonary disease. Am J Respir Crit Care Med 2008; 177(6):622–9.

17. Chin RC, Guenette JA, Cheng S, et al. Does the respiratory system limit exercise in mild chronic obstructive pulmonary disease? Am J Respir Crit Care Med 2013;187(12):1315–23.

18. Guenette JA, Chin RC, Cheng S, et al. Mechanisms of exercise intolerance in global initiative for chronic obstructive lung disease grade 1 COPD. Eur Respir J 2014;44(5):1177–87.

19. Elbehairy AF, Ciavaglia CE, Webb KA, et al. Pulmonary gas exchange abnormalities in mild chronic obstructive pulmonary disease. Implications for dyspnea and exercise intolerance. Am J Respir Crit Care Med 2015;191(12):1384–94.

20. Faisal A, Alghamdi BJ, Ciavaglia CE, et al. Common mechanisms of dyspnea in chronic interstitial and obstructive lung disorders. Am J Respir Crit Care Med 2016;193(3):299–309.

21. Simon PM, Schwartzstein RM, Weiss JW, et al. Distinguishable types of dyspnea in patients with shortness of breath. Am Rev Respir Dis 1990; 142(5):1009–14.

22. Wadell K, Webb KA, Preston ME, et al. Impact of pulmonary rehabilitation on the major dimensions of dyspnea in COPD. COPD 2013;10(4): 425–35.

23. Donesky D, Nguyen HQ, Paul SM, et al. The affective dimension of dyspnea improves in a dyspnea self-management program with exercise training. J Pain Symptom Manage 2014;47(4):757–71.

24. Banzett RB, Pedersen SH, Schwartzstein RM, et al. The affective dimension of laboratory dyspnea: air hunger is more unpleasant than work/effort. Am J Respir Crit Care Med 2008;177(12):1384–90.

25. Yorke J, Moosavi SH, Shuldham C, et al. Quantification of dyspnoea using descriptors: development and initial testing of the Dyspnoea-12. Thorax 2010;65(1):21–6.

26. Neder JA, Nery LE, Castelo A, et al. Prediction of metabolic and cardiopulmonary responses to maximum cycle ergometry: a randomised study. Eur Respir J 1999;14(6):1304–13.

27. Paintal AS. Mechanism of stimulation of type J pulmonary receptors. J Physiol 1969;203(3):511–32.

28. Aguggini G, Clement MG, Widdicombe JG. Lung reflexes affecting the larynx in the pig, and the effect of pulmonary microembolism. Q J Exp Physiol 1987; 72(1):95–104.

29. O'Donnell DE, Elbehairy AF, Webb KA, et al, Canadian Respiratory Research Network. The link between reduced inspiratory capacity and exercise intolerance in chronic obstructive pulmonary disease. Ann Am Thorac Soc 2017;14(Supplement_1): S30–9.

30. Jones NL, Makrides L, Hitchcock C, et al. Normal standards for an incremental progressive cycle ergometer test. Am Rev Respir Dis 1985;131: 700–8.

31. Henke KG, Sharratt M, Pegelow D, et al. Regulation of end-expiratory lung volume during exercise. J Appl Physiol (1985) 1988;64(1):135–46.

32. Wasserman K, Hansen JE, Sue DY, et al. Principles of exercise testing and interpretation. 3rd edition. Baltimore (MD): Lippincott Williams and Wilkins; 1999.

33. Ofir D, Laveneziana P, Webb KA, et al. Ventilatory and perceptual responses to cycle exercise in obese women. J Appl Physiol (1985) 2007;102(6): 2217–26.

34. Javaheri S, Sicilian L. Lung function, breathing pattern, and gas exchange in interstitial lung disease. Thorax 1992;47:93–7.

35. O'Donnell DE, Chau LK, Webb KA. Qualitative aspects of exertional dyspnea in patients with interstitial lung disease. J Appl Physiol (1985) 1998;84(6): 2000–9.

36. Schaeffer MR, Ryerson CJ, Ramsook AH, et al. Neurophysiological mechanisms of exertional dyspnoea in fibrotic interstitial lung disease. Eur Respir J 2018;51(1) [pii:1701726].

37. O'Donnell DE, Voduc N, Fitzpatrick M, et al. Effect of salmeterol on the ventilatory response to exercise in chronic obstructive pulmonary disease. Eur Respir J 2004;24(1):86–94.

38. O'Donnell DE, Hamilton AL, Webb KA. Sensory-mechanical relationships during high-intensity, constant-work-rate exercise in COPD. J Appl Physiol (1985) 2006;101(4):1025–35.

39. O'Donnell DE, Guenette JA, Maltais F, et al. Decline of resting inspiratory capacity in COPD: the impact on breathing pattern, dyspnea, and ventilatory capacity during exercise. Chest 2012;141(3):753–62.

40. Farina S, Bruno N, Agalbato C, et al. Physiological insights of exercise hyperventilation in arterial and chronic thromboembolic pulmonary hypertension. Int J Cardiol 2018;259:178–82.

41. Rolim JV, Ota-Arakaki JS, Ferreira EVM, et al. Inspiratory muscle weakness contributes to exertional dyspnea in chronic thromboembolic pulmonary hypertension. PLoS One 2018;13(9):e0204072.

42. Sun XG, Hansen JE, Oudiz RJ, et al. Exercise pathophysiology in patients with primary pulmonary hypertension. Circulation 2001;104(4):429–35.

43. Meyer FJ, Lossnitzer D, Kristen AV, et al. Respiratory muscle dysfunction in idiopathic pulmonary arterial hypertension. Eur Respir J 2005;25(1):125–30.

44. Neder JA, Ramos RP, Ota-Arakaki JS, et al. Insights into ventilation-gas exchange coupling in chronic thromboembolic pulmonary hypertension. Eur Respir J 2016;48(1):252–4.

45. Velez-Roa S, Ciarka A, Najem B, et al. Increased sympathetic nerve activity in pulmonary artery hypertension. Circulation 2004;110(10):1308–12.

46. Ramos RP, Arakaki JS, Barbosa P, et al. Heart rate recovery in pulmonary arterial hypertension:

relationship with exercise capacity and prognosis. Am Heart J 2012;163(4):580–8.

47. Porteous MK, Fritz JS. Hypoxemia in a patient with pulmonary arterial hypertension: getting to the heart of the matter. Ann Am Thorac Soc 2014;11(5): 836–40.

48. Neder JA, Ramos RP, Ota-Arakaki JS, et al. Exercise intolerance in pulmonary arterial hypertension. Ann Am Thorac Soc 2015;12(4):604–12.

49. Craig RJ, Selzer A. Natural history and prognosis of atrial septal defect. Circulation 1968;37(5):805–15.

50. Black LF, Hyatt RE. Maximal respiratory pressures: normal values and relationship to age and sex. Am Rev Respir Dis 1969;99(5):696–702.

51. Miller JM, Moxham J, Green M. The maximal sniff in the assessment of diaphragm function in man. Clin Sci (Lond) 1985;69(1):91–6.

52. Coleman RA, Stajich JM, Pac VW, et al. The ischemic exercise test in normal adults and in patients with weakness and cramps. Muscle Nerve 1986;9(3):216–21.

53. Voduc N, Webb KA, D'Arsigny CL, et al. McArdle's disease presenting as unexplained dyspnea in a young woman. Can Respir J 2004;11(2):163–7.

54. Neder JA, Hirai DM, Jones JH, et al. A 56-year-old, otherwise healthy woman presenting with light-headedness and progressive shortness of breath. Chest 2016;150(1):e23–7.

Printed and bound by CPI Group (UK) Ltd, Croydon, CR0 4YY

08/05/2025

01864745-0013